The Molecular Biology of Autoimmune Disease

NATO ASI Series

Advanced Science Institutes Series

A series presenting the results of activities sponsored by the NATO Science Committee, which aims at the dissemination of advanced scientific and technological knowledge, with a view to strengthening links between scientific communities.

The Series is published by an international board of publishers in conjunction with the NATO Scientific Affairs Division

A Life Sciences B Physics	Plenum Publishing Corporation London and New York
C Mathematical and Physical Sciences D Behavioural and Social Sciences E Applied Sciences	Kluwer Academic Publishers Dordrecht, Boston and London
F Computer and Systems Sciences G Ecological Sciences H Cell Biology	Springer-Verlag Berlin Heidelberg New York London Paris Tokyo Hong Kong

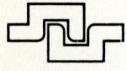

Series H: Cell Biology Vol. 38

The Molecular Biology of Autoimmune Disease

Edited by

Andrew G. Demaine
J-Paul Banga
Alan M. McGregor

Department of Medicine
King's College School of Medicine
Denmark Hill
London SE5 8RX, UK

Springer-Verlag Berlin Heidelberg New York
London Paris Tokyo Hong Kong
Published in cooperation with NATO Scientific Affairs Division

Proceedings of the NATO Advanced Research Workshop on Molecular Biology and Autoimmune Disease held in Athens, Greece, from April 16–20, 1989

ISBN 3-540-51771-5 Springer-Verlag Berlin Heidelberg New York
ISBN 0-387-51771-5 Springer-Verlag New York Berlin Heidelberg

Library of Congress Cataloging-in-Publication Data. NATO Advanced Research Workshop on Molecular Biology and Autoimmune Disease (1989: Athens, Greece) The molecular biology of autoimmune disease/ edited by Andrew G. Demaine, J-Paul Banga, Alan M. McGregor. p. cm.—(NATO ASI series. Series H, Cell biology; vol. 38) "Proceedings of the NATO Advanced Research Workshop on Molecular Biology and Autoimmune Disease, held in Athens, Greece, from April 16–20, 1989"—T.p. verso. "Published in cooperation with NATO Scientific Affairs Division."
ISBN 0-387-51771-5 (U.S.)
1. Autoimmune diseases—Molecular aspects—Congresses. 2. Immunogenetics—Congresses. I. Demaine, Andrew G., 1957– . II. Banga, J-Paul, 1953– . III. McGregor, Alan M., 1948– . IV. North Atlantic Treaty Organization. Scientific Affairs Division. V. Title. VI. Series. RC600.N38 1989 616.97—dc20 89-26236

Printed in Germany

Printing: Druckhaus Beltz, Hemsbach; Binding: J. Schäffer GmbH & Co. KG, Grünstadt
2131/3140-543210 – Printed on acid-free-paper

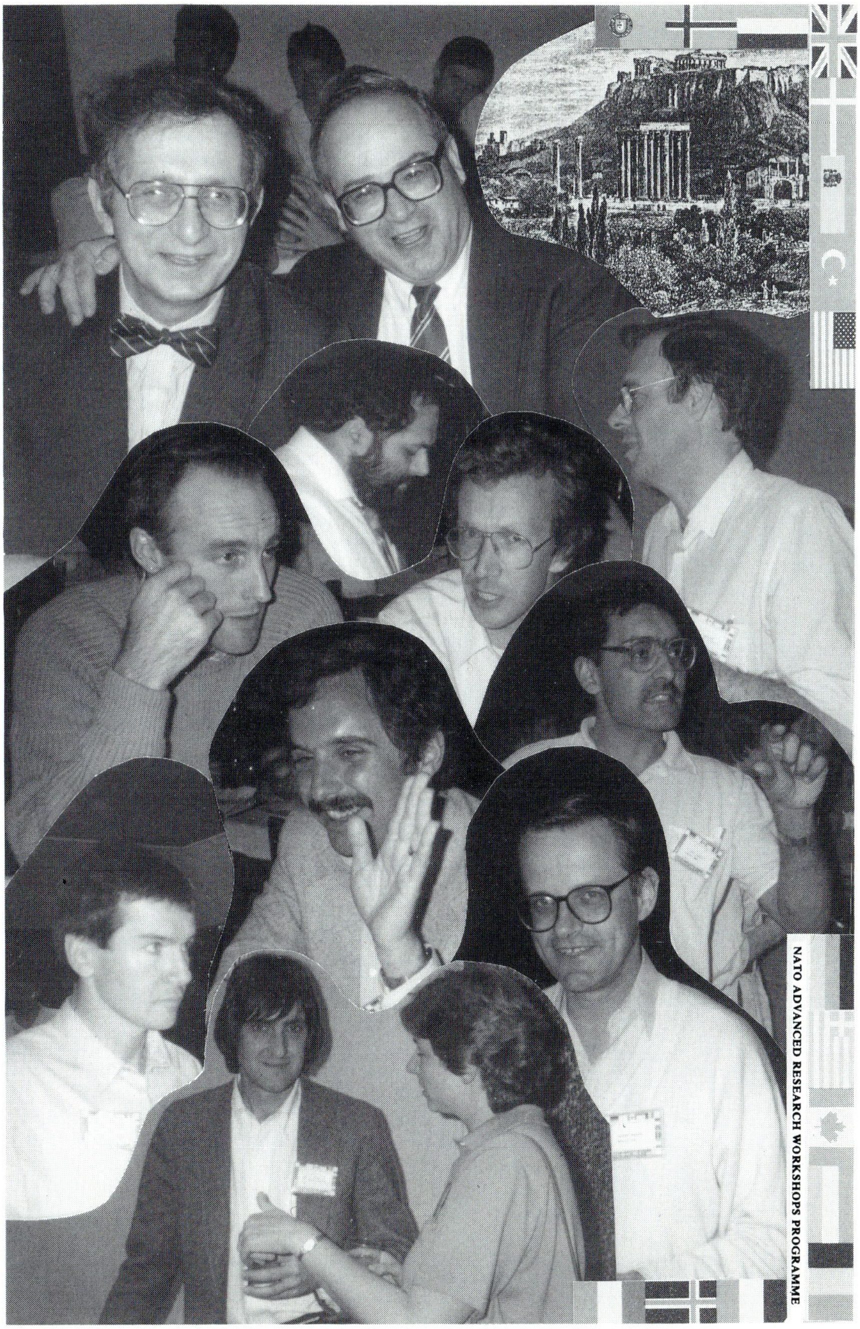

LEFT TO RIGHT IN ROWS: G.S. Eisenbarth, L.D. Kohn
S. Fling, R.C. Nayak, A. Lohse, G.Vassart
A.M. McGregor, G.T. Nepom, H. Wekerle, J-P Banga
P.M. Allen, A. Pullen

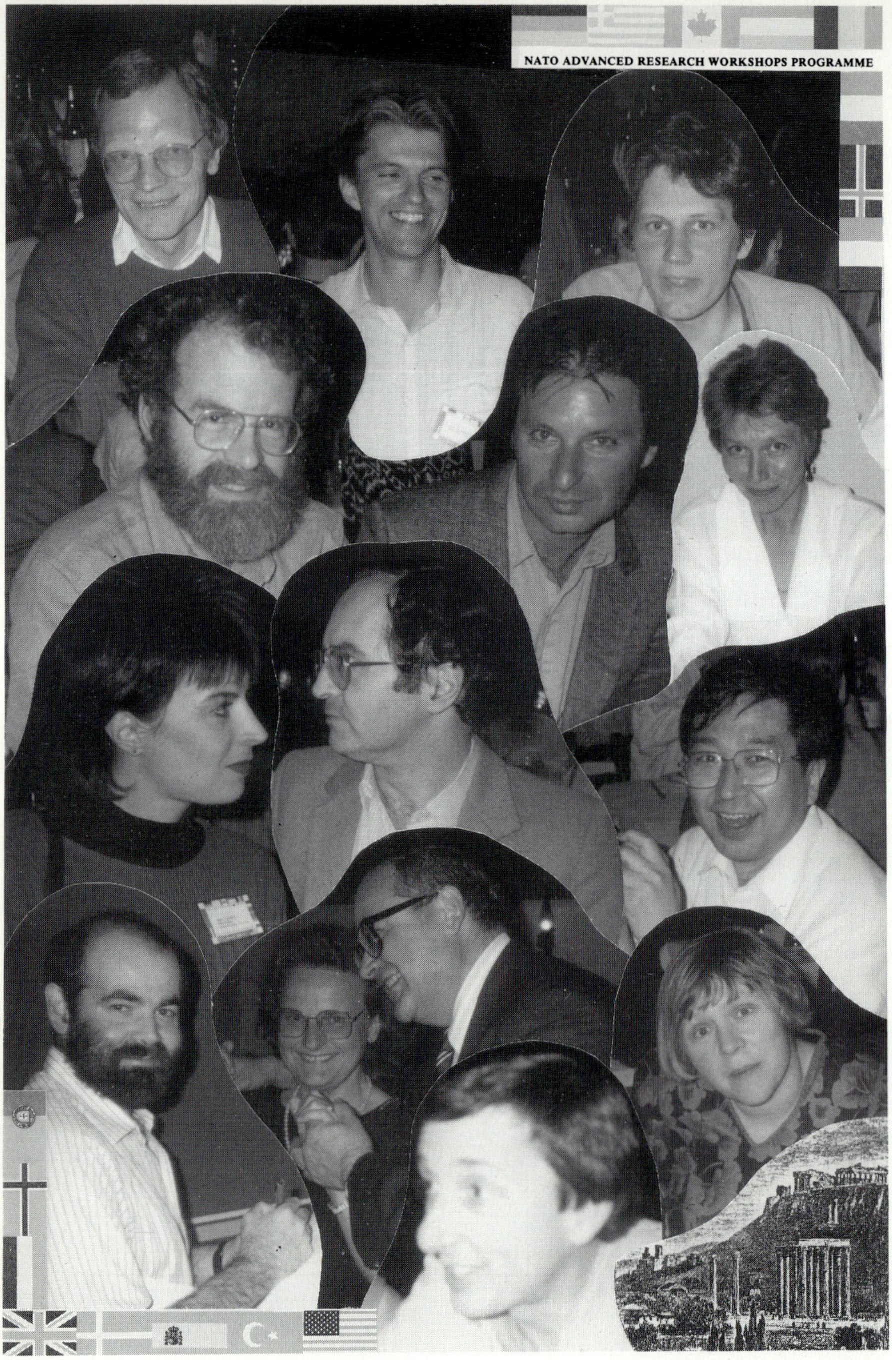

LEFT TO RIGHT IN ROWS: H.Bluthmann, T. Logtenberg, S. Buus
C.A. Janaway, H.A. Erlich, A. Cooke
T. Claudio, S. Tzartos, M. Hattori
A.G. Demaine, J. Charreire, L.D. Kohn, F. Gotch
J. Newsom-Davis

PREFACE

This publication represents the proceedings of a NATO Advanced Research Workshop which took place over 5 days in Athens, Greece in April of 1989. The aims of the meeting were to (i) highlight developments, particularly through recombinant DNA technology, in our understanding of the immune response and (ii) examine the implications of this new knowledge for autoimmunity and autoimmune disease.

The meeting was held as a Workshop of the 23rd Annual Scientific Meeting of the European Society for Clinical Investigation (ESCI). Sponsorship of the meeting, particularly from the NATO International Scientific Exchange Programme, but also from ESCI itself, Pharmacia Therapeutics AB (Sweden), Ortho Pharmaceutical Corporation (USA) and Napp Laboratories (UK) is gratefully acknowledged. In creating the scientific programme for the Workshop, Andy Demaine and I were helped enormously by our co-organisers Charles Janeway, Bernard Malissen, Terence Rabbitts and George Eisenbarth and their help too is gratefully acknowledged. A meeting and the resultant publication are only as good as those that contribute to them, both in terms of the scientific content of their presentation and the efficiency with which they then provide a manuscript for publication. In both senses, our contributors have been exemplary. I hope very much that the quality of their presentation and the enthusiasm which these generated will come over to the reader in the discussions which followed their presentations. In editing the book Andy and I were helped by our colleague, Paul Banga, and we thank him. Through lack of space, one of the highlights of our meeting does not appear in this publication and that was the abstracts for the Poster Sessions. The quality of the abstracts submitted was high and they attracted considerable discussion. For those wishing to see a record of these abstracts they can be found in the European Journal of Clinical Investigation in Part II of Volume 19, No. 2 - April 1989. The burden of making sense of the recorded discussions of the various papers and the typing and retyping of the discussion and of unsatisfactory manuscripts fell to Jacqui De Groote in the Department of Medicine, and she has responded magnificently. David Ewins from the Department ensured we captured the images of our invited speakers on film, and even if we have had to censor some of his creations to ensure the speakers retain their images, his contribution is gratefully acknowledged! Finally, and most importantly, I wish to thank Christine Edwards, also in the Department, whose direction of the Directors, organisation of the Organisers, persuasion of authors to produce manuscripts and running of the actual Workshop in Athens and every other odd job associated with the Workshop ensured its outstanding success. I am particularly indebted to her.

September 1989

Alan M McGregor
Department of Medicine
King's College Hospital
Medical School
London, UK

CONTENTS

ORGANIZATION AND EXPRESSION OF HUMAN V_H GENES

T. Logtenberg, J.E. Berman and F.W. Alt
The Howard Hughes Medical Institute
and Departments of Biochemisty and Microbiology
College of Physicians and Surgeons of Columbia University
701 W. 168th Street
New York, NY 10032

Introduction

The variable regions of immunoglobulin heavy chains are encoded by the three germline gene segments: V(ariable), D(iversity) and J(oining). These segments are joined during precursor B cell differentiation to form a functional V_HDJ_H variable region gene. In the mouse there are hundreds of different V_H gene segments that can be subdivided into families based on nucleotide sequence homology (reviewed in Alt, et al., 1987). Various studies of transformed and normal murine B lineage cells have shown that chromosomal position of V_H segments is a major determinant of their rearrangement frequency, resulting in a preferential rearrangement of V_H segments proximal to the cluster of J_H elements (Yancopoulos, et al., 1984, 1988; Reth, et al., 1986; Perlmutter, et al., 1985). This preferential rearrangement phenomenon leads to the biased expression of J_H-proximal V_H segments in primary B cell repertoires; for example, these gene segments are the major contributors to the Ig heavy chain mRNA produced by B lineage cells of the fetal liver (Yancopoulos, et al., 1988). In contrast, B cells in peripheral lymphoid organs of adult mice appear to utilize most V_H segments at equal frequency; that is the representation of different families in the peripheral Ig heavy chain mRNA repertoire correlates with the complexity of each family and is not related to chromosomal position (Yancopoulos, et al., 1988; Dildrop, et al., 1985). These findings led to the proposal that an initially biased repertoire is randomized, probably by cellular mechanisms, in the transition from primary to peripheral lymphoid tissues (Yancopoulos, et al., 1988).

Although the potential significance of the biased primary repertoire is not clear, it has been suggested that proximal V_H genes may have evolved specificities important early in development for the establishment of the repertoire (Rajewsky et al., 1987; Holmberg 1987). One way to

NATO ASI Series, Vol. H 38
The Molecular Biology of Autoimmune Disease
Edited by A. G. Demaine et al.

further analyze the significance of the preferential V_H gene rearrangement observed in mice is to determine whether similar phenomena exist in other mammalian species and, if so, to determine the nature of the antibodies encoded by proximal V_H genes. Recently, the general structure of the human Ig heavy chain variable region locus has been elucidated (Berman, et al., 1987; Kodaira et al., 1986). To begin to address the issues outlined above, we have studied the expression of V_H genes at different time points in B cell ontogeny and have correlated expression of the most J_H-proximal V_H segment with certain autoantibody specificities.

Organization of the human immunoglobulin heavy chain V_H locus

The human V_H locus contains 100-200 gene segments that have been grouped into 6 families (denoted V_H1-V_H6) that range in size from 1 member (V_H6) to more than 25 members (V_H3) (Berman, et al., 1987; Kodaira et al., 1986). In contrast to murine V_H organization patterns, members of the human V_H families are highly interspersed over the entire 2000 kb locus (fig. 1). We have employed pulsed field gel electrophoresis to demonstrate that the V_H locus begins within less than 90 kb of the J_H-$C\mu$ region with the V_H6 gene (a single membered family) being the most J_H-proximal human V_H gene segment (Berman, et al., 1987).

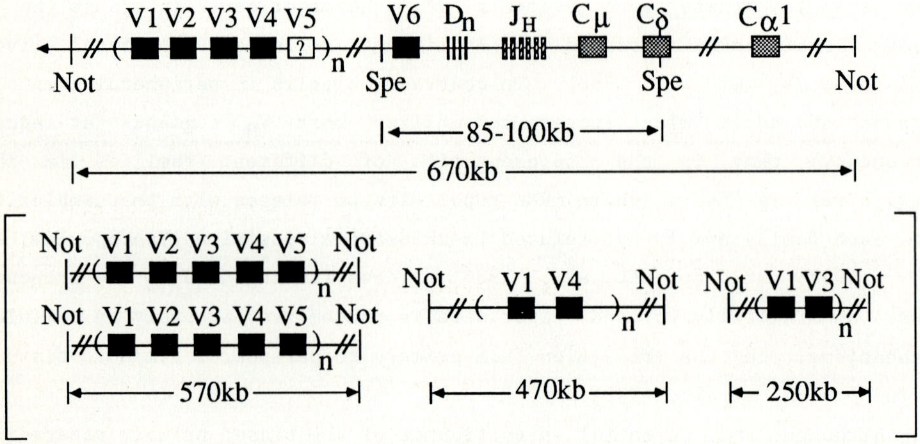

Figure 1. Organization of the human immunoglobulin V_H locus as determined by Pulse field gradient gel electrophoresis; for details see Berman et al., 1987.

Expression of Human V_H Genes in Primary and Peripheral Lymphoid Tissues

As an initial approach to assay the utilization frequency of V_H gene segments by surface Ig-positive B lymphocytes, we assayed the V_H family expressed by individual members of a collection of 187 monoclonal, IgM-secreting Epstein Barr virus (EBV)-transformed cell lines derived from adult and fetal tissues. The frequency of V_H family utilization by these lines roughly correlated with the complexity of the family (Table 1)--suggesting that the repertoire is randomized in the B lymphocytes that are the targets of EBV transformation. These results are reminiscent of those obtained with murine splenic hybridomas in which V_H utilization again correlated with family size.

	Tissue				
	adult periph. blood	19 week fetus liver	spleen	Total	Complexity no. of bands (%)
	(n=97)	(n=36)	(n=54)	(n=187)	
VH1	15	25	20	20	20-25 (33)
VH2	<5	<5	5	5	5-10 (11)
VH3	60	50	60	55	25-30 (40)
VH4	20	10	10	15	6-10 (11)
VH5	5	<5	10	5	2-3 (4)
VH6	<5	<5	<5	<5	1 (1)

Table 1. Frequency of V_H Gene Utilization in EBV-transformed Cell Lines. Total RNA from 187 monoclonal IgM-secreting EBV-transformed cell lines was analyzed in northern blotting experiments for hybridization to probes specific for each of the 6 V_H gene families. The data are presented as the percentage of the total number (n) of cell lines in a given collection that hybridizes to a V_H-specific probe.

To assay for the relative utilization of V_H gene families in primary and peripheral lymphoid cells, we used the Northern blotting assay previously described (Yancopoulos, et al., 1988). Briefly, in this assay, a standardized amount of Ig μ heavy chain mRNA is assayed for hybridization to family-specific V_H probes; the ratio of hybridization of each V_H to RNA from a primary lymphoid organ (in this case 16 and 24 week old fetal liver) to that of a peripheral organ (in this case, T cell-depleted peripheral blood; PBL) is analyzed. The data from this preliminary experiment are shown in figure 2.

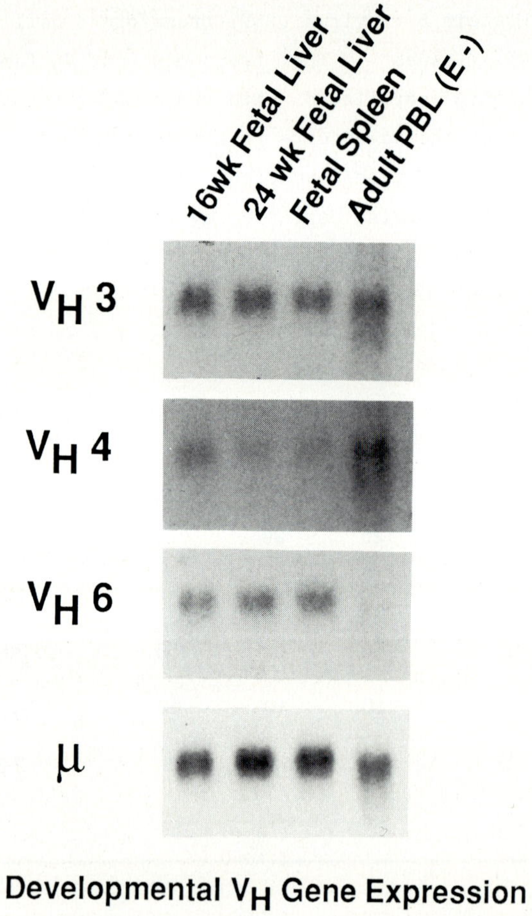

Figure 2. Biased V_H6 Gene Utilization in Early Development. RNA from two fetal livers (Lane 1 and 2), a fetal spleen (Lane 3) and adult peripheral blood non-T cells (Lane 4) was analyzed in Northern blotting experiments for hybridization to a V_H3, V_H4, V_H6 and $C\mu$-specific probe.

The V_H6 gene clearly hybridized much more intensely to the same amount of μmRNA from the fetal liver samples than to that from adult PBL. This result is very similar to that observed when the J_H proximal murine V_H81X gene is used to probe an equivalent amount of μmRNA from murine fetal liver and adult spleen (Yancopoulos, et al., 1988) and indicates that--like V_H81X in the mouse--the J_H proximal V_H6 gene segment in humans is much more abundantly represented in the fetal liver as opposed to the PBL repertoires. As opposed to V_H6, the V_H3 family appears to be equally represented in the fetal and adult repertoires, while the V_H4 family appears to be more abundantly expressed in adult repertoires. The findings with the V_H3 family are consistent with our previous observations that this is the largest gene family and that its members are interspersed across the entire V_H locus; therefore representation changes based on either rearrangement or cellular selection would be expected to be less apparent at the gross level of this assay (Yancopoulos, et al., 1988); but could be more obvious if individual members of the family were examined (Schroeder, et al., 1987; see below). In the context of our previous findings in the murine system, the increased representation of the intermediate sized V_H4 family in PBL as compared to fetal liver could be explained in various ways including a large number of functional members and or a more distal location (Yancopoulos, et al., 1988). Notably, we find that V_H utilization patterns in 24 week fetal spleen are similar to those of fetal liver (Figure 2); we have made similar findings in the mouse (Malynn, et al., submitted), and various analyses suggest that the bulk of the mRNA detected in these tissues at this stage may come from immature B lineage cells.

Together, the results of our analysis of V_H gene utilization in human B lineage cells are quite analogous to those obtained by similar studies of the murine system. These findings suggest that an initially position dependent repertoire is generated in differentiating human pre-B cells and that this repertoire is normalized in surface IgM-positive B lymphocytes. This normalization was evident even in our analyses of EBV-transformed B cells from 19 week old fetal tissues (Table 1), suggesting that normalization processes may act rapidly on the newly formed, sIgM-positive B cells. As noted above, none of our analyses permit detection of qualitative differences between the collections of V_H genes expressed from multi-membered families. In this regard, others found preferential expression of particular V_H1 and V_H3 genes in a cDNA library of 19 week old fetal liver (Schroeder, et al., 1987). It should be noted that the organization of families appears somewhat different in humans versus the mouse. Murine families tend to be relatively clustered as units whereas human families are highly interspersed. It will be of interest to determine if the V_H3 genes preferentially expressed in human fetal liver represent J_H-proximal members of that family.

Autoantibodies Encoded by the V_H6 Gene Family

Antigen-binding properties of IgM molecules secreted by the 187 EBV lines were assayed by screening culture supernatants in direct binding ELISA for reactivity against a panel of 24 antigens. A number of antibodies that employed heavy chains from families 1-5 bound to particular antigens within the panel; however, there was no obvious correlation between antigen-binding pattern and expression of these V_H families (not shown). In contrast, antibodies from each of the 4 V_H6-expressing cell lines in the collection bound to ssDNA and poly dT, regardless of the light chain expressed. In addition, V_H6 antibodies from individual cell lines displayed various patterns of binding activities with a limited number of antigens in the panel, notably dsDNA, cardiolipin, cytochrome C and hen egg lysozyme. Such polyreactivity is a characteristic of some monoclonal anti-DNA antibodies of both human and murine origin.

Clone #	origin	isotype	μg/ml of Ag required for 50% inhibition					
			ssDNA	nDNA	Card	PdT	CytC	Hel
A10[1]	adult PB	IgM,κ	5.0	0.02	0.1	0.02	-	0.02
A431[1]	adult PB	IgM,λ	5.0	0.3	0.2	5.0	2.0	-
L16[1]	130 d FL	IgM,λ	5.0	-	0.13	0.001	-	-
ML1[2]	130 d FS	IgM,κ	2.5	-	-	10.0	-	-

Table 2. Origin of V_H6-expressing EBV-transformed B Cell Lines and Properties of the Antibodies they Secrete. Liver and spleen cells from a 19 week old fetus and mononuclear peripheral blood cells from 3 adults were transformed with EBV under limiting dilution conditions. Supernatants from monoclonal, IgM-secreting lines were tested for reactivity against a panel of 24 antigens including haptens, protein (auto)antigens, polysaccharides and polynucleotides. Results obtained from the direct binding assays were confirmed in liquid phase inhibition ELISAs. Results are expressed as the concentration of competitor required for 50% inhibition of binding to solid-phase bound antigen. PB: peripheral blood. FL: fetal liver. FS: fetal spleen.

The molecular basis of the observed similarities and differences in antigen-binding patterns of these V_H-encoded autoantibodies was investigated by analyzing cDNA clones of the Ig heavy chain mRNA expressed by each cell line. The results demonstrated that both fetal tissue derived cell lines (L16 and ML1) expressed a germline V_H6 gene; the identical sequence has been observed in germline V_H6 genes from 5 different individuals (not shown). The V_H6 genes expressed in the adult tissue-derived cell lines A10 and A431 differed from the prototypic germline V_H6 nucleotide sequence by three and six nucleotides respectively. Eight out of these nine differences were confined to complementarity-determining regions 1 and 2, suggesting somatic mutations. Using the polymerase chain reaction, it was confirmed that the V_H6 sequence expressed in the A10 did not exist in the germline of the same donor (not shown). Antibodies from A10 and A431 bound with relatively high avidity to dsDNA, a property not displayed by germline V_H6-encoded antibodies.

To summarize, the V_H6 gene has many unique properties. It is remarkably well-conserved in the human population and represents the only single-membered V_H gene family. In addition, it is the J_H-proximal V_H gene segment and apparently contributes preferentially to the expressed early Ig heavy chain variable region repertoire. Finally, this V_H gene can encode antibodies that, regardless of light chain, have binding speicificities that are reminiscent of autoantibodies present in the sera of patients with systemic lupus erythematosus. In some of the antibodies studied, the expressed V_H6 genes show evidence for somatic mutation. Whether these antibodies actually contribute to the pathogenesis of SLE is at present unknown.

Acknowledgements

This study was supported by the Howard Hughes Medical Institute, the Netherlands Organization for the Advancement of Pure Research (ZWO) and NIH grants AI-20047 and CA-40427. T.L. and J.B. are fellows of the Howard Hughes Medical Institute.

REFERENCES

Alt FW, Blackwell TK, Yancopoulos GD (1987) Development of the primary antibody repertoire. Science 238: 1079-1087

Berman JE, Mellis SJ, Pollock R, Smith CL, Suh H, Heinke B, Kowal C, Surti U, Chess L, Cantor CR, Alt FW (1987) Content and organization of the human Ig V_H locus: definition of three new V_H families and linkage to the Ig C_H locus. EMBO J. 7: 727-738

Dildrop R, Krawinkel U, Winter E, Rajewsky K (1985) V_H-gene expression in murine lipopolysaccharide blasts distributes over the nine known V_H-gene subgroups and may be random. Eur. J. Immunol. 15: 1154-1156

Holmberg D (1987) High connectivity, natural antibodies preferentially use 7183 and QUPC 52 V_H families. Eur. J. Immunol. 17: 399

Kodaira M, Kinashi T, Umemura I, Matsuda F, Noma T, Ono Y, Honjo T (1986) Organization and evolution of variable region genes of the human immunoglobulin heavy chain. J. Mol. Biol. 190:529-541

Malynn BA, Yancopoulos GD, Barth JE, Bosma CG, Bosma MJ, Bona C, Alt FW Developmental expression of murine V_H gene families, submitted

Perlmutter RM, Kearney JF, Chang SP, Hood LE (1985) Developmentally controlled expression of immunoglobulin V_H genes. Science 227: 1597-1601

Rajewsky K, Forster I, Cumano A (1987) Evolutionary and somatic selection of the antibody repertoire in the mouse. Science 238: 1088

Reth MG, Jackson S, Alt FW (1986) V_HDJ_H formation and DJ_H replacement during pre-B differentiation: non-random usage of gene segments. EMBO J. 5: 2131

Schroeder Jr, HW, Hillson JL, Perlmutter RM (1987) Early restriction of the human antibody repertoire. Science 238: 791-793

Yancopoulos GD, Desiderio SV, Paskind M, Kearney JF, Baltimore D, Alt FW (1984) Preferential utilization of the most J_H proximal V_H gene segments in pre-B cell lines. Nature 311: 727-733

Yancopoulos GD, Malynn BA, Alt FW (1988) Developmentally regulated and strain-specific expression of murine V_H gene families. J. Exp. Med. 168:417-435

DISCUSSION

DEMAINE: How many functional or pseudo genes do you find on a single phage clone?

LOGTENBERG: _You can find either two functional, two pseudo or the mixture of both. Also, we find V genes as close together as 3kb and sometimes in phage clones as far apart as 20kb, so there is quite a variation in both what you can find in a single phage clone and how far these V genes are apart.

WILLCOX: Do you think that the VH6 clones that you describe where derived from CD5+ B cells?

LOGTENBERG: It is not easy to answer that question. A number of interesting observations have been made when we transform/select CD5+ B cells. First, we find that some of them lose their CD5 expression on the membrane, whilst retaining an RNA transcript for CD5 which we think is a non-spliced precursor. Other cells show no evidence at all of CD5 expression. In our VH6+ clones we have two that have this precursor RNA for CD5, and two which don't, so there is at least some evidence for CD5 expression. We never find this CD5 RNA in the CD5- B cells.

WILLCOX: It has previously been suggested that the expressed VH genes of CD5+ B cells do not mutate. Is this still true?

LOGTENBERG: I think all the evidence from the murine system, particularly lymphomas, shows that they remain germ line and non-mutated.

QUESTION: Which cells have the CD5 message?

LOGTENBERG: The two which have the CD5 message are the germ line ones from liver and spleen derived B cells.

There is no evidence for CD5 expression except in the two foetal tissue derived from the V6+ clones

GEARHART: Tom, can you refresh at least my memory on what is a CD5+ B-cell? Is it similar to an Lyl+ B-cell?

LOGTENBERG: Yes, as far as we can tell it is the same type of cell although its much better characterised in the murine system.

GEARHART: Can you elaborate on the characteristics of the CD5+ B-cells?

LOGTENBERG: In the murine system there is a separate population of CD5+ B cells which have an unusual tissue location. They are very abundant early in ontogeny and can account for up to 50% of foetal liver B cells. During development they move to the peritoneal cavity. What is interesting is that they contriibute mainly to the pool of natural autoantibodies, and the level of these B-cells are elevated in a number of mouse strains which develop autoimmune disease suggesting a role in autoimmunity. In man, I think the evidence is still scarce. Nobody knows where they come from and they may have a separate precursor lineage from conventional B cells, the length of their long lifespan is not known, nor the type of response which they participate in. It is clear that they are present in all CLL cell populations

NEPOM: One concept which was notable by its absence in your talk is that of germ line polymorphism and its contribution to autoantibody specificity - would you care to comment on this point, and the source of material for generating the clones.

<u>LOGTENBERG</u>: The collection of clones was derived from 8 individuals. The 1000 clones I described here were derived from 3 adults. We did not see any difference in the frequency of usage of VH genes between individuals. Interestingly, the VH6 gene is highly conserved in man. Also, certain VH3 genes keep being cloned in different laboratories throughout the world - Capra's and our own group repeatedly clone out the same VH3 genes and there is one particular gene which has been cloned 5 different times, each gene being 100% homologous. Therefore, it suggests that there is a very high degree of homology among individual VH genes in the human population. However, this may be biased because we are looking for certain VH genes because we have an interest in them and not trying to clone out all the VH genes. For instance, certain antibodies are interesting for a particular reason - you start to clone them and you find the same sequences as other people do. Therefore, whilst certain VH genes are very well conserved this may not be true for all VH genes.

<u>NEPOM</u>: Let me just mention that there is a manuscript or paper published in the Journal of Immunology which shows that using DNA probes to all the different CDR regions including CDR2 and CDR3 and going into germ line DNA there is a surprisingly high degree of germ line polymorphism for particular sequence cassettes of individual sub-members of each of these families.

<u>DIAMOND</u>: Is there any evidence for biased VH gene usage in conventional B cells at any stage of development which is a reflection of the development of the Lyl or CD5+ B cells?

LOGTENBERG: The only bias we have seen so far is when we look in very early tissues. 6-7 week old foetal liver has a very high expression of VH5 and VH6 and virtually no VH3 - similar to the murine system. There is no bias in CLL cells and normal CD5+ B cells.

DIAMOND: Are there any normal B cell precursors at the early stage

LOGTENBERG: Well of course we did not directly prove that and the only reason I can speculate is that they do seem to use similar restricted V genes but may be it goes a little far to say that they are the normal precursors

DIAMOND: Is there any bias of VH gene usage in the non-CD5+ B cells, assuming that these are going to develop into conventional B cells?

LOGTENBERG: If you deplete conventional CD5+ B cells you do have a bias utilisation of VH genes.

DIAMOND: No matter how early during development you look?

LOGTENBERG: We only looked in the cord blood.

JANEWAY: Its not exactly relevant to your presentation, but just out of curiosity, what is the structural or functional relationship between VH gene families of the mouse and VH gene families of man? For instance, is the size of the gene family similar, and are there any structural homologies and if so, do they correlate with family size and gene utilization?

LOGTENBERG: The VH families 1 to 3 do have counterparts in the murine system based on cross-hybridisation. One surprising thing, is that the J558 family which is the largest in the mouse, is a much smaller family in humans. The murine

S107 family is the one which is homologous to the VH3 family which is by far the largest in humans. In both the murine and human systems there is no evidence that retaining a certain V gene family confers selection advantage.

GEARHART: OK Tom, now I'm really confused, your results on the normal B cells from 19 week foetal spleens show no bias towards proximal VH genes, or positional bias, just a random utilisation and yet a proximal bias exsists in mice up until neonatal life, so what is going on in human system? Why is there randomisation so early in foetal life and at what point are these B cells expressing kappa or lambda light chain or are they also selected randomly?

LOGTENBERG: The cells express both light chains and make functional antibodies. What you are saying is correct, in the murine system the bias persists into neonatal life. We certainly don't see that in the human, which we found surprising, because we did expect to find that. A plausable explanation is that the 19 week old foetal liver may not be an important haemopoeitic organ and what you find is equivalent to that of a spleen of a normalised repertoire. We did see that bias very early in human life so there may be a similar process occurring in human foetal livers. Also, we cannot discriminate within a VH family, for example, is there is a biased utilisation in the VH3 gene family? One may find the recurrence of very restricted number of VH3 genes.

GEARHART: Did you look at pre-B cells at 19 weeks?

LOGTENBERG: No, these are all B cells.

<u>GEARHART</u>: If you had looked at pre-B cells you might expect to see that bias.

<u>LOGTENBERG</u>: Yes, but we have very few of them so it is very hard to do the analysis.

<u>GEARHART</u>: Have you checked adult bone marrow?

<u>LOGTENBERG</u>: No.

<u>DEMAINE</u>: Has anyone looked at the VH gene organisation of wild type mice compared to the inbred strains? Do you still find segregation of VH families or are they are interspersed?

<u>LOGTENBERG</u>: No, I don't know if anyone has looked.

<u>GEARHART</u>: You have mentioned that you and others keep cloning out the same variable genes, a VH3 gene, and you had also given an estimate of the number of VH genes in the human to be around 100 to 200. Does this mean that most of them are pseudo genes that are not being used and how large would you estimate is the actual repertoire of functional VH genes in human?

<u>LOGTENBERG</u>: That is mainly from the work of Jeff Berman, he cloned out about 30 germ line V genes - what he found is that roughly 50% of them are pseudo genes so if you want to look at the functional VH gene repertoire that is about half of the 100 to 200 genes. Again that is a very rough estimate because using different approaches you derive different numbers as has been done for the murine system but it is at least a number we can go by although half of them may be pseudo genes.

IMMUNOGLOBULIN KAPPA VARIABLE GENE SEGMENT USAGE DURING ONTOGENY

A. Lawler and P. Gearhart
Department of Biochemistry
Johns Hopkins University School of Hygiene and Public Health
615 N. Wolfe Street
Baltimore, Maryland 21205

The immunoglobulin repertoire is initially generated by the rearrangement of discrete gene segments encoding the heavy and light chains. Heavy chain genes are composed of a variable gene segment (V_H), a diversity (D) gene segment and a joining (J_H) gene segment, and kappa light chain genes contain variable (V_K) and joining (J_K) gene segments. In developing B cells, the gene segments are independently selected from pools of several hundred V_H and V_K gene segments, 12 D gene segments, and four J_H or J_K gene segments, creating a diverse population of immunoglobulins. The V_H gene segments are grouped into nine subfamilies which contain gene segments that share 80% or greater homology, and span a region between 500 and 2500 kilobasepairs (kb) that is located several hundred kb upstream of the D and J_H gene segments on chromosome 12 (Brodeur PH, Riblet R, 1984; Brodeur PH, 1987). V_K gene segments have been grouped into at least 18 subfamilies and are located upstream of the J_K gene segments on chromosome 6 (Potter M, et al, 1982). Addition and deletion of nucleotides at the junctions of the gene segments creates greater diversity in the third hypervariable region in each gene. The repertoire generated by gene rearrangements can be modified by interactions between immunoglobulins expressed on the B-cell surface and endogenous antigens leading to the expansion or inhibition of certain antibody specificities.

We have examined the patterns of V_H and V_K gene segments used in fetal and neonatal pre-B and B cells in order to define the initial repertoire of immunoglobulins as well as to characterize the rearrangement process which activates gene segments dispersed over large chromosomal regions.

V_K usage is more diverse than V_H usage in fetal and neonatal B cells. V_H expression in fetal and neonatal pre-B and B cells from BALB/c mice has been examined in many systems including Abelson virus-transformed cell lines (Yancopoulos GD, et al, 1984; Lawler AM, et al, 1987), lines that rearrange in culture (Yancopoulos GD, et al, 1984; Reth MG, et al, 1986), B cell hybridomas (Perlmutter RM, et al, 1985), pre-B and B cell colonies (Wu GE, Paige CJ, 1986), total RNA from neonatal liver (Yancopoulos GD, et al, 1988) and *in situ* hybridization to fetal liver B cells (Jeong HD, Teale JM, 1988). All of the studies have observed frequent use of the V_H7183 and V_HQ52 subfamilies which are located closest to the J_H gene segments, suggesting that the J_H-proximal gene segments are more available for rearrangement than the rest of the locus. To compare the pattern of V_K rearrangements to

NATO ASI Series, Vol. H 38
The Molecular Biology of Autoimmune Disease
Edited by A. G. Demaine et al.

	CELL LINE	V_K SUBFAMILY	V_K GENE	SIZE (kbp)
HYBRIDOMAS	DA4–6	1	V105	3.3
	ID3–2	1	1.60	6.0
	MD2–16	4	4.58	5.8
	4–1	4	H1	3.0
	45–1	4	4.68	6.8
	15–56–1	9	9.42	4.2
	GB3–1	10	10ArsA	3.2
	BC2–5–12	12	K2	4.8
	BM32–1–6	21	21E1.5	5.3
	BC2–5–12	21	21E1.6	12.0
18–81 SUBCLONES	1H6A	1	V105	2.7
	T17B	4	H13	2.2
	T17B	4	4.30	3.0
	T17B	4	R11	4.6
	T29B5–2	4	H9	3.4
	1H6A	10	10ArsA	3.8
	T4B20	19	19.34	3.4
	T24B	23	23.32	3.2
	16C	24	A5	4.8
	1H6A	24	M167	7.5
	2E5A	24	24.23	2.3

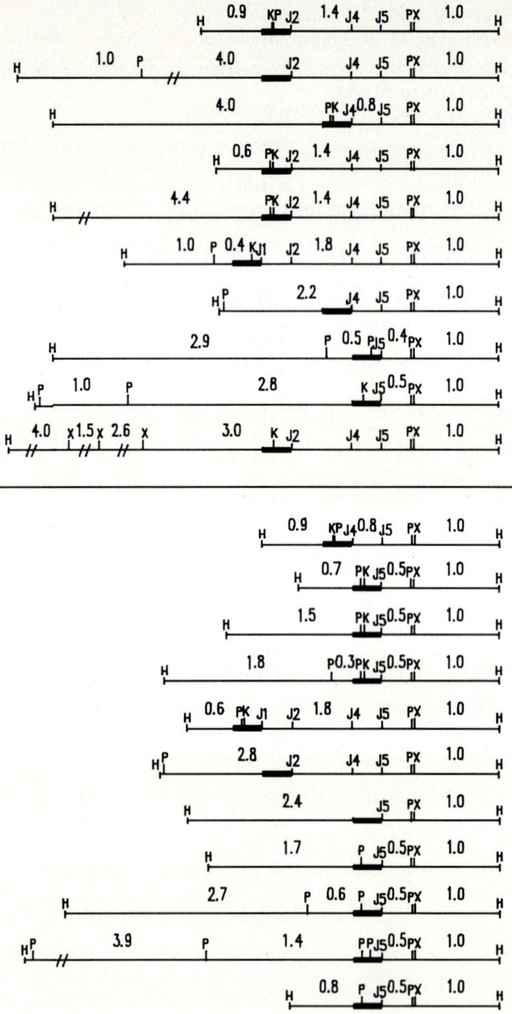

Figure 1. Restriction enzyme maps of V_K rearrangements from B cell hybridomas and 18-81 subclones. Sizes indicate the length of the cloned HindIII fragment in kb. Solid bars depict the V_K coding segments. J_K gene segments are shown as a line. The distance in kb between restriction sites is shown above each map. Distances that are not drawn to scale are represented as two diagonal lines. H = HindIII, K = KpnI, P = PstI, X = XbaI.

V_H rearrangements, we identified the V_K gene segments in two cell populations: (1) fetal and neonatal B cell hybridomas, and (2) subclones of a Abelson virus-transformed pre-B cell, 18-81, that rearranged V_K gene segments during culture. Each rearrangement was cloned from genomic DNA and sequenced to identify individual gene segments. Restriction enzyme maps of the rearranged genes are shown in Figure 1. Twelve V_K rearrangements from the hybridomas were distributed over six different V_K subfamilies: 1, 4, 9, 10, 12, and 21. Similarly, the 13 V_K rearrangements from six 18-81 subclones contained gene segments from an overlapping set of six V_K subfamilies: 1, 4, 10, 19, 23, and 24. A recent map of the V_K locus (D'Hoostelaere LA, et al, 1988) indicates that these subfamilies are distributed throughout the locus, indicating that early V_K rearrangements are more heterogeneous than V_H rearrangements. Several processes may contribute to the diverse V_K repertoire as compared to the biased pattern of V_H rearrangements. The V_K genes may be in a chromatin structure that allows the recombination enzymes to reach the entire locus whereas the V_H locus may be in a conformation in which the J_H-proximal subfamilies are more accessible for rearrangement than the rest of the locus. Alternatively, initial rearrangements to J_K-proximal V_K gene segments may be replaced by secondary rearrangements (Lewis S, et al, 1982; Fedderson RM, et al, 1985; Shapiro MA, Weigert M, 1987). Secondary rearrangements of variable genes which can occur on the kappa locus but not on the heavy chain locus (Figure 2), may facilitate rearrangement to upstream V_K gene

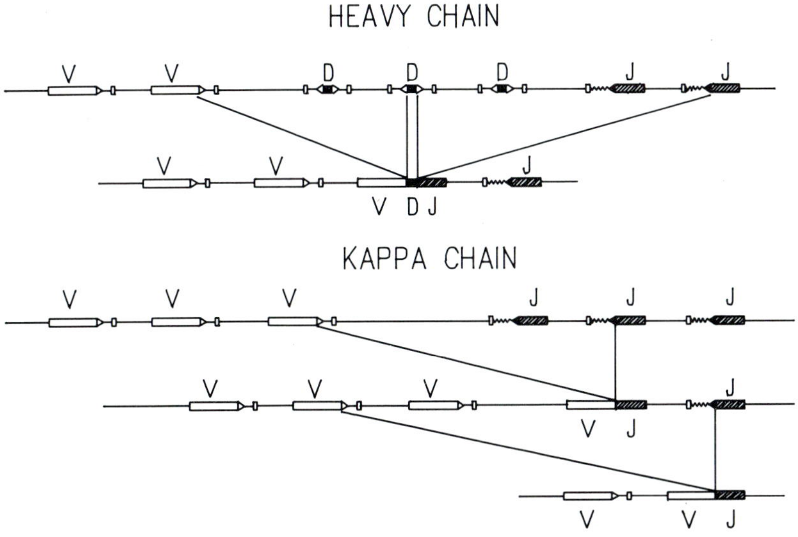

Figure 2. Secondary variable gene rearrangements can occur on the V_K locus but not on the V_H locus. Deletion of the DNA between the D and J_H gene segments and the V_H and D gene segments during heavy chain rearrangements prevents secondary V_H rearrangements. On the kappa locus, upstream germline V_K gene segments can rearrange to downstream J_K gene segments, deleting or inverting the initial VJ rearrangement.

subfamilies. Secondary rearrangements may have contributed to the a frequency of J_K5 gene segments used in the 18-81 subclones. Since some initial rearrangements would be lost by a secondary rearrangement that occurs by deletion, the pattern of initial rearrangements and the contribution of secondary rearrangements to the final repertoire has not been measured.

VJ junctions in 18-81 subclones. The sequences of the VJ junctions in the 25 rearrangements are shown in Figure 3. In several cases, i.e., V_K1.60, V_KH1, V_K4.30, V_KR11, V_KH9, V_K23.32, V_KM167, and V_K24.23, extra nucleotides were detected in the junctions between the V_K and J_K gene segments. The extra nucleotides may be encoded by germline V_K gene segments, or alternatively, they may be added *de novo* by terminal transferase during joining (Desiderio SV, et al, 1984). Although normally found in the junctions of V_H rearrangements, extra nucleotides are not usually observed in V_K rearrangements.

Figure 3. VJ junctions of rearrangements from hybridomas and 18-81 subclones.

V_K Subfamily	Cell Line	V_K Gene				
			90			
(1)	DA4-6	V_KV105	CAA AGT ACA CAT GTT CCC A		TGTACACGT	J2
	IH6A		--- --- --- --- --- --		ATTCACGT	J4
	ID3-2	V_K1.60	CAA GGT ACA CAT TTT CCT	CAT	ACGT	J2
(4)	MD2-16	V_K4.58	CAG TGG AGT AGT TAC CCA		TTCACGT	J4
	4-1	V_KH1	CAG TAC AGT GGT TAC CCA	TCA	ACGT	J2
	45-1	V_K4.68	CAG TGG AGT AGT TAC CC		GTACACGT	J2
	T17B	V_KH13	CAG TGG AGT AGT AAC CCA	A	TCACGT	J5
	T17B	V_K4.30	CAG TGG AGT AGT AAC CCA	CGGC	GCTCACGT	J5
	T17B	V_KR11	CAG TGG AGT GGT TAC CCA	CCCATGC	CACGT	J5
	T17B	V_KH9	CAG CGG AGT AGT TAC CCA	TGA	TCACGT	J4
	T29B5-2		--- --- --- --- --- -		ACGT	J1
(9)	15-56-1	V_K9.42	CAG TAT GAT AAT CT		GTGGACGT	J1
(10)	134-1	V_K10ArsA	CAG GGT AAT ACG CTT CC		GTACACGT	J2
	IH6A		--- --- --- --- --- --		--------	J2
	GB3-1		--- --- --- --- --- --TCC		ATTCACGT	J4
(12)	BC2-5-12	V_KK2	CAT TTT TGG AGT ACT CC		GCTCACGT	J5
(19)	T4B20	V_K19.34	CAA CAT TGG AAT TAT C		CTCACGT	J5
(21)	BM32-1-6	V_K21E1.5	CAC AGT AGG GAG CTT CC		TCACGT	J5
	BFL14		--- --- --- --- --- --C		ATTCACGT	J4
	BC2-5-12	V_K21E1.6	CAC AGT TGG GAG ATT CC		GTACACGT	J2
(23)	T24B	V_K23.32	AAT GGT CAC AGC TTT CCT	CCG	TCACGT	J5
(24)	T17B	V_KA5	CAA AAT CTA GAA CTT CC		GCTCACGT	J5
	16C		--- --- --- --- --- --		--------	J5
	IH6A	V_KM167	CAA CTT GTA GAG G	A	CACGT	J5
	2E5A	V_K24.23	CAA CTG CTA GAA CTC CCC	TT	CTCACGT	J5

Repeated rearrangements of variable gene segments suggest gene targeting. Of the 25 V_K gene segments identified, four were repeated twice and one was repeated three times. Repeated V_H gene segment rearrangements have also been observed in Abelson-transformed pre-B cell lines (Yancopoulos GD, et al, 19844; Lawler AM, 1987), suggesting that certain V_K and V_H gene segments are inherently more susceptible to rearrangement than others. Targeting of individual gene segments may result from a higher binding affinity of the recombination enzymes for DNA sequences flanking the gene segments. Some gene segments could be favored by variations in local chromatin structure that increases their accessibility to recombination enzymes. The chromatin structure may also place some V_K gene segments in a position relative to the J_K gene segments that facilitates rearrangement (Cockerill PN, et al, 1986).

Comparison of early V_H and V_K rearrangements with the autoimmune repertoire. Studies of variable gene segments in rheumatoid factors and other autoantibodies revealed predominant use of the V_H7183, V_HQ52 and V_HJ558 subfamilies and the V_K1, 4, 10 and 19 subfamilies (Bona C, 1988). V_K8 gene segments were also used frequently in the group of rheumatoid factors (Shlomchik M, et al, 1987). Table 1 compares the usage of these subfamilies in fetal and neonatal pre-B and B cells with the repertoire of autoantibodies and rheumatoid factors. Although V_H usage in fetal and neonatal B cells is biased towards the V_H7183 and V_H Q52 subfamilies, rheumatoid factors and autoimmune antibodies use these

Table 1. Comparison of variable gene subfamilies used most frequently in early B cells and autoimmune antibodies.

	V_H Subfamily Usage (%)		V_K Subfamily Usage (%)		
	7183+Q52	J558	1,4,10,19	8	21,24
Fetal and Neonatal B cell Hybridomas[1]	61	4	58	0	25
Adult Spleen[2]	35	37	ND[5]	ND	ND
Autoimmune Antibodies[3]	40	46	68	7	0
Rheumatoid Factors[4]	35	47	61	3	5

[1] Current study and Perlmutter, RM, et al, 1985.
[2] Jeong HD, Teale JM, 1988.
[3] Bona C, 1988.
[4] Shlomchik MD, et al, 1987.
[5] Not done

subfamilies at frequencies seen in the adult. V_K usage is similar between the early hybridomas and autoimmune antibodies or rheumatoid factors in that roughly 60% of the repertoire is represented by the four subfamilies of V_K1, 4, 10, and 19. Clearly, the population of variable genes found in fetal and neonatal B cells is capable of expressing many autoimmune antibodies and rheumatoid factors, although the importance of these immunoglobulins on the development of tolerance has not been defined.

REFERENCES

Bona C (1988) V Genes Encoding Autoantibodies: Molecular and Phenotypic Characteristics. Ann. Rev. Immunol. 6:327-358.

Brodeur PH, Riblet R (1984) The Immunoglobulin Heavy Chain Variable Region (Igh-V) Locus in the Mouse I. One Hundred Igh-V Genes Comprise Seven Families of Homologous Genes. Eur J Immunology 14:922-930.

Brodeur P (1987) Genes Encoding the Immunoglobulin Variable Regions. In: Calabi F, Neuberrger MS (eds) Molecular Genetics of Immunoglobulin. Elsevier Science Publishers, New York, 1987.

Cockerill PN, Garrard WT (1986) Chromosomal Loop Anchorage of the Kappa Immunoglobulin Gene Occurs next to the Enhancer in a Region Containing Topoisomerase II Sites. Cell 44:273-282.

Desiderio SV, Yancopoulos GD, Paskind M, Thomas E, Boss MA, Landau N, Alt FW, Baltimore, D (1984) Insertion of N Regions into Heavy-chain Genes is Correlated with Expression of Terminal Deoxytransferase in B Cells. Nature 311:752-755.

D'Hoostelaere LA, Huppi K, Mock B, Mallett C, Potter M (1988) The IgK Chain Allelic Groups Among the IgK Haplotypes and IgK Crossover Populations Suggest a Gene Order. J Immunology 141:652-661.

Feddersen RM, Van Ness BG (1985) Double recombination of a single immunoglobulin K-chain allele: Implications for th mechanism of rearrangement. Proc Natl Acad Sci USA 82:4793-4797.

Jeong HD, Teale JM (1988) Comparison of the Fetal and Adult Functional B Cell Repertoires by Analysis of V_H Gene Family Expression. J Exp Med 168:589-603.

Lawler AM, Lin PS, Gearhart, PJ (1987) Adult B-cell reperotire is biased toward two heavy-chain variable-region genes that rearrange frequently in fetal pre-B cells. Proc Natl Acad Sci USA 84:2454-2458.

Lewis S, Rosenberg N, Alt W, Baltimore D (1982) Continuing Kappa-Gene Rearrangement in a Cell Line Transformed by Abelson Murine Leukemia Virus. Cell 30:807-816.

Perlmutter RM, Kearney JF, Chang S, Hood LE (1985) Developmentally Controlled Expression of Immunoglobulin V_H Genes. Science 227:1597-1600.

Potter M, Newell JB, Rudikoff S, Haber E (1982) Classification of Mouse V_K Groups Based on the Partial Amino Acid Sequence to the First Invariant Tryptophan: Impact of 14 New Sequences from IgG Myeloma Proteins. Molecular Immunology 19:1619-1630.

Reth MG, Jackson S, Alt FW (1986) V_HDJ_H Formation and DJ_H replacement During Pre-B Differentiation: Non-random Usage of Gene Segments. EMBO J. 5:2131-2138.

Shapiro MA, Weigert M (1987) How Immunoglobulin V_K Genes Rearrange. J Immunology 139:3834-3839.

Wu GE, Paige CJ (1986) V_H Gene Family Utilization in Colonies Derived from B and Pre-B Cells Detected by the RNA Colony Blot Assay. EMBO J 5:3475-3481.

Yancopoulos GD, Desiderio SV, Paskind M, Kearney JF, Baltimore D, Alt FW (1984) Preferential Utilization of the Most J_H-proximal V_H Gene Segments in Pre-B-cell Lines. Science 311:727-733.

Yancopoulos GD, Malynn BA, Alt FW (1988) Developmentally Regulated and Strain-specific Expression of Murine V_H Gene Families. J Exp Med 168:417-435.

DISCUSSION

DEMAINE: In your model of replacement/silent mutations, how do you correct for the nonsense mutations as these will not be expressed in the cDNA clones? You are assuming that the rate of mutation is independent of the production of cDNA clones? Nonsense mutations may prevent you from reading through your transcripts, there may be mutations which are lethal and these would not be represented as cDNA which has been primed by an IgC gamma oligomer.

GEARHART: Thats a good point, all these were in frame and we would have totally missed the nonsense mutations. Even though both alleles can be rearranged and transcribed the productive allele has a lot more transcription than the non-productive allele, so if one prepares cDNA the productive allele is always represented, so the mutation rate might even be even higher.

JANEWAY: The 597 bases that you looked at, did you identify only the sense strand?

GEARHART: All the information is recorded from the sense strand.

JANEWAY: Sense is judged by what in the pseudo gene?

GEARHART: Sense is the top strand in the 5' and 3' orientation of these genes.

JANEWAY: How do you know the orientation of a pseudo gene?

GEARHART: You don't, but it does not make any difference because even if you looked at the other strand you would still have the same ratio.

<u>JANEWAY</u>: But may be I'm being dense but it seems to me if you don't know which is the coding strand then you don't know which way to turn them when you put the 5' one on top, therefore, you may never see a segregation.

<u>GEARHART</u>: It doesn't matter for the pseudo genes because those frequencies are equal. It would be important for the immunoglobulin genes that we studied in symmetry you are bound to know which strand it was occurring on, but the pseudo genes it was equal on both strands so it doesn't matter which strand you are taking the data from.

<u>McGREGOR</u>: Looking at your immunised mice I wasn't sure whether the message you were giving is that in any mouse the same mutation would probably occur against a particular autoantigen? Would you expect different people to have a variety of mutations or do you think that in one disease the same mutation is always occurring?

<u>GEARHART</u>: What is known about mutation is that it occurs randomly and our data showed more random mutation at the early stage followed later by selection against its specific antigen. There might be a higher probability of seeing the same mutation because of selection but these mutations are likely to be generated randomly.

<u>McGREGOR</u>: If you investigate 8 mice, and you immunise them with phosphorylcholine do you get the same pattern of mutation in the antibodies that are generated in these 8 mice?

<u>GEARHART</u>: There are some repeated amino acid changes in hyper variable regions but in general it is heterogeneous, but there are certain cases of repeated amino acid in the hypervariable regions which indicates contact points with antigen.

MOLECULAR ANALYSIS OF T LYMPHOCYTE RECOGNITION

B. Malissen, D. Blanc, D. Couez, J. Gabert, C. Gregoire, I. Hue, F. Letourneur, M. Malissen and J. Trucy.
Centre d'Immunologie INSERM-CNRS de Marseille-Luminy, Case 906 13288 - Marseille Cédex 9 France

The mouse T cell clones that have been previously analyzed for allelic exclusion of T cell receptor genes were known to be either reactive to antigen-derived peptides bound to self major histocompatibility complex (MHC)-encoded molecules or alloreactive, that is able to recognize intraspecies allelic variants of self MHC molecules in the absence of exogenously added antigen. However, many T cell clones selected to respond to antigens in the context of self MHC molecules express a concomitant reactivity for allogeneic MHC molecules. Two main hypotheses have been proposed to explain the molecular basis of dual reactivity. The first states that dual reactive T cell clones possess a single αβ T cell receptor heterodimer that detects cross-reactive determinants shared by allogeneic MHC products and self MHC products complexed to foreign antigens. The second hypothesis considers that T cell clones with dual specificity violate allelic exclusion and express two different αβ T cell receptor heterodimers on their surface, one reacting with foreign antigen bound to syngeneic MHC products and the second with allogeneic MHC products. In order to distinguish between these two hypotheses and reveal whether the principle of allelic exclusion holds true for dual reactive T cells, we have analyzed all the T cell receptor α - and β - chain rearrangements present in a dual reactive T clone. Furthermore, in other experiments we have analyzed the contribution of the CD8 molecule to T-cell recognition.

1. A T cell clone expresses two T cell receptor α genes but uses one αβ heterodimer for allorecognition and self MHC-restricted antigen recognition

(Malissen et al. Cell, 55, 49-59, 1988)

We have identified by Southern blot analysis and subsequently cloned and sequenced all of the α- and β-chain gene rearrangements that have occured in a dual reactive helper T cell clone provided by F.W. Fitch. This clone, denoted A10, originates from a B10.A mouse and reacts both to hen egg ovalbumin (OVA) presented by A^k-bearing cells and to the alloantigen A^s in the absence of OVA. This clone exhibits allelic exclusion of its β-chain genes in that only one of the two alleles is productively rearranged. Unexpectedly, it displays two productive Vα-gene rearrangements, denoted A10αA and A10αB, which are both transcribed into 1.5 kb mRNA. The contribution of each of the two productive α genes to the dual recognition was analyzed by gene transfer. To this end, each of the two α genes was separately transfected with the single productively rearranged β gene. Transfer of only one of the two αβ combinations restored both allogeneic MHC recognition and self MHC-restricted antigen recognition. Thus, T cell dual recognition results from the cross-reactive recognition of an allo-MHC product by a single antigen-specific and MHC-restricted αβ T cell receptor.

Furthermore, the presence of two productively rearranged α-chain genes in a T cell clone raises questions concerning the level at which allelic exclusion operates in T cells. The α gene rearrangements in A10 cells can be envisioned as having occured according to a model similar to

NATO ASI Series, Vol. H 38
The Molecular Biology of Autoimmune Disease
Edited by A. G. Demaine et al.

the one previously elaborated for the immunoglobulin K-chains. Thus, one can imagine that the rearrangement resulting in A10αB occured first. This gene was not able either to contribute to the formation of an αβ dimer expressed at the cell surface or to saturate the intracellular A10β chains, and accordingly, the V-J recombination machinery remained active and subsequently produced A10αA on the homologous chromosome. Since the A10αA product was able to form a functional αβ heterodimer, the A10 cell was picked out to a further differentiation step and the V-J recombination process was thereafter shut off. Alternatively, the mechanisms regulating α gene rearrangement may be tentatively coupled to the selection of T cell repertoire in the thymus (see Figure 1, in fine). In such instances, the A10αB product may be expected to properly pair with the A10β chain, but the resulting A10αB/A10β receptor may have subsequently failed to be positively selected in the thymus. Accordingly, the A10 cell in its primary configuration was not allowed to mature to a differentiation step devoid of recombinase activity but was thereafter rescued by a second α rearrangement resulting in the production of a compatible T cell receptor able to recognize antigen plus self-MHC but not self-MHC alone in the periphery. In this model, the presence of a major αβ combination at the surface of the A10 cells may be accounted for by the preferential surface expression of the A10αA/A10β pair.

Interestingly, we have found a second T cell clone (denoted BM 3.3 and provided by A-M. Schmitt-Verhuls) which displays two productive Vα-gene rearrangements. In order to sort out between the above models, we have constructed a mouse T cell recipient lacking functional α - and β-chains. Transfer of the A10αB/A10β combination and analysis of its ability to be properly expressed at the cell surface is under investigation.

2. Analysis of the function of the CD8 molecule by in vitro mutagenesis and DNA-mediated gene transfer

The T cell receptor α and β chain genes donated by an H-2 class I-specific, CD8-dependent cytotoxic T cell clone were transfered, alone or in combination with the Ly-2 (CD8α) gene, into a class II-restricted, CD4+ T cell hybridoma. Two important points emerged. First, the α and β T cell receptor genes endowed the recipient with the H-2 class I specificity of the donor only if the same cell had also been transfected with the Ly-2 gene. Second, the functional Ly-2 molecule was expressed on the transfected cells in the absence of the Ly-3 (CD8β) polypeptide. These results demonstrate that, besides the T cell receptor, the Ly-2 polypeptide is the only subset-specific molecule required to retarget a class II-reactive, CD4+ T cell line toward H-2 class I molecules.

More recently we have introduced mutations in the CD8 α polypeptide and analyzed their effects on T-cell recognition (see figure 2, in fine). In the first mutant, the amino-acids corresponding to the cytoplasmic tail have been deleted. In the second one, the transmembrane and cytoplasmic domains of CD8 α have been substituted by the transmembrane and cytoplasmic domains originating from the H-2 K^k class I MHC molecule. In both instances, following transfection, the mutated CD8 α polypeptides are expressed in high level at the surface of the DO-11.10 T cell hybridoma. These mutations appear to affect partially the accessory role of the CD8 α polypeptide.

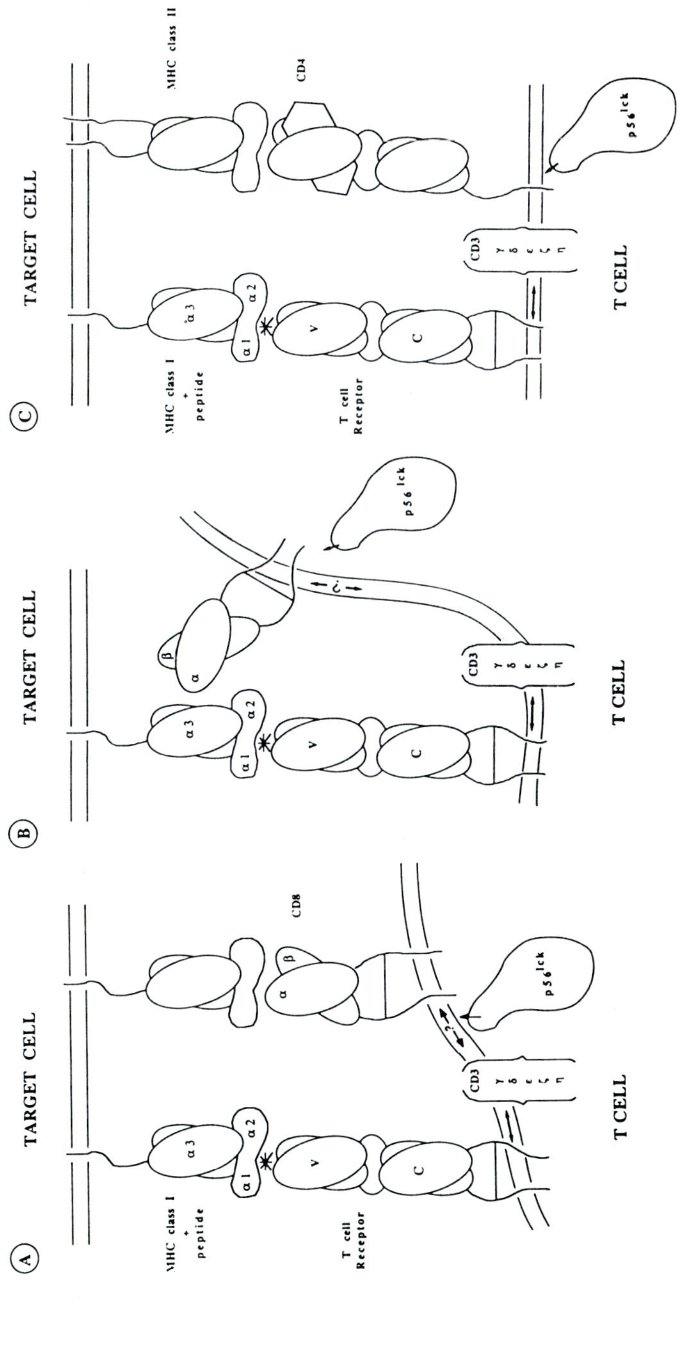
A
TARGET CELL
MHC class I + peptide
α1
α2
α3
V
C
T cell Receptor
CD8
α
β
CD3
γ δ ε ζ η
p56lck
T CELL
B
TARGET CELL
α1
α2
α3
V
C
α
β
CD3
γ δ ε ζ η
p56lck
T CELL
C
TARGET CELL
MHC class I + peptide
α1
α2
α3
V
C
T cell Receptor
MHC class II
CD4
CD3
γ δ ε ζ η
p56lck
T CELL

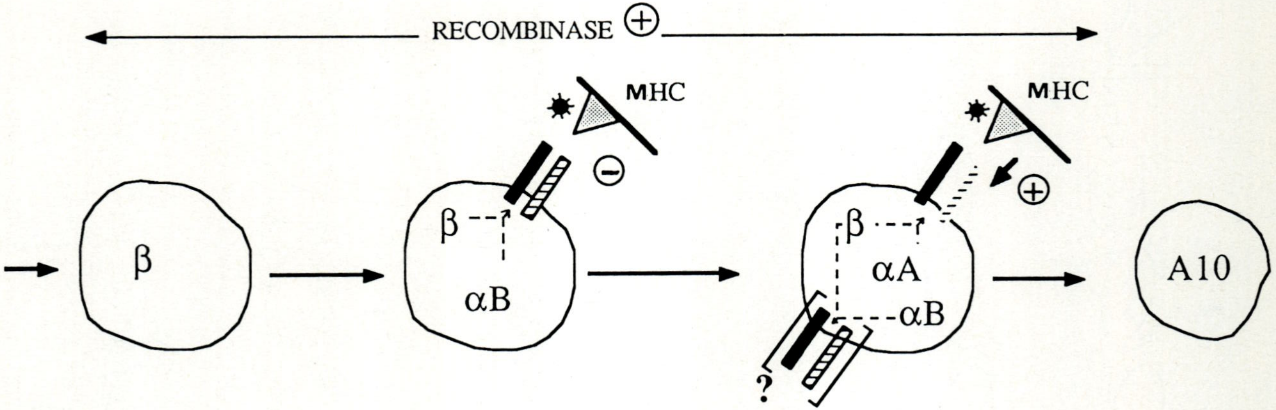

- no signalling through αB/β
- clone not allowed to mature to a step devoid of recombinase activity.

- cell clone rescued by a second α chain gene rearrangement.
- A10 picked out to a further stage of differentiation.

DISCUSSION

JANEWAY: Bernard, have you checked any of your transfectants for their ability to bind to class I MHC which may also vary when you change the cytoplasmic domain. The interaction of the cytoplasmic domain may change lateral mobility and alter binding in ways that you don't anticipate.

MALISSEN: No, the only way it would be possible would be to use some kind of system similar to the one that was worked out by Strominger to look at CD4 and, more recently, by Parham & Lipman for the CD8 molecule which they have overexpressed in Cos cells. We should be able to use this system because we have the native and mutated forms of cDNA for this molecule. We have used many monoclonal antibodies which are specific for the CD8 V domain and have been carrying out Scatchard analysis on molecules with mutated forms of the cytoplasmic tail to assess the effect on the structure of the variable domain.

MOUTSOPOULOS: I have two questions. First, concerning the site directed mutagenesis which you have done with the low molecular weight, constant components of the T cell receptor. When you change the lysine to an arginine you still see transduction - would that not argue that charge alone is not a necessary component but that there is something in addition to charge perhaps molecular configuration that is necessary since arginine and lysine are both positively charged?

MALISSEN: I think the molecular configuration is very important. I don't think anybody has been successful in reversing the polarity of salt bridges and from a biophysical point of view it is a completely crazy idea. It is very important for the protein to have the structure of the salt bridge established. Initially we thought that if we mutated the alpha chain genes and identify those that are not expressed and try and select second site mutants which may be in the alpha chain or in the CD3 complex. This should immediately map which CD3 component is interacting with the alpha chain.

MOUTSOPOULOS: Second question, assuming that the CD8 molecule in some way associates with class I MHC perhaps via a non-polymorhic determinant, is there any evidence that a soluble class I MHC molecule will bind to CD8 molecules.

MALISSEN: That's a very good question, I think the only evidence which has been reported was from Dan Lipman, but they have not been able to test the system in a soluble phase in spite of the fact that they have soluble CD8 and probably soluble CD4 molecules. They have been unable to demonstrate direct binding of soluble CD4 to MHC which may be due the low affinity between CD4 and class II and of CD8 and class I. This may be overcome if you overexpress the CD8 molecule and in the paper of Lipman they claim that in their transfectants the level of CD8 expression is 200 times higher than the normal expression on the surface of normal peripheral B lymphocytes. Once you have a high level expression of CD8 at the surface of B cells they become adherent and form a monolayer. They can be cloned with EBV transformed cell line which are presenting HLA class I or some mutant of HLA class I. By measuring the binding of EBV cell line to the monolayer it is possible to conclude that at least in this system the third domain of CD8 is important for its binding to MHC class I.

<u>JANEWAY</u>: In your transmembrane receptor mutation system the S35 methionine gel which you showed looked as though the molecule was extremely poorly glycosalyted. Do you know why?

<u>MALISSEN</u>: No we don't. Perhaps something is going wrong in the assembly process.

<u>JANEWAY</u>: Do the mutated molecules assemble with any of the CD3 proteins?

<u>MALISSEN</u>: It assembles with some CD3 proteins because when you run a gel there is still some components of CD3 but we are not sure which one.

T CELL DEVELOPMENT IN T CELL RECEPTOR TRANSGENIC MICE

Horst Blüthmann[1], Michael Steinmetz[1]
and Harald von Boehmer[2]

[1] Central Research Units
F. Hoffmann-La Roche & Co. Ltd.
CH-4002 Basel, Switzerland

[2] Basel Institute for Immunology
CH-4005 Basel, Switzerland

NATO ASI Series, Vol. H 38
The Molecular Biology of Autoimmune Disease
Edited by A. G. Demaine et al.

Introduction

During T cell development in the thymus genes coding for the α and ß chains of the T cell receptor (TCR) are assembled from the respective gene segments (for review see Kronenberg et al. 1986). Combinatorial joining of different α and ß gene segments leads to a diverse spectrum of TCR specificities on developing thymocytes which are positively selected for self-MHC recognition and negatively for self tolerance during further maturation (Fink and Bevan 1978, Zinkernagel et al. 1978). The enormous diversity of the T cell repertoire, however, makes it difficult to follow a T cell with a given specificity during T cell development.

Recently it was discovered that certain Vß regions show an intrinsic affinity to certain alloantigens (Kappler et al. 1987; Kappler et al. 1988; MacDonald et al. 1988; Pullen et al. 1988). T cells expressing these Vß regions were drastically reduced among CD4 or CD8 single positive thymocytes and peripheral T cells in mice expressing the corresponding antigen. It was concluded that autospecific T cells are clonally deleted in the thymus.

Transgenic mice offer an alternative way to study T cell development. Molecular analysis of T cell clones from normal mice have shown that in most cases only one of the two ß gene alleles is productively rearranged (Goverman et al. 1985, Chou et al. 1986, Dembic et al. 1986, Fink et al. 1986, Malissen et al. 1986). On the other hand a T cell clone with two productively rearranged α genes and a thymoma with ongoing α gene rearrangement have been described (Marolleau et al. 1988, Malissen et al. 1988). Analysis of mice transgenic for a TCR ß gene showed that the rearranged ß gene exerts allelic exclusion and suppresses rearrangement of endogenous ß genes (Uematsu et al. 1988). The transgenic mice express the transgenic ß chain on virtually all of their T cells and facilitate the analysis of TCR gene expression during T cell development with the help of specific antibodies.

Positive selection in TCR-transgenic mice specific for H-Y/D^b in the absence of nominal antigen

To study acquisition of self-MHC restriction and tolerance induction during T cell development transgenic mice were generated containing productively rearranged TCR α and ß genes in germline DNA (Blüthmann et al. 1988). The transgenic α and ß genes were isolated from a cytotoxic T cell clone specific for the male antigen H-Y and restricted by the MHC class I molecule D^b. Expression of the α and ß transgenes was detected by the two monoclonal antibodies T3.70 (Teh et al. 1989) and F23.1 (Staerz et al. 1985), respectively.

The αß TCR-transgenic founder Tg71 of $H\text{-}2^{b/d}$ haplotype was crossed with strain C57L($H\text{-}2^b$) to establish the transgenic line Tg71($H\text{-}2^b$) expressing the restriction element D^b, and also to strain DBA/2($H\text{-}2^d$) in order to establish the D^b negative line Tg71($H\text{-}2^d$). Positive selection in the thymus was then studied in female αß transgenic mice (i.e. in the absence of the nominal antigen H-Y) by comparing T cell development in the presence and absence of the D^b MHC molecule (Teh et al. 1988; Kisielow et al. 1988).

The results showed that in both lines almost all $CD4^+8^+$ thymocytes expressed the transgenic TCR. $CD4^-8^+$ single positive T cells of the transgenic phenotype, however, were deteced only in D^b positive transgenic mice. The preferential selection of such cells in these mice changed the ratio of $CD4^+8^-$ to $CD4^-8^+$ thymocytes to 1:2 as opposed to about 4:1 in normal mice. $CD4^+8^-$ cells that developed in these mice expressed high levels of the transgenic ß chain but low levels of the transgenic α chain. They probably had rearranged endogenous α chains thus creating new TCR specificities selectable by class II MHC molecules during development in the thymus. In D^b negative mice, on the other hand, no bias for $CD4^-8^+$ thymocytes was found and both single positive subpopulations expressed only low levels of the transgenic α chain.

The bias for $CD4^-8^+$ thymocytes of transgenic idiotype in $H\text{-}2^b$ and the absence of such cells in $H\text{-}2^d$ mice strongly argue that the development of single positive thymocytes from their double positive precursors is strictly dependent on the specificity of the TCR for either class I or class II MHC molecules. This specificity determines the CD4/CD8 phenotype of the mature T cell.

In agreement with our results Sha et al. (1988a) reported the selective expression of an alloreactive $H\text{-}2^b$ restricted TCR on $CD4^-8^+$ T cells in αß transgenic mice of $H\text{-}2^b$ haplotype.

Tolerance induction in male TCR transgenic mice

Tolerance induction to self antigens was analysed in male αß transgenic mice of $H\text{-}2^b$ haplotype (Kisielow et al. 1988). Male transgenic mice were found to develop a very small thymus containing only about 5-10% of the normal amount of thymocytes due to the deletion of most of their $CD4^+8^+$ cells. Thymocytes spared by the deletion process were of $CD4^-8^-$ phenotype or expressed only low amounts of the CD8 accessory molecule. Both subpopulations expressed the transgenic receptor (Teh et al. 1989) but could not be stimulated by syngeneic male target cells (Kisielow et al. 1988). This argues that the low expression of the CD8 molecule on their surface prevented these cells from being autoreactive. A small proportion of $CD4^{+}8^{-}$ cells also developed in the thymus of male transgenic mice. These cells expressed on the surface high amounts of the transgenic β chain but only low amounts of the transgenic α chain and had probably rearranged endogenous α chains.

The results show that one way to establish self tolerance is through deletion of autospecific cells in the thymus at their immature double positive stage. The accessory molecule CD8 plays an essential role in this process by contributing to the avidity of the T cell for its target. Recently, W. Sha et al. (1988b) also observed a deletion of auto-specific T cells in their TCR transgenic mice at or before the $CD4^{+}8^{+}$ stage in thymic development.

T cell development in αβ transgenic SCID mice

The transgenic line Tg71($H-2^{b}$) was further crossed with C.B-17 scid ($H-2^{d}$) mice (Bosma et al. 1983) and mice homozygous for this mutation and transgenic for the αβ TCR on $H-2^{b/d}$ or $H-2^{d}$ background selected. The scid mutation renders, in its homozygous state, developing B and T cells largely unable to productively rearrange their Ig and Tcr genes (Schuler et al. 1986). Scid mice develop only a thymic rudiment containing very few $Thy1^{+}$ cells which are of $CD4^{-}8^{-}$ phenotype. Upon introduction of productively rearranged α and β TCR genes into the germline of these mice, a normal sized thymus developed regardless of the H-2 haplotype expressed (Scott et al. 1989). Like in normal mice they were mostly of $CD4^{+}8^{+}$ phenotype and virtually all of them carried receptors encoded by the transgenes. Significant numbers of $CD4^{-}8^{+}$ thymocytes (about 15%)

with high levels of the transgenic receptor, however, were found only in mice of the compatible (b) haplotype. $CD4^{+}8^{-}$ thymocytes could not be detected in neither of them. These results demonstrate that the development of double positive thymocytes from their double negative precursors requires the productive rearrangement of α and/or ß TCR loci. The presence of γδ cells is not necessary for this maturation step. The results also confirm our earlier finding that differentiation of $CD4^{+}8^{+}$ thymocytes into single positive ones requires the interaction of TCR molecules with "permissive" thymic MHC molecules.

Despite the development of $CD4^{-}8^{+}$ cells in the thymus of D^{b}-positive transgenic <u>scid</u> mice, the number of peripheral T cells remains as small as in non-transgenic <u>scid</u> mice (Scott et al. 1989). This result indicates that peripheral expansion of transgenic T cells requires stimulation by other T or B cells which are severely depleted in <u>scid</u> mice. In D^{b}-positive transgenic <u>scid</u> mice the majority of the peripheral T cells were of $CD4^{-}8^{+}$ phenotype expressing the transgenic receptor. The major population in D^{b}-negative mice, on the other hand, were $CD4^{-}8^{-}$ cells which also carried the transgenic receptor. These double negative cells might be derived from thymocytes that had left the thymus without being positively selected.

Although $CD4^{+}8^{-}$ T cells could not be detected in significant numbers in the thymus of αß transgenic <u>scid</u> mice of either haplotype, they clearly accumulated in the periphery of both of them. In both cases virtually all of them expressed the transgenic ß chain but only a fraction of them expressed the transgenic α chain (Scott et al., 1989). These cells probably stem from very rare thymocytes that manage to rearrange endogenous α genes and thus create new selectable receptors.

In male αβ transgenic *scid* mice of H-$2^{b/d}$ haplotype the same drastic deletion of $CD4^+8^+$ immature thymocytes was found as in normal αβ transgenic mice (Kisielow et al. 1988). This demonstrates that the deletion process operating during tolerance induction is not anti-idiotypic and does not require other regulatory cells that express complementary TCRs.

Conclusion

The transgenic mouse model with defined TCR specificities has added strong experimental support for the concept of positive and negative selection leading in the thymus to a T cell repertoire that is both self MHC-restricted and self tolerant. In combination with the *scid* mutation it was shown that positive and negative selection events can take place in the absence of other regulatory T cells. However, other experimental approaches indicate that anti-idiotypic interactions in the periphery might also control self-reactive T cells (Kakimoto et al. 1988, Sun et al. 1988). Again the transgenic mouse will be a useful model to study these anti-idiotpyic interactions and their relevance with respect to self-tolerance. In addition, the development of $CD4^+8^+$ from $CD4^-8^-$ thymocytes can be studied in TCR transgenic *scid* mice. A separate introduction of rearranged α or β transgenes into these mice will reveal whether expression of TCR α and/or β chains is required for this maturation step to occur.

Acknowledgement

We thank Ms. A. Iff for expert preparation of the manuscript. The Basel Institute for Immunology was founded and is supported by F. Hoffmann-La Roche & Co. Ltd., Basel, Switzerland.

References

Blüthmann H, Kisielow P, Uematsu Y, Malissen M, Krimpenfort P, Berns A, von Boehmer H, Steinmetz M (1988) T-cell-specific deletion of T-cell receptor transgenes allows functional rearrangement of endogenous α- and ß-genes. Nature 334, 156-159

Bosma GC, Custer RP, Bosma MJ (1983) A severe combined immunodeficiency mutation in the mouse. Nature 301, 527-530

Chou HS, Behlke MA, Godambe SA, Russel JH, Brooks CG, Loh DY (1986) T cell receptor genes in an alloreactive CTL clone: implications for rearrangement and germ line diversity of variable gene segments. EMBO J. 5, 2149-2155

Dembic Z, Haas W, Weiss S, McCubrey J, Kiefer H, von Boehmer H, Steinmetz M (1986) Transfer of specificity by murine α and ß T cell receptor genes. Nature 330, 232-238

Fink PJ, Bevan MJ (1978) H-2 antigens of the thymus determine lymphocyte specificity. J. Exp. Med. 148, 766-774

Fink PJ, Matis LA, McElligott DL, Boodman M, Hedrick SM (1986) Correlations between T-cell specificity and the structure of the antigen receptor. Nature 321, 219-226

Goverman J, Minard K, Shastri N, Hunkapiller T, Hansburg D, Sercarz E, Hood L (1985) Rearranged ß T cell receptor genes in a helper T cell clone specific for lysozyme: no correlation between Vß and MHC restriction. Cell 40, 859-867

Kakimoto K, Katsuki M, Hirofuji T, Iwata H, Koga T (1988) Isolation of T cell line capable of protecting mice against collagen-induced arthritis. J. Immunol. 140, 78-83

Kappler JW, Roehm N, Marrack P (1987) T cell tolerance by clonal elimination in the thymus. Cell 49, 273-280

Kappler JW, Staerz U, White J, Marrack PC (1988) Self-tolerance eliminates T cells specific for Mls-modified products of the major histocompatibility complex. Nature 332, 35-40

Kisielow P, Blüthmann H, Staerz UD, Steinmetz M, von Boehmer H (1988) Tolerance in T-cell-receptor transgenic mice involves deletion of nonmature $CD4^{+}8^{+}$ thymocytes. Nature 333, 742-746

Kisielow P, Teh HS, Blüthmann H, von Boehmer H (1988) Positive selection of antigen-specific T cells in thymus by restricting MHC molecules. Nature 335, 730-773

Kronenberg M, Siu G, Hood LE, Shastri N (1986) The molecular genetics of the T-cell antigen receptor and T-cell antigen recognition. Ann. Rev. Immunol. 4, 529-591

MacDonald HR, Schneider R, Lees RK, Howe RC, Acha-Orbea H, Festenstein H, Zinkernagel RM, Hengartner H (1988) T-cell receptor V_{β} use predicts reactivity and tolerance to Mls^{a}-encoded antigens. Nature 332, 40-45

Malissen M, McCoy C, Blanc D, Truy J, Devaux C, Schmitt-Verhulst AM, Fitch F, Hood L, Malissen B (1986) Direct evidence for chromosomal inversion during T-cell receptor ß gene rearrangements. Nature 319, 28-33

Malissen M, Truy J, Letourneur F, Rebai M, Dunn DE, Fitch FW, Hood L, Malissen B (1988) A T cell clone expressed two T cell receptor α genes but uses one αß heterodimer for allorecognition and self MHC-restricted antigen recognition. Cell 55, 49-59

Marolleau JP, Fondell JD, Malissen M, Trucy J, Barbier E, Marcu KB, Cazenave PA, Primi D (1988) The joining of germ-line Vα by Jα genes replaces the pre-existing Vα-Jα complex in a T cell receptor αß positive T cell line, Cell 55, 291-300

Pullen AM, Marrack P, Kappler JW (1988) The T-cell reportoire is heavily influenced by tolerance to polymorphic self antigens. Nature 335, 796-801

Scott B, Blüthmann H, Teh HS, von Boehmer H (1989) The generation of mature T cells requires an interaction of the αß T cell receptor with major histocompatibility antigens. Nature 338, 591-593

Sha W, Nelson CA, Newberry RD, Kranz DM, Russell JH, Loh DY (1988a) Selective expression of an antigen receptor on CD8-bearing T lymphocytes in transgenic mice. Nature 335, 271-274

Sha W, Nelson CA, Newberry RD, Kranz DM, Russell JH, Loh DY (1988b) Positive and negative selection of an antigen receptor on T cells in transgenic mice. Nature 336, 73-76

Schuler W, Weiler IJ, Schuler A, Phillips RA, Rosenberg N, Mak TW, Keerney JF, Perry RP, Bosma MJ (1986) Rearrangement of antigen receptor genes is defective in mice with severe combined immune deficiency. Cell 46, 963-972

Staerz U, Rammensee H, Benedetto J, Bevan MJ (1985) Characterization of a murine monoclonal antibody specific for an allotypic determinant on T-cell antigen receptor. J. Immunol. 134, 3994-4000

Sun D, Qin Y, Chluba J, Epplen JT, Wekerle H (1988) Suppression of experimentally induced autoimmune encephalomyelitis by cytolytic T-T cell interactions. Nature 332, 843-845

Teh HS, Kisielow P, Scott B, Kishi H, Uematsu Y, Blüthmann H, von Boehmer H (1988) Thymic MHC antigens and the specificity of the αß T cell receptor determine the CD4/CD8 phenotype of T cells. Nature 335, 229-233

Teh HS, Kishi H, Scott B, von Boehmer H (1989) Deletion of autospecific T cells in T cell receptor (TCR) transgenic mice spares cells with normal TCR levels and low levels of CD8 molecules. J. Exp. Med. 169, 795-806

Uematsu Y, Ryser S, Dembic Z, Borgulya P, Krimpenfort P, Berns A, von Boehmer H, Steinmetz M (1988) In transgenic mice the introduced functional T cell receptor ß gene prevents expression of endogenous ß genes. Cell 52, 831-841

Zinkernagel RM, Callahan GN, Althage A, Cooper S, Klein PA, Klein J (1978) On the thymus in the differentiation of "H-2 self-recognition" by T cells: evidence for dual recognition? J. Exp. Med. 147, 882-892

DISCUSSION

JANEWAY: I think the failure of these cells to accumulate in the periphery is extremely interesting. I wonder if the cells ever do anything once they leave the thymus, have you tried putting a male skingraft on these transgenic mice?

BLUTHMANN: Not with these mice.

NEPOM: That's a very fascinating presentation. The results that you presented in which a particular T cell receptor was sufficient for positive selection, whilst the CD8/CD4 plays a role in the acquisition of negative selection helps to explain the usual pathway but what about all those double negative cells? Does that imply that no negative selection is operating on the double negative population at all?

BLUTHMANN: The double negative cells express the T cell receptor, including those mice with the wrong haplotype. They are able to reach the periphery with out being selected, and they are not reactive as they cannot be stimulated with male target cells.

NEPOM: You don't think there is any negative selection operating on that population?

BLUTHMANN: It is not necessary because they are not reactive - they accumulate somehow in the male mouse but they also accumulate in the female mice of the wrong haplotype and there is no negative selection for these mice.

NEPOM: I just wonder about that, it doesn't seem very cost effective from the body's point of view?

BLUTHMANN: Thats true, but that's the thymic system

JANEWAY: Another question about the double negative population. I was struck by the suggestion that the double negative peripheral population only accumulates in the mice of the wrong haplotype and is missing in the mice in the right haplotype - now if that's a shunt it ought to operate independently of H-2?

BLUTHMANN: You also have to bear in mind the total cell numbers in the different mice which were of similar numbers in the periphery

JANEWAY: I was wondering if you think that positive selection in these transgenic mice can in some way influence the double negative population?

BLUTHMANN: Yes, its hard to comment on that. It is still not known how this population manages to go into the periphery, and whether any escape selection or other influences which may favour their appearance in mice with the wrong haplotype.

MALISSEN: Your experiment may suggest that there is a scheme where the cells first go through an alpha beta positive stage which then leads to the induction of expression of the CD4 antigen

BLUTHMANN: That is right, whether it needs to be alpha and beta positive is not known. It might be that the rearrangement of the beta chain gene and/or the internal appearance of the beta chain might be sufficient to induce the expression of CD4/CD8. Our beta chain transgenic mice will show whether there is any possibility for the beta chain alone to appear on the surface with a CD3 molecule and some extra molecule which remains to be detected, or more likely, that an alpha-beta T cell receptor appears on the surface and that is a signal for CD4/CD8 expression.

<u>WILCOX</u>: Have you tried to test which cell types are responsible for the positive and the negative selection in the thymus

<u>BLUTHMANN</u>: We know that T helper cells are not necessary as they don't appear there, but positive and negative selection is still going on

<u>MALISSEN</u>: Could you tell me what the latest news is on gamma delta receptors?

<u>JANEWAY</u>: Will you pay my life insurance policy, Bernard? Some of the things that I know I'm maybe not free to say, none of the work is my own. There are a number of gamma delta transgenic mice around and I'm so involved thinking about these mice that my mind is a bit of blank right now. Basically these gamma delta transgenic mice are showing some very unexpected things concerning allelic exclusion. To summarise, I think they effectively rule out, along with the experiment published a couple of weeks ago by Esther Winoto and David Baltimore, that the alpha beta lineage and the gamma delta lineage arise sequentially, in that alpha beta arises through a failure to rearrange gamma delta properly. That is to say, the number and representation of alpha beta bearing cells in gamma delta transgenic mice is indistinguishable from the normal. Having a gamma delta transgene does not affect the alpha beta lineage detectably and there is a surprisingly modest increase in gamma delta bearing cells. Also, in the alpha beta cells they have not lost the gamma delta transgene

but both genes are silent suggesting that the lineage split is based on some kind of transcriptional signal. Another aspect which is very interesting, is if you look at the endogenous gamma genes of gamma delta receptors (you cannot really look at delta in the alpha beta lineage), they do rearrange in the alpha beta lineage suggesting that it is permissive for some rearrangement of the gamma locus. However, you cannot make a complete receptor as you've deleted delta. In contrast, in the gamma delta lineage where the transgenes are being transcribed gamma rearrangement is completely suppressed, and delta is also in the germ line configuration - you can now assay for it. If you make a functional gamma delta rearrangement then you shut down everything. If the rearrangement is non-functional then you get alpha betas. However, based on Esther Winoto's data is seems that you don't actually rearrange gamma and delta, at least not delta. If you are going to be an alpha beta then you go straight to rearranging alpha and beta suggesting some influence independent of the receptor and independent of rearrangements which tell individual T cells to be alpha beta or gamma delta. One other point is that homing into the epithelia is independent of the nature of the receptor even though when you look at the epithelia you see restricted V gene usage. Therefore gamma deltas will home to epithelia even though they bear the 'wrong receptor'. The presence of restricted receptors in epithelia must be based on some something else.

TARGET SEQUENCES AND ACCESSIBILITY FOR CHROMOSOMAL TRANSLOCATIONS INVOLVING T-CELL RECEPTOR GENES

T H Rabbitts, T Boehm, A. Forster, I. Lavenir and L. Mengle-Gaw*

Medical Research Council
Laboratory of Molecular Biology
Hills Road
Cambridge CB2 2QH
England

* Present Address: Monsanto Company, 700 Chesterfield Village Parkway, St Louis, Missouri 63198, USA

NATO ASI Series, Vol. H 38
The Molecular Biology of Autoimmune Disease
Edited by A. G. Demaine et al.

Summary

The human T cell receptor δ/α and β genes are frequent sites for chromosomal translocation found in T cell tumours. The formation of these abnormalities requires two components; target sequences for the recombination events and chromosomal accessibility for the enzymes involved. The examination of sequences at and near the junctions of chromosomal translocations reveals the underlying recognition processes leading to the inter-chromosomal exchange resulting in translocation.

The T cell receptor α/δ genes are frequently involved in chromosomal abnormalities

The TCRD/A locus in man is found on chromosome 14 at the band 14q11 and many chromosomal translocations and inversions have been shown to have breakpoints within this locus (recently reviewed by Rabbitts *et al.*, 1989). These abnormalities included translocations to chromosome 11 (t(11;14)(p13;q11); t(11;14)(p15;q11)); chromosome 8 (t(8;14)(q24;q11) and to chromosome 14 itself (t(14;14)(q11;q32)). This latter abnormality has an analogous inversion 14 (inv(14) (q11;q3)) with similar breakpoints.

The location of some of these breakpoints and a diagram of the arrangement of the human δ and α genes is shown in Figure 1.

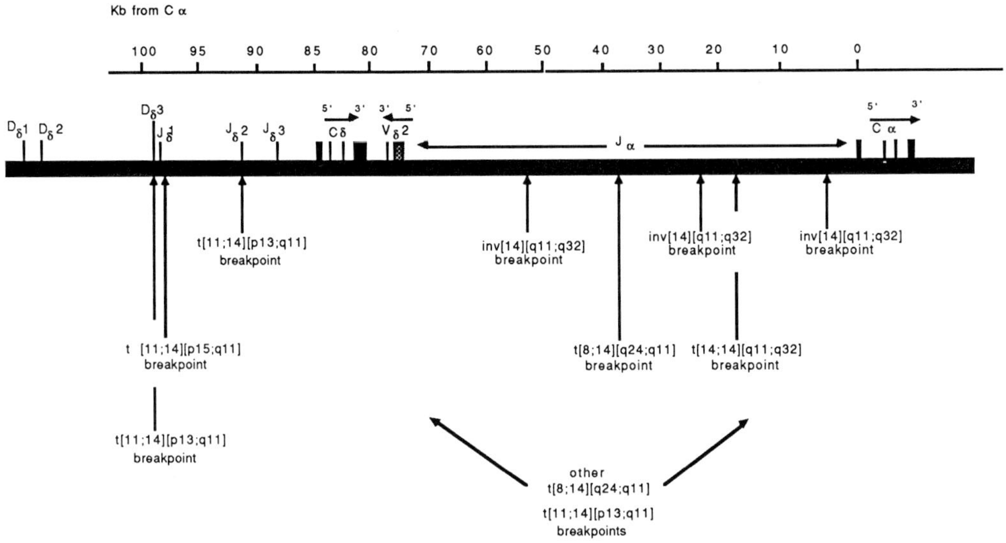

Figure 1. Chromosome abnormalities within the human TCRD/A locus. A diagram of the TCR δ and α genes is shown (the long region within many Jα elements is indicated). The vertical arrows represent breakpoints of the indicated translocations.

There is a general but not absolute correlation between the occurrence of TCRD breakpoints in the immature T cell acute leukaemias (T-ALL) and TCRA breakpoints in the mature T cell chronic leukaemias (T-CLL). However, in all cases thus far studied, the chromosomal abnormality breakpoint occurs at the 5' end of a D or a J segment within TCR D or TCR A (this is also true of a translocation t(7;10)(q35;q24) involving TCR B). This fact (illustrated in Figure 2) is, in itself, strongly suggestive of a direct involvement of the V-D-J recombinase in the process of chromosomal translocation or inversion.

Does the V-D-J recombinase recognise signal-like sequences on both chromosomes in the translocation process?

The fact that so many lymphoid tumours have translocations involving the rearranging genes (immunogloblulin genes in B cell tumours and T cell receptor genes in T cell tumours) intuitively implicates the V-D-J recombinases in the process of creating the abnormal chromosome. This view is considerably supported by the observed abutting of translocation junctions with D or J elements of TCR D/A or TCR B (i.e. the normal position for incoming V segment). Thus it is an obvious question to

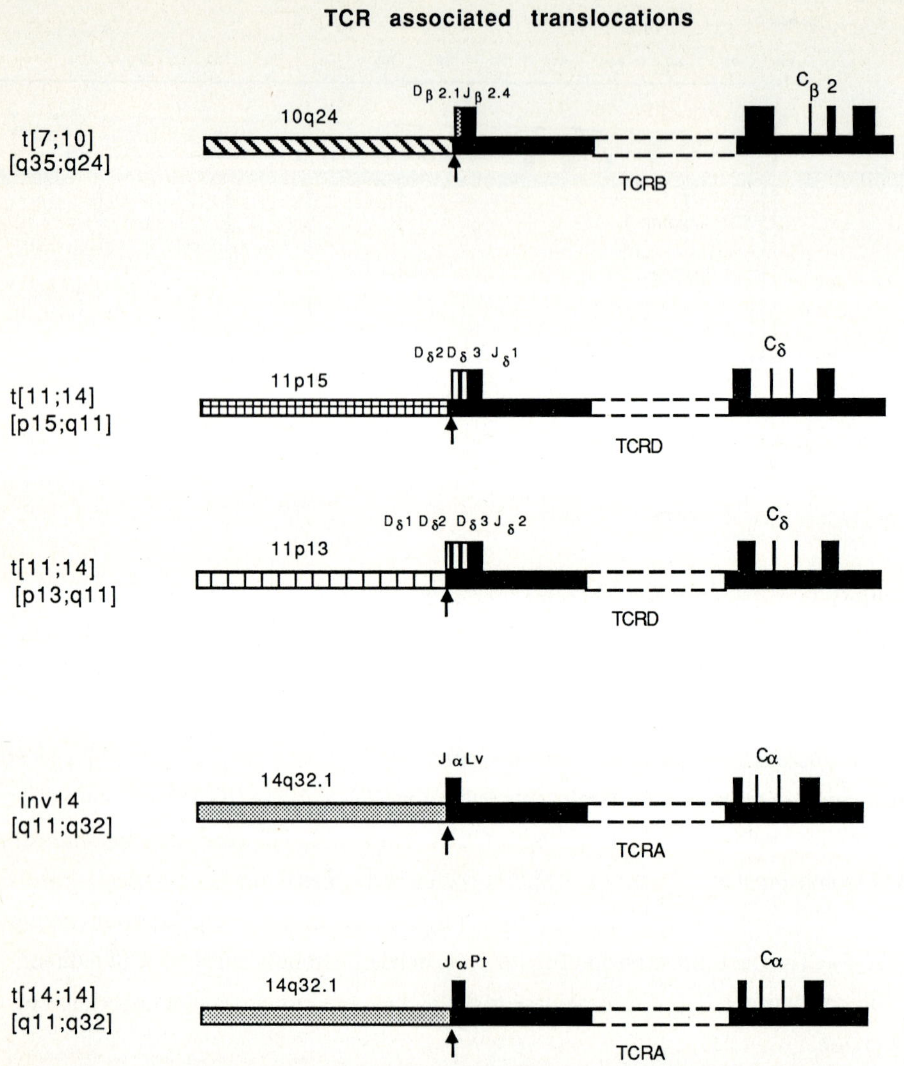

Figure 2. T cell receptor associated translocations. Various TCR-associated abnormalities are illustrated with the relevant D-J organisation at the chromosome junctions.

ask whether, since recombinase apparently cuts one chromosome in the translocation process, does it cut both chromosomes, and further does it recognise its target sequence on the second chromosome?

For an understanding of this, a brief description of the target sequence for V-D-

J joining by recombinase is necessary. The recombinase in its simplest form recognise a short element (7 mer and 9 mer sequences) downstream of all V-segments on either side of D-elements and upstream of J elements (Figure 3).

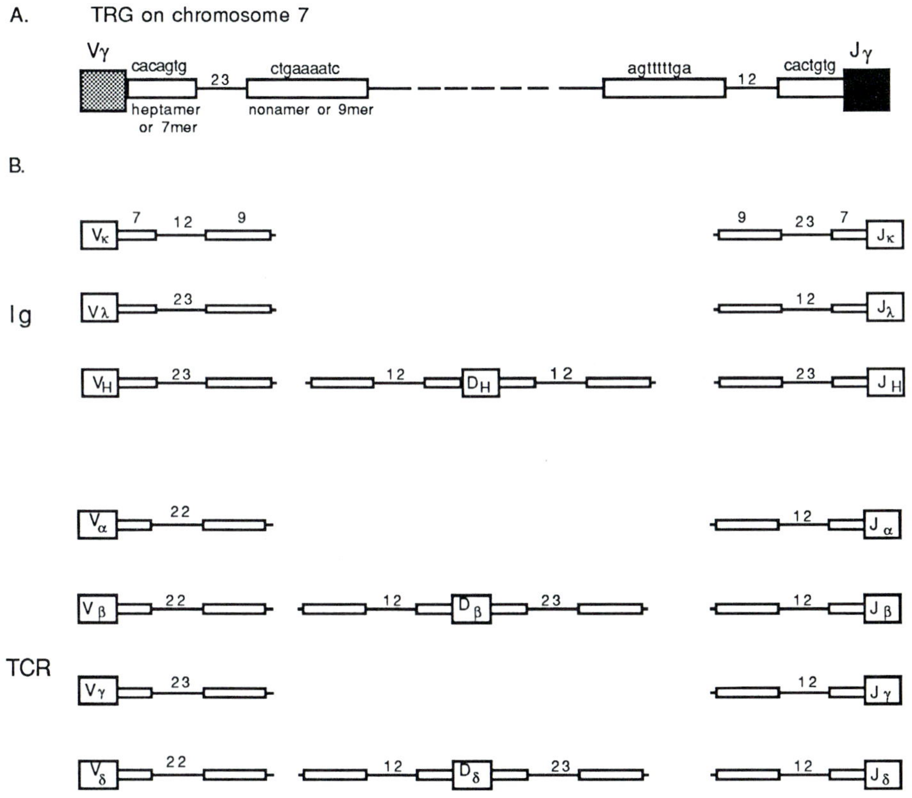

Figure 3. V-D-J recombinase signal sequence of Ig and TCR genes.

A. The 7 and 9 mer sequences near the elements of the human TRGγ gene. Canonical 7 and 9 mers are shown downstream of Vγ and upstream of Jγ.

B. Organisation of V, D and J elements of the human Ig gene (top section) and TCR genes (bottom section). Spacing of 7 and 9 mer at 12 or 23 are shown.

Since these are inverted with respect to each other (i.e. 7-9 and 9-7 on either side of prospective join), they can allow the dual recognition needed for successful V-D, D-J or V-J joining. Thus the rearranging elements of both Ig and TCR genes have these conserved signal sequence, a feature which endorses the view that a single recombinase exists in B and T cells.

The consistent occurrence of 7 and 9 mers at recombinase recognition sites has been the basis of the 12-23 rule which says that only joins with 7 and 9 mers separated by 12 basepairs on one side and 23 base pairs of the other can be legitimate (Tonegawa, 1983). Recently, occurrence of apparently 7 mer-only recognition joins have been described in TCRA (Baer *et al.*, 1988) so that sometimes the 9 mer would appear dispensable (see also below). Presumably, however, 7-9 mer mediated joins are the most efficient and certainly they are the most common.

The involvement of recombinase by site-specific joining can be assessed simply by examination of sequences at translocation junctions. This has been done in a number of instances (Croce, 1987) and supports the notions that recombinase is involved in some translocations by recognition of signal-like sequences. A clear example of this exists in the T-ALL-associated translocation t(11;14)(p13;q11) (Boehm *et al.*, 1988a). One such tumour, designated 8511, has been shown to involve TCRD on chromosome 14q11 and a sequence from chromosome 11p13 which bears a perfect match to a 7-mer sequence (viz. CACGGTG) but no 9-mer-like sequence. Recombinase error is thus very likely in this case, causing the interchromosomal exchange. The model for the creation of the 8511 chromosome translocation is shown in Figure 4. Thus, normal D_δ-D_δ and D_δ-J_δ joins can be seen at the interchromosomal junction and the Vδ element is simply replaced by 11p13 DNA; the whole event apparently mediated by recombinase error by utilising 7 and 9 mer from Dδ2 and the 7-mer-like element in chromosome 11.

However, not all such translocations seem to work in this way. For example, another t(11;14) breakpoint occurs only 800 bp away from that of the 8511 tumour, but in this instance, no heptamer or nonamer homology can be seen at the junction. Furthermore it can be said that the '8511 7-mer' was ignored in the creation of the latter translocation. Other clear examples which lack signal-like sequence have also been found in inv(14) chromosome (Mengle-Gaw *et al.*, 1988).

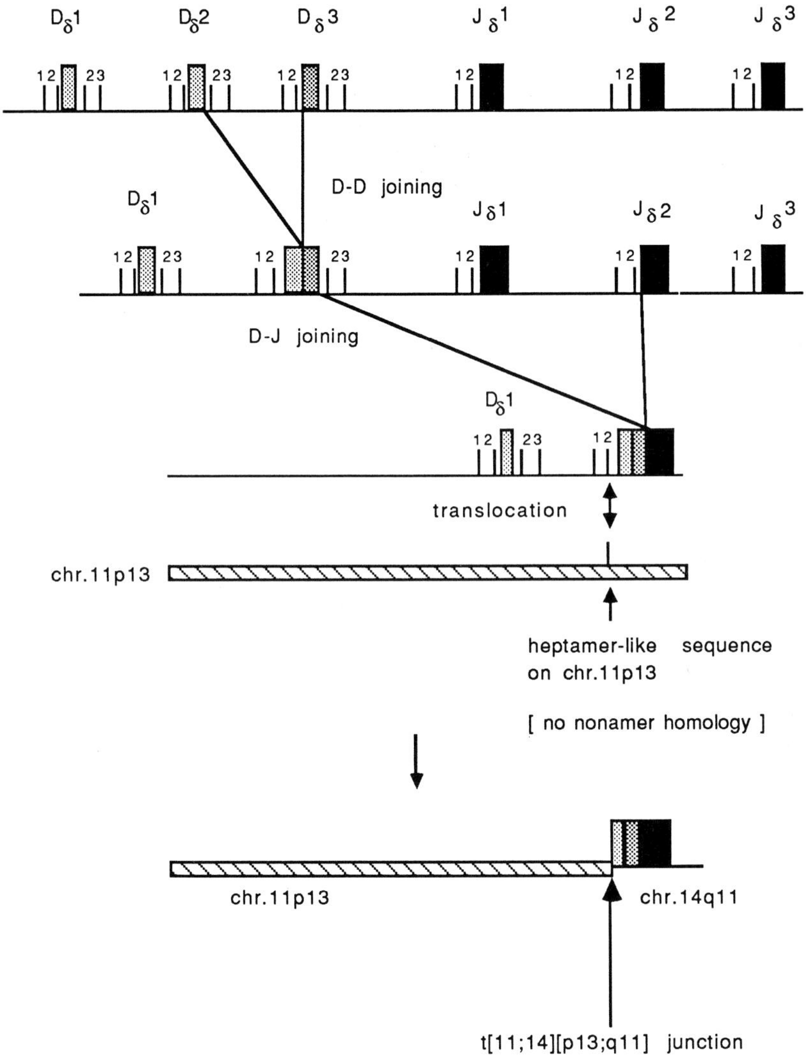

Figure 4. Model for the translocation t(11;14)(p13;q11) in the tumour 8511. Only the D-J δ region of human TCR δ is diagrammatically shown with the indicated joins and the translocation. The various events are not necessarily in the order implied by the diagram.

Accessibility for chromosome translocation

The hypothesis of Alt and co-workers (Yancoupolos and Alt, 1985) suggest that prior transcription of elements to undergo rearrangement allows recombinase accessibility. An example of this is the inversion chromosome 14 abnormality in T cells. In one case, this involved the IgH and TCRA loci where transcription of both IGH and TCRA apparently predisposes the chromosome to the inversion process (Baer *et al.*, 1987). However, in several well characterised translocations, no evidence for transcriptionally activity near to the chromosomal breakpoints can be found (Boehm *et al.*, 1989). In such cases, it might be supposed that something intrinsic to the local DNA sequence might be important.

One such putative sequence found near the junction of four different chromosomal abnormalities is a stretch of alternating purine-pyrimidine (in all cases, the residues TG). These are diagrammatically illustrated in Figure 5, in which the various chromosome breakpoint positions are shown relative to the purine-pyrimidine stretch. Such potential Z-DNA stretches might allow perturbation of the chromatin in their locality, thereby allowing recombinase access to the DNA. Thus, rearrangement would be allowed merely as a consequence of DNA sequence and not by prior gene activity.

Conclusion: a model for chromosomal translocation

We would assume that most, but not necessarily all, chromosome abnormalities are somatically acquired mutations which confer growth immortality on cells which acquire them. The lymphoid series of tumours have a propensity to carry abnormalities directly involving the rearranging antigen receptor genes. Recombinase may sometimes act at both sites of breakage by sequence specific recognition. Access for this enzyme can be provided either by transcriptional activity or apparently by some feature of the DNA sequence itself causing chromosome perturbation. Thus, for example, it is possible that a transcriptionally silent gene may be placed in a new environment after translocation by the action of recombinase at a chromatin site, containing a 7-mer like sequence, made accessible by a long stretch of alternating purine and pyrimidine base pairs. Such a new environment may cause transcriptional activation of this gene which thus leads ultimately to tumour formation. In this context the continued study of the gene, now designated the rhombosin gene, located near to potential Z-DNA stretch of the translocation t(11;14)(p15;q11) breakpoint (Boehm *et al.*, 1988b) will be important.

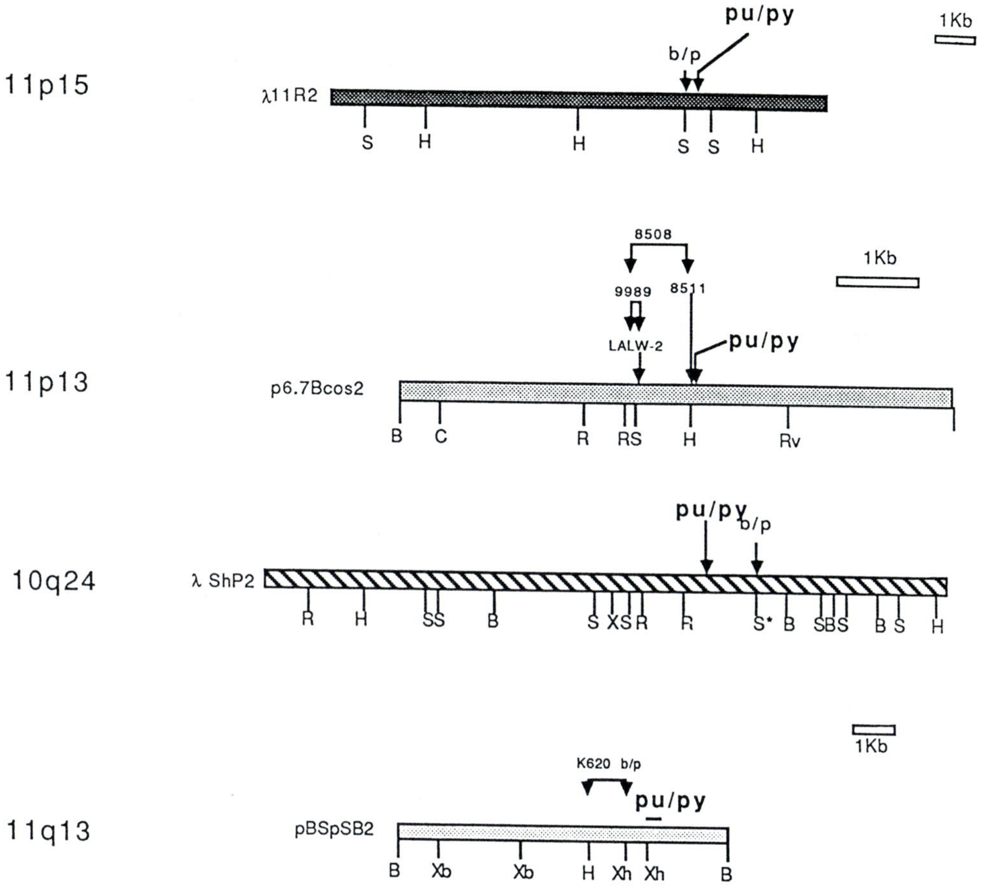

Figure 5. Putative Z-DNA near to junctions of chromosome abnormalities. The abnormalities shown are for:

(a) 11p15: t(11;14)(p15;q11) T-ALL
(b) 11p13: t(11;14)(p13;q24) T-ALL
(c) 10q24: t(7;10)(q35;q24) T-ALL
(d) 11q13: t(8;11)(?;q13) B-myeloma

Each line represents a partial restriction map of the relevant region with the potential Z-DNA indicated as pu/py and abnormality breakpoints indicated.

References

Baer, R., Boehm, T., Yssel, H., Spits, H. and Rabbitts, T.H. (1988) Complex rearrangements within the human Jδ-Cδ/ Jα-Cα locus and aberrant recombination between J alpha segments. EMBO J., 7: 1661-1668.

Baer, R., Forster, A. and Rabbitts, T.H. (1987) The mechanism of chromosome 14 inversion in a human T cell lymphoma. Cell, 50: 97-105.

Boehm, T., Buluwela, L., Williams, D., White, L. and Rabbitts, T.H. (1988a) A cluster of chromosome 11p13 translocations found via distinct D-D and D-D-J rearrangements of the human T cell receptor δ chain gene. EMBO J., 7: 2011-2017.

Boehm, T., Baer, R., Lavenir, I., Forster, A., Waters, J.J., Nacheva, E.and Rabbitts, T.H. (1988b) The mechanism of chromosomal translocation t(11;14) involving the T cell receptor Cδ locus on human chromosome 14q11 and a transcribed region of chromosome 11p15. EMBO J., 7: 385-394.

Boehm, T., Mengle-Gaw, L., Kees, U.R., Spurr, N., Forster, A. and Rabbitts, T.H. (1989) Potential Z-DNA tracts may promote chromosomal translocations seen in a variety of human lymphoid tumours. Submitted for publication.

Croce, C.M. (1987) Role of chromosome translocations in human neoplasia. Cell, 49: 155-156.

Mengle-Gaw, L., Albertson, D.G., Sherrington, P.D.and Rabbitts, T.H. (1988) Analysis of a T-cell tumour-specific breakpoint cluster at human chromosome 14q32. Proc. Natl. Acad. Sci. USA, 85: 9171-9175.

Rabbitts, T.H., Boehm, T.and Mengle-Gaw, L. (1988) Chromosomal abnormalities in lymphoid tumours: mechanism and role in tumour pathogenesis. Trends Genet., 4: 300-304.

Tonegawa, S. (1983) Somatic generation of antibody diversity. Nature, 302: 575-581.

Yancopoulos, G.D.and Alt, F.W. (1985) Developmentally controlled and tissue-specific expression of unrearranged VH gene segments. Cell, 40: 271-281.

INTRODUCTION BY H A ERLICH TO SESSION ON THE STRUCTURE AND FUNCTION OF THE MHC AND ITS GENES:

As you know in humans the general polymorphisms are HLA DR DQ and DP and perhaps one thing that we can think about - is there any different functions to these different alpha beta heterodimers. As you know, many species have DR and DQ analogues but do not have DP analogues so another question is - are there any different functions that can be attributed to these different alpha beta heterodimers'.

There are now up to 23 alleles as HLA DP beta. Obviously the development of PCR technology has facilitated the study of allele diversity quite significantly. Anyway it is clear that most of the beta chains are extremely polymorphic. The beta one locus clearly has many alleles, then there is another locus which is sometimes called beta 3 which has 52a 52b 52c, and then the beta 4 locus which in fact appears to be a different locus and not an allele. The alpha loci with the exception of DQ alpha are not polymorphic. Another thing is what selective forces determine the extent of polymorphism in different class II genes and why, for instance, is DQ alpha the only polymorphic alpha chain. What is the functional significance of structural polymorphism with respect to autoimmunity. Also, there are some evolutionary issues surounding the enormous polymorphism that has been observed in the contemporary human population. One of the things that genetists, evolutionary biologists and immunologists have been speculating about is, how is the polymorphism generated, how is it maintained, and what is its functional significance? Although I think these two explanations are not really

NATO ASI Series, Vol. H 38
The Molecular Biology of Autoimmune Disease
Edited by A. G. Demaine et al.

mutually exclusive, they represent alternative poles of evolutionary explanations. One is that polymorphism was generated recently and I think for many people this was the current view. Until quite recently they were seduced by the gene conversions in the bm12 mouse and assumed that polymorphism was generated rapidly by mutation and gene conversion and that diversity was being selected for. An alternative view is that in fact allelic diversities observed in the human population are in fact ancient and preceded speciation and present in ancestral species and that various alleles have been maintained in the population by selection. In meetings on evolution people will discuss these two as if they are mutually exclusive models and you will have people standing up arguing bitterly with each about who suggested what first and which of these models is correct. I think they need not be mutally exclusive and that for some loci I think one can clearly show that this model explains the pattern of evolution of polymorphism by far the best but for other class II loci, particularly the beta chain, it appears that there are certain residues that appear ancient and selected and maintained over 5 and 20 million years whereas other ones appear to have been generated much more recently. The other observation that suggests that DP might be different is that the distribution of alleles in the population is very different from that of DR and DQ, at least at the beta chain locus which is, as you know, very polymorphic but the allelic distribution is quite even - you don't find one major allele and a number of minor ones, they are actually all fairly evenly distributed which, from a population genetics point of view, clearly excludes neutrality. The kind of distribution of polymorphic alleles you see of DR and DQ is consistent with strong selection. In our studies of HLA DP and its probably true for the studies using PLT typing, is that the distribution of alleles is very different, that is, in caucasions there is at least one allele which we call DP 4.1 that is present in about 40 or 50% and then you have several alleles that are present in about 10%, and then a great number of alleles that are present at around 1-2% and are quite rare. Therefore the distribution of alleles suggests a different kind of selection to the one attributed to DR and DQ. I am not aware of any functional data but in some species one doesn't find an homologous DP locus, and that the distribution of DP alleles suggests the possibility that they may have a slightly different function from DR and DQ. With respect to its role in autoimmune susceptibility some people have made the point that because there is in general a linkage equilibrium between say DR and DP that is because there is no evidence for linkage disequilibrium and they are about 2 centemorgans apart people have suggested that DP may not play a role in autoimmunity. What they actually meant to say was that DP cannot account for the observed DR associations so a number of people have dismissed DP as contributing to genetic susceptibility to autoimmunity and explaining the HLA disease associations. However, you can demonstrate DP associations with disease that are totally independent of linkage to DR so the fact that they are not in linkage disequilibrium with DR means that you can't use the DP polymorphism to account for the DR association which is instead independent. I think DP contribute very significantly to a variety of autoimmune diseases and that is one of things that we will discuss in the genetics of autoimmunity.

<u>QUESTION:</u> Could you give an explanation for having the DP 4.1 allele, is it linked to another important gene?

<u>ERLICH</u>: Although in different populations it looks as if there is another allele, for instance in the Japanese population the frequency of DP 4.1 is very low and the frequency of DP5 allele is very high. Since we are talking about DP and DR, I should point out that we have been doing DP typing using the PCR method so that we have identified the number of alleles and therefore made it much more easy to look at linkage disequilibrium. In general there is no linkage disequilibrium between DR, DQ and DP. Certain haplotypes show quite a strong linkage disequilibrium, and for instance on the B8 DR3 haplotype about 50% of the haplotypes are DP1 whereas DP1 has only a 10% allele frequency in general so that there are certain haplotypes in which the linkage disequilibrium extends all the way down to DP. This suggests that there may be haplotypes with specific recombinational hot spots whilst others have cold spots. That is one of the reasons why we are very interested in this method of genetic mapping, using individual gametes and PCR because that is really the only way one can determine the recombination distances between 2 linked loci from an individual because conventional gene mapping really just averages over a large number of individuals with

family data. But if one can look at a 1000 sperm from individuals of different HLA haplotypes one can in fact accurately measure individual differences in recombination rates.

STRUCTURE OF HUMAN MAJOR HISTOCOMPATIBILITY COMPLEX CLASS II GENES

Lars Rask, Ann-Kristin Jonsson, Stefan Lundgren and Leif Andersson
Department of Cell Research, Department of Animal Breeding and Genetics, Swedish University of Agricultural Sciences and Uppsala University
Box 596
S-751 24 Uppsala
Sweden

The class II antigen molecule

Class II histocompatibility antigens, which are encoded by the Major histocompatibility complex (HLA in man) are expressed mainly by cells belonging to the immune system. They are composed of two dissimilar protein chains, both spanning the cell membrane. The two chains, denoted α and β, and with approximate m.w. of 35,000 and 28,000, respectively, interact non-covalently. The extra-cellular portion of each chain is composed of two domains, each consisting of approximately 90 amino acid residues. A stretch of approximately 20 hydrophobic or non-charged amino acid residues spans the cell membrane. On the cytoplasmic side of the cell membrane fairly short peptide segments are located, composed of 10 to 22 residues. The membrane-proximal domain (2nd domain) of the two chains displays sequence similarity to immunoglobulin constant domains, whereas the amino-terminal domain (1st domain) lacks this similarity. A salient feature of class II antigens is their polymorphism. The amino acid replacements, which create the corresponding sequence variability, are almost exclusively located in the 1st domain of the β chain and in some isotypes of class II antigens also in the 1st domain of the α chain (Rask et al. 1985). A schematic picture of a class II molecule and its corresponding genes is shown in Fig. 1.

In man, three main isotypic forms of class II antigens have been defined, DP, DQ, and DR. Each isoform is composed of a separate set of α and β chains. The three different α and the three different β chains, respectively, are highly similar in amino acid sequence but can nevertheless easily be distinguished from each other.

Organization of human class II genes

The genes encoding the class II α and β chains are organized with separate exons corresponding to the different portions of the proteins: Thus, the signal peptide is coded for by exon 1, 1st and 2nd domain by exons 2 and 3, respectively. In the α gene exon 4 corresponds to the membrane-spanning, the cytoplasmic segment and part of the 3'-untranslated sequence. Exon 4 of the β gene encodes the membrane-spanning portion of the β chain and part of its cytoplasmic segment. The remaining part of the cytoplasmic segment is coded for by exons 5 and 6.

NATO ASI Series, Vol. H 38
The Molecular Biology of Autoimmune Disease
Edited by A. G. Demaine et al.

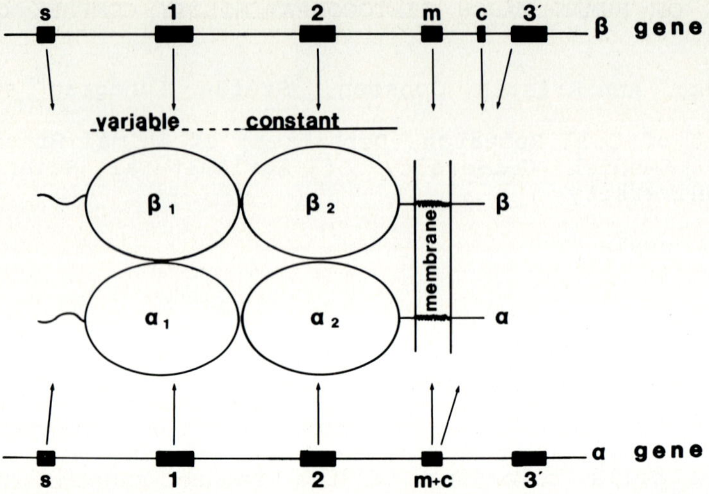

Fig. 1. Schematic picture of the class II antigen α and β chains and their corresponding genes. s denotes the exon encoding the signal sequence. 1 and 2 indicate the exons coding for the 1st and 2nd domains, respectively. m, c and 3' are the assignments for the exons encoding the membrane-spanning portion, the cytoplasmic segment and the 3'-untranslated region.

The last exon also contains the coding information for the 3'-untranslated sequence (Fig. 1).

The Major Histocompatibility Complex in man, HLA, is located on the short arm of chromosome 6 in segment 21.3. Within the HLA-region the class II genes are situated centromeric to the complement genes and the class I genes. Molecular cloning has shown that six α and six to nine β genes are present. However, all these genes are not functional (see below). In contrast to the situation in the mouse, the human class II region has not yet in its entirety been isolated in overlapping cosmid and phage clones. Three main clusters of genomic clones containing four DP-, four DQ-, and four to five DR-genes have been constructed. By the use of pulsed-field gel electrophoresis and Southern blotting it has been possible to estimate the distances within the HLA class II region with reasonable accuracy (Hardy et al. 1986). The DP-locus, which is located towards the centromere is approximately 400 kb apart from the DQ-locus. The distance between this locus and the DR-locus, which is situated closest to the complement genes, is approximately 250 kb (Fig.2).

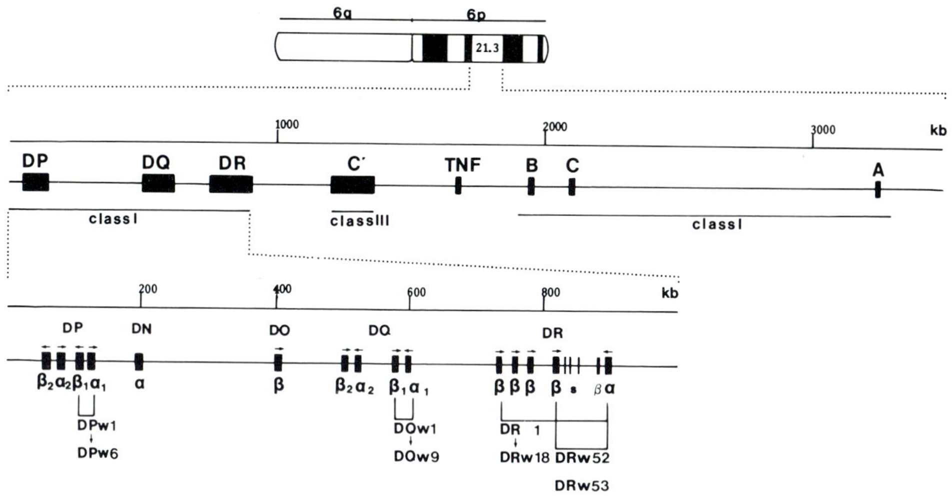

Fig.2. Partial map of the short arm of human chromosome six. Organization of the human MHC. TNF denotes the genes encoding the tumor necrosis factor and C' indicates the complement genes. Organization of the genes within the class II region. s denotes free signal sequence exons and β represents a single β gene 1st domain exon.

The DP locus

The DP-genes are like many other class II genes, e.g. DQ-genes (see below) organized as two α-β gene pairs. In contrast to the latter genes the DP-gene pair has its promoter regions in close proximity to each other. The DP α and β genes are also transcribed from the opposite strand compared with the DQ and DR α and β genes. These features of the DP-genes are probably of no functional significance and may be the result of a series of gene duplications, contractions and inversions (Gustafsson et al. 1987). Of importance is, however, the fact that two of the DP-genes, DPA2 and DPB2, are pseudogenes. DPA2 contains a larger number of deleterious mutations than DPB2 and has diverged more from DPA1 than DPB2 has from DPB1. It is conceivable that both DP-gene pairs once have been expressed and that DPA2 mutated into a non-functional gene at an earlier time-point than DPB2. There is no evidence for the presence of a higher or lower number of DP-genes in any human individual and in the investigated individuals only the two polymorphic DPA1 and DPB1 are expressed.

The DQ-locus

The number of DQ genes in man seems to be invariantly four. The four DQ-genes have been sequenced and found to be highly similar. No pseudocriteria whatsoever have been identified in these genes (Jonsson et al. 1987). The only conspicuous difference between the DQ β genes is a mutated acceptor splice junction at exon 5 of DQB1, causing this exon to be spliced out. In spite of this, no indications exist that DQA2 and DQB2 (formerly called DXα and DXβ) are transcribed. Both DQA1 and DQB1 are polymorphic.

The DR-locus

In all human individuals investigated, a single α gene DRA, has been found in the DR locus. In contrast, the number of β genes varies between different individuals. In DR-homozygous individuals carrying the DR-specificities 3, 5, and w6 three DR β genes are present, whereas those carrying the DR-specificities 4,7, and 9 have four DR β genes. The DR-specificity 1 most probably corresponds to two DRβ genes and the DRw8 specificity to a single DRβ gene (Böhme et al. 1985). Southern blotting analysis showed that the DR-loci corresponding to DR 3, 5, and w6 are closely related, as are those corresponding to 4, 7, and 9. This notion is consistent with the fact that from each of these DR-loci two different DR-molecules are encoded. In addition to the DR-antigen carrying the DR 3, 5, or w6 specificity, a second DR molecule containing the DRw52 epitope(s) is encoded from these loci. Likewise, from each of the DR4, 7, and 9 loci transcripts corresponding to two DR antigens are produced, one with the DR4, 7, or 9 specificity, and the other with the DRw53 specificity. Accordingly, the DR3, 5, w6 and DR4, 7, 9 are denoted DRw52 and DRw53 supertypic loci, respectively.

Detailed molecular maps are available for the DR3 and 4 loci (Rollini et al. 1985; Spies et al. 1985; Andersson et al. 1987). The DR3 region contains the three β genes DRB1, DRB2, and DRB3, in order from the centromere. DRB1 and DRB3 encode the β chains carrying the DR3 and DRw52 specificities, respectively. DRB2 is a pseudogene with a deleted exon 2. Telomeric to DRB3 a free 5'-end of a β gene is present (Rollini et al. 1985). The organization of the DR4 locus is similar, with the main exception that a second pseudogene,DR4β pseudo 1, is inserted between DRB1 and DRB2. DRB2 is probably a pseudogene as it lacks exon 2 (Andersson et al. 1987). DRB4 encodes the DRw53 molecule. DRB1, DRB3, and DRB4 are polymorphic, whereas DRA is invariant. The DR4 locus is the only one where all DR β genes have been sequenced. A careful comparison of the restriction maps and patterns of deletions and insertions revealed that the four β genes of the DR4 locus look like patchwork of each other, which indicates that these genes have exchanged sequence information during evolution. It was from these data not possible to suggest how the DR4 region has evolved. Serologically, DRw52 and DRw53 have been regarded as belonging to the same allelic series. This notion was recently questioned, since a comparison of the restriction map and the DNA sequence of the DRB4 gene with those of DRB1, DRB2, and DRB3 of DR3 suggested that DRB4 is more related to DRB2 than to DRB3 (Gorski et al. 1987). These authors proposed a model where the DRw52 and DRw53 supertypic loci have evolved independently by duplication of two ancestral β genes (Fig. 3). This hypothesis has gained further support from sequence comparison by a parsimony computer program of DR β chain nucleotide sequences where it was found that DR4β pseudo 1 belonged to the same branch of the dendrogram as the sequences corresponding to the chains carrying the DRw53-epitope (Jonsson et al. 1989). In the DRw53 supertypic DR loci several separate signal sequences and a free exon 2 are located between DRB4 and DRA. Several of these structures have been sequenced (Meunier and Trowsdale, 1986, Widmark et al. to be published). They are, however, most probably of no functional significance since they all contain pseudogene criteria in the form of frame-shift mutations and premature stop-codons.

The DOB and DNA genes

In addition to the DP,DQ, and DR genes two other human class II genes have been described, DOB and DNA (Servenius et al. 1987; Trowsdale and Kelly 1985). DOB is the homologue of an earlier characterized murine class II β gene, $A\beta_2$, accidentally isolated due to its close proximity to Aβ (Larhammar et al. 1985). DOB has recently been mapped 100 kb centromeric of DQB2 (Hardy et al. 1989). This gene is transcribed at a low rate (1/10 to 1/30 of DRB1) in EBV-transformed B-cells (Jonsson and Rask 1989). In spite of this no protein product corresponding to this gene has been detected in any cell or tissue. No pseudogene criteria are apparent in the sequence (Servenius et al. 1987).

DNA (formerly called DZα) has been mapped to the telomeric side of the DP locus (Hardy et al. 1986) (Fig. 2). Also this gene is expressed at a low level in EBV-transformed B-cells (Jonsson and Rask 1989). Neither in this case has any DNA-related protein been detected. Nevertheless, the sequence of the gene has the general characteristics of class II α genes with no apparent pseudogene criteria.

Class II genes and autoimmune diseases

It is well established that the frequency of certain class II alleles is higher than expected in patients suffering from several diseases of known or suspected autoimmune etiology (Tiwari and Terasaki 1985). Many aspects of class II molecules and their genes need to be elucidated in order to understand their role in these diseases. There is no evidence for the class II genes being deleted or inactivated in patients with autoimmune diseases. On the contrary, in several instances ectopic expression of class II antigens has been reported in the affected tissues. It is, however, probable that this is due to an activation of the genes by local production of lymphokines and not to an abberant structure of the class II gene promoters as such.

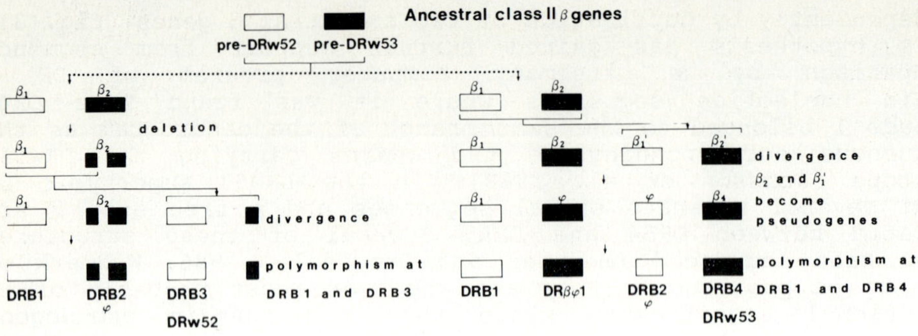

Fig. 3. Schematic representation of the evolution of the DR genes in the DRw52 and DRw53 supertypic groups.

The association between diseases and class II specificities might be related to the function of the class II antigens in antigen presentation. If this is the case, the attention should be directed towards the involvment of specific class II alleles in this process, like the DQw3.2 allele in insulin dependent diabetes mellitus (Böhme et al. 1986).

Might class II genes that usually are considered to be non-functional like DOB, DNA, DQA2 and DQB2 be involved in autoimmune diseases? Of these four genes DOB should be considered most seriously. Homologues to this gene are present in several mammals like the mouse ($A\beta_2$), rat, and cattle (Andersson and Rask 1989). It is extremely well conserved within the species. RFLP analyses revealed only limited polymorphism in man (Servenius et al. 1987) and mouse (Larhammar et al. 1985). Three DOB exon sequences are available which are 99.8% identical (Jonsson and Rask 1989). Further, DOB homologues seem to be highly conserved also between species. Thus, the gene pair DOB/$A\beta_2$ is more similar than DQB/Aβ and DRB/Eβ (Servenius et al. 1987). The conservation of DOB is most easily explained by the gene being expressed. As discussed above, no DOB protein product has been identified and there is no obvious candidate for a corresponding α chain although DNα has been discussed. DNA is also relatively well conserved in man (Jonsson and Rask 1989) and displays only limited polymorphism in RFLP analysis of cattle (Andersson et al. 1989). Accordingly, it may be rewarding to investigate other cells and tissues than B-cells for DOβ and DNα chains. Extensive efforts have been made to find transcripts of DQA2 and DQB2 in B-cells, all with negative results. Both these genes seem to display little sequence variability. The fact that they are lacking in at least some species like the mouse indicates that they do not have a unique function among the class II genes. It is not known whether DQA2 and DQB2 might be activated under certain conditions. Accordingly, the possibility that some disease associations of DR and DQ specificities actually are explained by the involvment of highly linked genes as DOB, DQA2, and DQB2 should not be overlooked. In this context it should be pointed out that hitherto unidentified non-class II genes might exist intermingled with the class II genes. Such genes if they exist might also be important for the occurence of the disease associations of class II specificities.

Acknowledgment

Work cited from the authors' laboratory was supported by grants from the Swedish Cancer Society and the Swedish Medical Research Council.

References

Andersson,G, Larhammar D, Widmark E, Servenius B, Peterson PA Rask L (1987) Class II genes of the human major histocompatibility complex. Organization and evolution of the DRβ genes. J.Biol.Chem. 262:8748-8758

Andersson L, Lundén A, Sigurdardottir S, Davies CJ, Rask L (1988) Linkage relationships in the bovine MHC region. High recombination frequency between class II subregions. Immunogenetics 27:273-280

Andersson L, Rask L (1988) Characterization of the MHC class II region in cattle. The number of DQ genes varies between haplotypes. Immunogenetics 27:110-120

Böhme J, Andersson M, Andersson G, Möller E, Peterson PA, Rask L (1985) HLA-DR β genes vary in number between different DR specificities whereas the number of DQ β genes is constant. J.Immunol. 135: 2149-2155

Böhme J, Carlsson B, Wallin J, Möller E, Persson B, Peterson PA, Rask L (1986) Only one DQ-β restriction fragment pattern of each DR specificity is associated with insulin-dependent diabetes. J.Immunol. 137:941-947

Gorski J, Rollini P, Mach B (1987) Structural comparison of the genes of two HLA-DR supertypic groups: The loci encoding DRw52 and DRw53 are not truly allelic. Immunogenetics 25: 397-402

Gustafsson K, Widmark E, Jonsson A-K, Servenius B, Sachs DH, Larhammar D, Rask L, Peterson PA (1987) Class II genes of the human major histocompatibility complex: Evolution of the DP region as deduced from nucleotide sequences of the four genes. J.Biol.Chem. 262:8778-8786

Hardy DA, Bell JI, Long EO, Lindsten T, McDevitt HO (1986) Mapping of the class II region of the human histocompatibility complex by pulsed-field gel electrophoresis. Nature 323:453-455

Jonsson A-K, Andersson L, Rask L (1989) A cellular and functional split in the DRw8 haplotype is due to a single amino acid replacement ($DR\beta^{ser57-asp57}$). Immunogenetics (in press)

Jonsson A-K, Hyldig-Nielsen JJ, Servenius B, Larhammar D, Andersson G, Jörgensen F, Peterson PA, Rask L (1987) Class II genes of the human major histocompatibility complex: Comparisons of the DQ and DX α and β genes. J.Biol.Chem. 262:8768-8777

Jonsson A-K, Rask L (1989) Human class II DNA and DOB genes display low sequence variability. Immunogenetics (in press)

Larhammar D, Hammerling U, Rask L, Peterson PA (1985) Sequence of gene and cDNA encoding murine major histocompatibility complex class II gene $A\beta_2$. J.Biol. Chem. 260: 14111-14119

Meunier HF, Carson S, Bodmer WF, Trowsdale J (1986) An isolated β_1 exon next to the DRα gene in the HLA-D region. Immunogenetics 23:172-180

Rask L, Gustafsson K, Larhammar D, Ronne H, Peterson PA (1985) Generation of class II antigen polymorphism. Immunological Reviews 84: 123-143

Rollini P, Mach B, Gorski J (1985) Linkage map of three HLA-DR β-chain genes: Evidence for a recent duplication event. Proc. Natl. Acad. Sci. USA 82: 7197 -7201

Servenius B, Rask L, Peterson PA (1987) Class II genes of the human major histocompatibility complex: The DOβ gene is a divergent member of the class II β gene family. J.Biol. Chem. 262: 8759-8766

Spies T, Sorrentino R, Boss JM, Okada K, Strominger JL (1985) Structural organization of the DR subregion of the human major histocompatibility complex. Proc. Natl. Acad. Sci. USA 82: 5165-5169

Tiwari JL, Terasaki P (1985) HLA and disease association. Springer-Verlag, New York

Trowsdale J, Kelly A (1985) The human class II α gene DZα is distinct from genes in the DP, DQ, and DR subregion. EMBO J. 4:2231-2237

DISCUSSION

ERHLICH: In the nomenclature that you use for the DR4 haplotype and the DR3 haplotype you use the same term DR beta 2 to describe loci on these haplotypes - are they in fact the same gene?

RASK: It is not my own. I don't like the nomenclature but it has been proposed at the Workshop.

ERHLICH: We have also identified a gene which at one time we also called DR beta 2, just to make things more confusing, that's only present on DR1, DR2 and DR10 haplotypes. The second question I have regards your suggestion that DO beta might be involved in autoimmunity - it seems to me that since the genetic susceptibility and disease associations have to do with polymorphic haplotypes, some haplotypes are susceptible and some are not and would require that a gene contributing to susceptibility would have to be polymorphic because if it weren't then you wouldn't get those associations

RASK: You don't always get a pathological expression of the genes. Also, under certain conditions there might be interference with the assembly of other class II proteins.

DISSECTION OF THE ROLES OF SPECIFIC CLASS II ANTIGENS AND ACCESSORY MOLECULES IN ANTIGEN PRESENTATION

Daniel M. Altmann, David Wilkinson, Hitoshi Ikeda and John Trowsdale

Human Immunogenetics Laboratory,

Imperial Cancer Research Fund,

Lincolns Inn Fields,

Holborn, London

NATO ASI Series, Vol. H 38
The Molecular Biology of Autoimmune Disease
Edited by A. G. Demaine et al.

KEYWORDS/ABSTRACT:HLA-DR,DQ,DP/class II/transfectants/ monoclonal antibodies/T cells/ICAM-1/Accessory molecules/antigen presentation

This paper reviews our experiments using mouse cells transfected with human HLA class II sequences to study several aspects of antigen presentation,including: the production and screening of monoclonal antibodies; the roles of different HLA-DR2 class II loci products in presenting an *M.leprae* antigen to T cells; and, using transfectants super-transfected with ICAM-1, the effect of this accessory molecule on the T cell response.

Introduction

It is now generally accepted that antigen presentation to a CD4-positive T cell involves presentation of a peptide fragment in association with a class II molecule (Shimonkevitz at al 1983). The characteristics of binding between peptides and class II molecules are being analysed in some detail particularly since a structural model for the antigen binding cleft of HLA molecules has been proposed (Babbitt et al 1985, Brown et al 1988, Bjorkman et al 1988).

In view of this model it is now important to examine the roles of different class II products and to determine the rules for binding of peptides to them. However, this has been difficult in the past because human cells express HLA products from a number of loci. To overcome this problem we have introduced human HLA genes, and cDNA clones in appropriate expression vectors, into heterologous cells which do not express HLA products. These reagents permit us to investigate the functions of single HLA products in isolation. This paper summarises some of the recent observations using this approach.

Transfectants

Early experiments from the laboratory involved the use of genomic clones but more recently we have obtained more consistent, high levels of expression using full-length cDNA clones expressed from viral promoters (Austin et al 1985, Wilkinson et al 1988). Recipient cell lines have included mouse L cells, mouse mastocytoma P815 cells and a human class II-negative B lymphoblastoid cell line. Two types of cDNA expression vectors have been used. In an example of the first type, cDNA's for the α chain and β chain of DR2 were cloned separately into the vector pJ4Ω in which the sequences are driven off the mouse moloney leukemia virus LTR. An alternative approach has been to link the α and β chains, each coupled to SV40 early promoters, on one DNA molecule, multiple copies of which are then packaged in a cosmid vector. The advantage of this system is that when a dominant selectable marker is incorporated, high level expression transfectants may be obtained without the need for FACS sorting (Ikeda et al 1988).

Monoclonal Antibodies

The transfectants have proved invaluable in assigning specificities to the large number of monoclonal antibodies to HLA class II producs, using ELISA binding assays (Altmann et al 1989). In addition, they are being used to generate new monoclonal reagents by immunising syngeneic mice. In this system, all of the immunising cell proteins except for the transfected gene product are self, so the immune system of the animal is focussed onto the particular HLA product. This approach has been used to generate monoclonal antibodies against DPw4 transfectants. The resulting antibody was DPα specific, but bound only to cells expressing DPw4 or DPw2. Apparently, binding to the constant α chain is influenced by structural constraints of the accompanying β chain (Heyes et al 1986, Young et al 1988). More information about transfectants being used in HLA typing and monoclonal antibody characterisation may be found in recent reviews from this laboratory (Altmann et al 1989, Wilkinson et al 1989).

Antigen presentation.

One of the most interesting areas of research using the transfectants are concerns questions of genetic restriction during antigen presentation to T cells. By studying an antigen presenting cell in which the only human product is the functional HLA molecule one can address questions about the level of class II needed for presentation, the nature of antigen processing, the handling of various antigens by specific class II molecules and the roles of other molecules in these processes. Below, we give an example of these studies in which we have been examining the functions of the two different class II molecules of the HLA DR2Dw2 haplotype.

In these experiments, cDNA clones for the two different DRβ chains of the DR2Dw2 haplotype were isolated (Lock et al 1988). The two clones were then introduced individually into mouse L cells along with DRα chains, all in cDNA expression vectors as described above (Wilkinson et al 1988). Products of the two loci were clearly distinguishable by two-dimensional electrophoresis as sets of more acidic (DR2a) or more basic (DR2b) polypeptides. A series of DR2-restricted T cell clones and lines have been stimulated using the transfectants in antigen-presentation assays. The conclusion from these data is that the DR2a product is by far the most commonly used DR2 restricting element. So far, less than five per cent of antigen-specific T cell clones and lines restricted to DR2 utilise the DR2b product, and this proportion could become much smaller as more studies are done. Why one of the expressed products should be so poorly represented in the T cell repertoire is unclear, particularly since both chains are functional, as judged by their ability to stimulate an MLR-like response (Altmann et al 1989).

An interesting aspect of this work was the fact that the L cell transfectants were capable of processing antigens. For example, using a T cell clone specific to *M. leprae* , synthetic peptide, whole protein and even intact mycobacteria could be processed. The fact that cells of diverse lineages may act as antigen presenting cells for T cell stimulation is of key importance in consideration of autoimmune disease although the involvement of cells other than those classically in the immune system in these processes *in vivo* is not well understood (Botazzo et al 1983, Londei et al 198 ,Marmann et al 1988).

Accessory Molecules

So far, we have been discussing the nature of antigen presentation through the HLA molecule - a fascinating example of biological design which fulfils a specific function. However, it is now becoming clear that other aspects of the presenting cell may be important in determining the strength or specificity of a particular response and the precise cells that are stimulated. Various antigen-independent interactions such as those between CD4 and HLA-class II, LFA-1 and ICAM1, and LFA3 and CD2 may play a role in the process since antibodies against these molecules partially or totally inhibit presentation.

Our work showed that presentation to *M. leprae* specific T cells was inhibited by antibodies against LFA-1 when the antigen presenting cell was a B cell but not with the L cell transfectants (Altmann et al 1989). To investigate this further, we supertransfected HLA-DR transfectants with a cDNA clone for the accessory molecule ICAM-1, which is a member of the integrin family of molecules of 80-114kDa and whose ligand is LFA-1 Marlin et al 1987, Simmons et al 1988). A panel of transfectant cell lines has now been constructed in which ICAM-1 is expressed in the presence of high or low levels of HLA classII molecules. The transfectants were then used to stimulate T cell lines of both cytotoxic and helper varieties. The outcome of these experiments is that ICAM-1 was shown to enhance T cell stimulation, particularly when the level of class II was low. Thus, a transfectant with low levels of DR7 was efficiently killed by a cytotoxic alloreactive T cell line but only if the presenting cells expressed ICAM-1. Similar reconstitution of antigen presenting cell function was demonstrable in MLR-like responses to low levels of DR and in presentation of recall antigens to freshly isolated T cells. These experiments showed that ICAM-1 can be a decisive factor in determining whether a T cell response will result.

Using transfectants it should now be possible to examine the roles of various accessory molecules in activation and signal transduction in T cells. The interaction between LFA-3 and CD2 is of particular interest in this regard (Springer et al 1987). The lysis of some Burkitt's lymphoma lines by anti-EBV CTL showed that accessory molecules were involved in the process but their importance remains to be elucidated clearly (Barbosa et al 1986, Gregory et al 1988).

Conclusions

In summary, the transfection of HLA and accessory molecule sequences is proving an invaluable tool for dissecting antigen presentation. Future work will undoubtedly involve *in vitro* mutagenesis of the sequences before transfection to probe the interaction between peptide, class II and the T cell receptor. Coupled with the availability of transgenic mice in the near future the coming years should yield considerable advances in our understanding of antigen presentation in humans.

References.

Altmann DM,Wilinson D,Ikeda H,Trowsdale J (1989)Analysis of antigen presentation using HLA transfectants. *In press.*

Austin P, Trowsdale J,Rudd C,Bodmer W,Feldmann M,Lamb J. (1985) Functional expression of HLA-DP genes transfected into mouse fibroblasts. Nature 313:61-64.

Babbit BP,Allen PM, Matsueda G,Haber E,Unanue ER (1985) Binding of immunogenetic peptides to Ia histocompatiblity molecules. Nature 317:359-361.

Barbosa JA,Mentzer SJ,Kamark ME, Hart J,Biro PA, Strominger JL, Burakoff SJ (1986) Gene mapping and somatic cell hybrid analysis of the role of human lymphocyte function-associated antigen-3 (LFA-3) in CTL-target cell interactions. J Immunol 136:3085-3091.

Botazzo GF,Pujol-Borrell R,Hanafusa T,Feldmann M (1983) Role of aberrant HLA-DR expression and antigen presentation by endothelial cells. Lancet ii:1115-1119.

Brown JH, Jardetsky T,Saper MA,Samraoui B,Bjorkman PJ,Wiley DC (1988) A hypothetical model of the foreign antigen binding site of class II histocompatibility antigens Nature 332:845-847.

Bjorkman PJ,Saper MA,Samraoui B,Bennett WS, Strominger JL,Wiley DC (1988) The foreign antigen binding site. Nature 329:512-518.

Gregory CD,Murray RJ, Edwards CF, Rickinson AB (1988) Downregulation of cell adhesion molecules LFA-3 and ICAM-1 in Epstein-Barr virus-positive Burkitt's lymphoma underlies tumor cell escape from virus specific T cell surveillance. J Exp Med 167:1811-1824.

Heyes J,Austin PJ,Bodmer J,Bodmer WF,Madrigal A Mazzilli M, Trowsdale J (1986) Monoclonal antibodies to HLA-DP transfected mouse L cells. Proc Natl Acad Sci USA 83:3417-3421.

Ikeda H, Trowsdale J, Saito I. (1988) Mulcos:a vector for amplification and simultaneous expression of two foreign genes in mammalian cells. Gene 71:19-27.

Lock CB,So AKL,Welsh KI,Parkes JD, Trowsdale J (1988) MHC class II sequences of an HLA-DR2 narcoleptic. Immunogenetics 27:449-455.

Londei M,Lamb JR,Botazzo GF,Feldmann M (198) Epithelial cells expressing aberrant MHC class II determinants can present antigen to cloned human T cells. Nature 312:639-641.

Markmann J,Lo D, Naji A, Palmiter RL,Brinster RL Heber-Katz (1988) Antigen presenting function of class II MHC expressing pancreatic beta cells. Nature 336:476-479.

Marlin S,Springer TA (1987) Purified intercellular adhesion molecule-1 (ICAM-1) is a ligand for lymphocyte function-associated antigen 1(LFA-1). Cell 51:813-819.

Shimonkevitz RJ, Kappler JW, Marrack P, Grey H (1983) Antigen recognition by H-2 retricted T cells.1.Cell-free antigen processing. J Exp Med 158:303.

Simmons D,Makgoba MW,Seed B. (1988) ICAM, an adhesion ligand of LFA-1 is homologous to the neural crest adhesion molecule NCAM. Nature 331:624-627.

Springer TA,Dustin ML,Kishimoto TK,Marlin SD (1987) The lymphocyte function associated LFA-1,CD2 and LFA-3 molecules: cell adhesion receptors of the immune system. Ann Rev Immunol 5:223-252.

Wagner CR,Vetto RM,Burger DR (1984) The mechanism of antigen presentation by endothelial cells. Immunobiol 168:453-469.

Wilkinson D,de Vries RRP,Madrigal JA,Lock CB,Trowsdale J, Altmann DM (1988) Analysis of HLA-DR glycoproteins by DNA-mediated gene transfer. Definition of DR2β gene products and antigen presentation to T cell clones from leprosy patients. J Exp Med 167:1442-1458.

Wilkinson D,Altmann DM,Ikeda H,Trowsdale J (1989) Analysis of HLA-classII products by DNA-mediated gene transfer. In press.

Young JAT,Lindsay J,Bodmer JG, Trowsdale J (1988)Epitope recognition by a DPa chain specific monoclonal antibody (DP11.1) is influenceed by the interaction between the DPa chain and its polymorphic partner. Hum Immunol 23:37-44.

DISCUSSION

JANEWAY: John, have you looked at the allo reactive potential or stimulating potential of your alpha transgenic mice, for instance the DR alpha transgenics? If you put them together with the B10.5R mouse strain which has basically the same MHC but uses an E alpha instead of DR alpha, do you get some lymphocyte reactivity?

TROWSDALE: We haven't done that yet.

NEPOM: Along the same lines, what was the antigen in the case where you deleted reactivity in responder mouse strains with the DR alpha transgene, have you any ideas about that?

TROWSDALE: The antigen was TGL. I think the answer's going to be that you have wiped out the set of T cell clones - its going to be difficult to sort out what's going on. I think there are a number of other groups that have transgenic mice with different DR specificities and the question is what is the T cell repertoire in these mice and how has it altered by having a human class II transgene.

DEMAINE: I've got a couple of questions. First, do you think the low level of class II expression and ICAM-1 may have a role in the aberrant class II expression proposed in models of autoimmunity. Second, is there any difference in the level of expression of MHC class II molecules between the two haplotypes of a heterozygous phenotype such as the DR3,4 phenotype associated with diabetes?

TROWSDALE: First question, I think ICAM 1 could play a role if its expression was induced in the same pancreatic islet cells. I haven't looked, but I think there is a very good

THE FINE SPECIFICITY OF RECOGNITION OF INFLUENZA VIRUS PROTEINS BY HUMAN CYTOTOXIC T CELLS

Frances M. Gotch
Institute for Molecular Medicine,
John Radcliffe Hospital,
Headington,
Oxford. OX3 9DU

NATO ASI Series, Vol. H 38
The Molecular Biology of Autoimmune Disease
Edited by A. G. Demaine et al.

Influenza specific, MHC restricted cytotoxic T cells have been shown to be of importance during the in vivo response to Influenza A virus infection in mouse and man (Lin et al 1981, McMichael et al 1983.) It has been possible to map the virus specificity of such CTL raised in vitro from immune individuals using recombinant vaccinia viruses which express single influenza viral proteins in appropriate target cells. Thus CTL have been shown to recognise the conserved internal proteins of Influenza A virus - nucleoprotein (NP), basic polymerase (PB2) and matrix protein (M1) (Gotch et al 1987a). Peptides derived from influenza proteins have been identified that were recognised by virus specific human CTL in association with MHC class I molecules (Townsend et al 1986 and Gotch et al 1987b). Thus it seems likely that viral antigens are processed inside infected cells and peptides representing discrete entities from individual antigens are presented on the surface of the target cell specifically bound to class I MHC molecules. CTL recognition and destruction of virally infected targets may therefore be thought of as a tripartite interaction between peptide, MHC molecule and T cell receptor, and it was of considerable interest to elucidate further the nature of this tripartite complex and to understand the interactions involved. Such information would facilitate the prediction of peptide epitopes from other viruses for interaction with HLA molecules. Our strategy has been to look at this interaction in several different ways, some of which are discussed below.

We have performed experiments where HLA-A2 together with Influenza A matrix peptide 57-68 was the restricting element in CTL recognition (Gotch et al 1987b). The three-dimensional structure of HLA-A2 has been resolved (Bjorkman et al 1987a,b) revealing a groove on the surface of the molecule between two long alpha helices (alpha 1 and alpha 2) lying across an eight stranded beta pleated sheet. Thus our results can be visualised in terms of the 3-dimensional structure of the HLA-A2 molecule.

We here report experiments in which we examined recognition of target cells by CTL when certain parameters were changed. Firstly alterations were made or occurred naturally within the A2 molecule. Secondly we made alterations to the peptide. Finally we describe novel assays where binding of purified MHC molecules to peptides are visualised in vitro.

Experiments with naturally occurring variants of HLA-A2 and deliberately constructed mutants of HLA-A2 containing single amino-acid changes (Santos-Aguado et al 1987) have identified residues within the groove of the HLA-A2 molecule that may be important for binding the influenza matrix peptide. Table 1A shows recognition of matrix peptide by influenza specific CTL with normal and variant A2 molecules. Influenza virus specific CTL from 15 donors were established by culture of peripheral blood mononuclear cells with virus for seven days. These CTL included 5 from donors with HLA-A2.1; 7 with variant A2 molecules; one with HLA AW68 and two with HLA AW69 (which has a natural exon shuffle replacing the alpha-1 domain of the HLA A2.1 with that of AW68 (Holmes et al 1985). It may be seen that CTL from all donors with HLA A2.1, as defined by isoelectric focussing (Gotch et al 1985), recognised the matrix peptide. In contrast, Influenza A virus specific CTL from donors with variant HLA-A2 molecules, HLA-AW68 and HLA-AW69 failed to recognise the peptide but did recognise influenza A virus infected autologous target cells.

Table 1E shows recognition of matrix peptide with mutant A2 molecules by A2.1 CTL lines. The RDA2 cell lines expressing mutant HLA-A2 molecules constructed by site-directed mutagenesis have been described previously (Santos-Aguado et al 1987) and included point mutations at positions 9. 43, 152 and 156 as well as changes at positions 107, 66, 70 and 74. A double mutant at positions 62 and 63 and a mutant with six changes

TABLE 1A

HLA A2 VARIANTS STUDIED

VARIANT	CELLS	SUBSTITUTION	ORIENTATION[1]	RECOGNITION OF AUTOLOGOUS TARGET CELLS		
				AX31	peptide	O
A2.1	JM, AT, GP, IH, KW			+	+	-
A2.2F	AD, JJ	43 Q→ R 95 V→ L 156 L→ W	O * *	+	-	-
A2.2Y	AM, WT49 FM	9 F→ Y 43 Q→ R 95 V→ L 156 L→ W	* O * *	+	-	-
A2.3	DEW	149 A→ T 152 V→ E 156 L→ W	↑ * *	+	-	-
A2.4	TR	9 F→ Y	*	+	-	-
AW68	DC	63 E→ N 66 K→ I 97 R→ I 114 H→ R 116 Y→ D 156 L→ W	* * * * * *	+	-	-
AW69	IDF, WI	9 F→ Y 62 G→ R 63 E→ N 66 K→ N 70 H→ Q 74 H→ D	* ↑ * * * *	+	-	-

[1]Symbols indicate the orientation of the residue on the HLA A2 crystal as determined by Bjorkman.
O - position away from groove.
* - pointing into the groove.
↑ - pointing towards the T cell receptor.

TABLE 1B

HLA A2 MUTANTS STUDIED

	CELLS	SUBSTITUTION	ORIENTATION[1]	RECOGNITION OF TARGETS BY JM CTL	
RD mutants				peptide	O
	RD9Y	9F→ Y	*	±	-
	RD43R	43Q→ R	O	+	-
	RD62/63RN	62G→ R 63E→ N	↑ *	±	-
	RD66I	66K→ I	*	-	-
	RD70Q	70H→ Q	*	±	-
	RD74D	74H→ D	*	+	-
	RD107G	107W→ G	O	+	-
	RD152E	152V→ E	*	-	-
	RD156R	156L→ R	*	-	-
	RD70-80	70H→ Q 74H→ D 76V→ E 77D→ S 79G→ R 80T→ N	* * ↑ * O *	-	-

[1]Symbols indicate the orientation of the residue on the HLA A2 crystal as determined by Bjorkman.
O - position away from groove.
* - pointing into the groove.
↑ - pointing towards the T cell receptor.

between residues 70 and 80 were also studied. It may be seen that peptide treated HLA-A2 mutant target cells with differences at positions 66, 152 and 156 were not recognised by A2.1 CTL lines. Recognition of the 62/63 mutant was greatly impaired and mutants with changes at positions 43, 107 and 74 were recognised. Mutants at positions 9 and 70 gave discrepant results in different experiments which were shown to be due to differing clonal composition in the T cell lines.

From these results it was concluded that the long alpha-helices of HLA-A2 make important contact with the peptide at positions 66, 152 and 156. Different amino acids at position 9, which is in the floor of the peptide binding groove of HLA-A2, and position 70, may modulate the fine orientation of the peptide so that some T cell clones react and others do not.

The second set of experiments describe the use of analogue peptides, each containing a single amino acid point substitution to identify critical residues for binding the matrix peptide to HLA-A2, and thus to determine the conformation and orientation of the peptide within the peptide binding groove of the A2 molecule. These experiments could distinguish between residues necessary for recognition by the antigen receptor of the T cell, and those needed to bind the restriction element. Figure 1 shows CTL recognition of autologous B lymphocytes in the presence of 55 analogue peptides with single amino acid substitutions indicated. Lysis is given as a percentage of specific lysis with the 57-68 index matrix peptide. Thus a core of five amino acids 61-65, where one or more changes completely abrogated recognition was revealed. The glycine at position 61 was the only residue where no substitution was tolerated. Analogue peptides that did not induce CTL-mediated lysis were tested as competitors with the natural peptide and those with substitutions at positions 60, 64 and 65 inhibited thus identifying residues that possibly interact with the TCR. A second approach to the identification of residues in the peptide that point towards the TCR was the analysis of recognition by CTL clones. Marked differences in recognition by individual CTL clones were observed

Fig 1

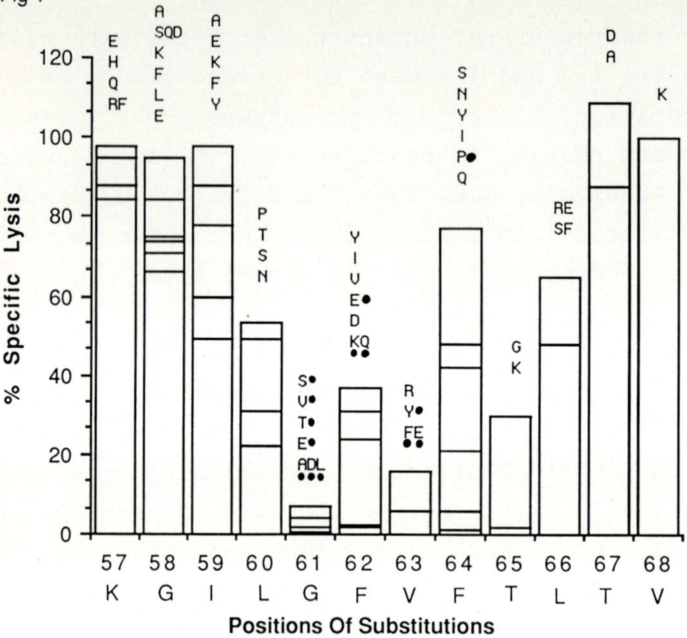

CTL recognition of Autologous B lymphocytes in the presence of 55 analogue peptides with single amino acid substitutions indicated. Peptides were used at 10μM final concentration in the assay. The killer:target ratio was 5:1. Lysis is given as a percentage of specific lysis with the 57-68 index matrix peptide (45-60%)

● complete failure to bind in all assays.

for several substituted peptides, in particular those with substitutions at positions 59, 60, 62, 64, 65 and 66.

The data presented indicates that most of the analogue petides in fact bind to the HLA-A2 molecule. The peptide interaction with HLA-A2 is obviously fairly permissive although it should be remembered that each analogue has only a single amino acid change and the eleven remaining amino acids are constant. HLA-A2 must bind to any analogue that stimulates one or more T cell clones, and variant peptides that abrogate response but compete must also bind. Thus of 55 analogue peptides tested only 14 failed to bind, thirteen of which were substituted at positions 61-63, which three positions we suggest must make critical contact with HLA-A2. A substitution for proline at position 64 also totally abrogated binding.

Fig 2

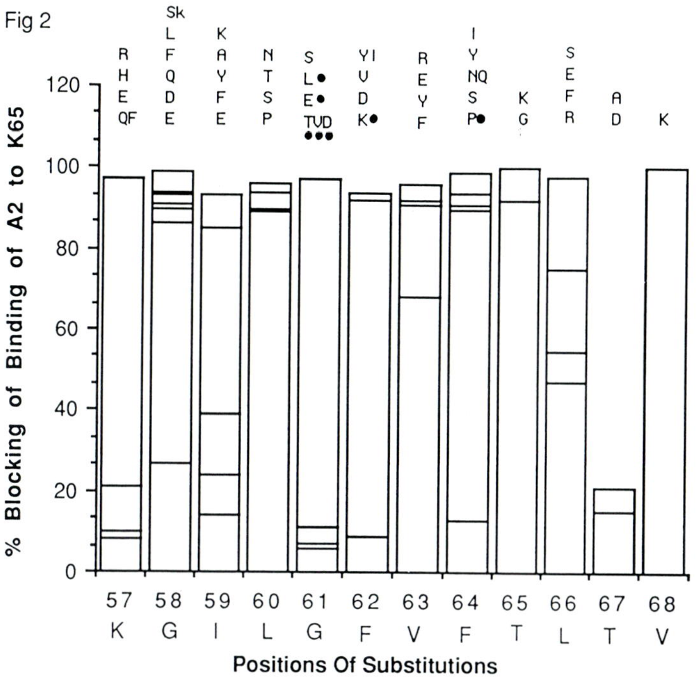

Binding of 51 analogue peptides with single amino acid substitutions indicated to radiolabelled A2. Peptides were used at 15μg/ml. Binding of analogue peptides is here visualised by blocking of binding of A2 molecules to plastic plates coated with the analogue peptide K65.

● peptides which also did not bind in CTL assay.

In a third set of experiments we have examined the physiscal association between HLA-A2.1 molecules and the matrix peptide. The method used has been previously described by Bouillot et al 1989. Binding of purified radiolabelled A2 to analogue peptides was directly measured and attempts were made to correlate results with those obtained in the functional assays described above. The results are shown in figure 2. Of the 14 analogue peptides which did not compete in the functional assay, those substituted at position 61 (with the exception of S61) also failed to bind in this assay further demonstrating the critical importance of this position. Those peptides substituted at position 62 which were not recognised by CTL, did not bind well, but the three peptides with substitutions at position 63 which did not compete in functional assays bound well. Also peptides with substitutions at positions 57 and 67 which have been shown to bind in functional assays did not bind here. This was found to be a function of solubility, peptides with substitutions at positions 57 and 67 were relatively insoluble in PBS, but when dissolved in 10% DMSO they bound. It is, of course, possible that the peptide may be further processed by target cells prior to presentation and recognition on the surface of the target cell, and the fact that physical binding of a synthetic peptide to a purified, radiolabelled and immobilised MHC molecule does not correlate completely with functional data is not suprising. It should be noted that a proline substitution at position 64 which completely abrogates recognition in the functional assay also results in an analogue peptide which does not physically bind to HLA-A2.

The results presented suggest a complex picture where individual peptides from viral proteins bound to MHC molecules in a highly specific fashion - we have only found one peptide from the influenza A virus which is recognised together with HLA-A2.1 although others have been demonstrated from influenza B (Robbins et al 1989) and HIV (Nixon et al 1988). However, analogue peptides, based on the matrix peptide which interacts with HLA-A2.1, appear to bind in a relatively permissive fashion although there are clearly some constraints on size and sequence. These peptides only differ from one another in one amino acid and it does not seem suprising if the general pattern of their binding is similar to that of the native peptide. Recognition by the TCR of virus specific CTL is exquisitely specific indicating that discrimination between peptides from viral proteins lies to a great extent with the TCR.

Bjorkman P J, Saper M A, Samraoui B, Bennett W S, Strominger J L, Wiley D C (1987a) The structure of human class I histocompatibility antigen HLA-A2. Nature 329: 506-512

Bjorkman P J, Saper M A, Samraoui B, Bennett W S, Strominger J L, Wiley D C. (1987b) Structural Identification of the foreign antigen binding site and T cell recognition regions of class I histocompatibility antigens. Nature 329: 512-518

Bouillot M, Choppin J, Cornille F, Papo T, Gomard E, Fournie-Zaluski M-C, Levy J-P. (1989) Physical association between MHC class I molecules and immunogenic peptides. Submitted for publication.

Gotch F M, Kelly C, Ellis S A, Wallace L, Rickinson A B, Van der Poel J J, Crumpton M J, McMichael A J, (1985) Characterisation of the HLA A2.2 subtype: T cell evidence for further heterogeneity. Immunogenetics 21: 11-23

Gotch F M, McMichael A J, Smith G, Moss B, (1987a) Identification of viral molecules recognised by influenza specific human cytotoxic T lymphocytes. J Exp Med 165: 401-416

Gotch F M, Rothbard J, Howland K, Townsend A P M, MxMichael A J, (1987b) Cytotoxic T lymphocytes recognise a fragment of influenza virus matrix protein in association with HLA A-2. Nature 326: 881-882

Holmes N, Parham P, (1985) Exon shuffling in vivo can generate novel HLA class I molecules. EMBO Journal 4: 2849-2854

Lin Y L, Askonas B A, (1981) Biological properties of an influenza A virus specific killer T cell clone. J Exp Med 154: 225-230

McMichael A J, Gotch F M, Noble G R, Beare P A S. (1983) Cytotoxic T cell immunity to influenza. N Eng J Med 309: 13-17

Nixon D F, Townsend A R M, Elvin J, Rizza C R, Gallwey J, McMichael A J M, (1988) HIV-1 gag-specific cytotoxic T lymphocytes defined with recombinant vaccinia virus and synthetic peptides. Nature 336: 484-487

Robbins P A, Lettice L A, Santos-Aguado J, Rothbard J, McMichael A J, Strominger J L, (1989) Definition of a discrete location within HLA-A2 for an influenza B virus nucleoprotein peptide. Submitted for puplication.

Santos-Aguado J, Biro P A, Fuhrmann V, Strominger J, Barbosa J. (1987) Amino acid sequences in the alpha 1 domain and not glycosylation are important in HLA-A2/beta 2 microglobulin association and cell surface expression. Mol and Cell Biol 73: 982-990

Townsend A R M, Rothbard J, Gotch F M, Bahadur G, Wraith D, McMichael A J. (1986) The epitopes of influenza nucleoprotein recognised by cytotoxic T lymphocytes can be defined with short synthetic peptides. Cell 44: 959-968.

DISCUSSION

NEPOM: I just wanted a little clarification on the MHC class I binding assay, what is the indicator compound that's on the plate, is it a peptide?

GOTCH: Its a peptide.

NEPOM: Has it got some kind of spacer arm?

GOTCH: It has no spacer on it, we just fix it to the plastic plate.

NEPOM: The 11mer or 12mer which is stuck on the plastic is successful in competition. Are you not surprised by that?

GOTCH: I was extremely skeptical about this assay altogether until I did it for myself and found it works. I can't explain how it is possible to recognise a peptide stuck onto a plastic dish.

NEPOM: How is the class I radiolabelled?

GOTCH: Its iodinated in the normal way.

NEPOM: Where are the iodinated tyrosines, are they in the groove?

GOTCH: I don't know.

NEPOM: Did you find long specific regions in the peptide?

GOTCH: This assay works perfectly well if we use other peptides on the dish, if we use the index peptide, for example, but it does work better if we use it long.

ALLEN: If you do the assay backwards by radiolabelling the peptide, does it still work?

GOTCH: I haven't done that. We have never radiolabelled the peptide.

<u>ALLEN</u>: A lot of people have had difficulty getting binding of soluble class I with peptide, because you have one peptide on the plate and one in solution do you think there may be problems?

<u>GOTCH</u>: Well we can in fact do direct binding onto the plate. There is nothing to stop one putting all the peptides under test onto the plate and just putting on radiolabelled class I. But this method is perhaps a little bit more sensitive and works perfectly well.

<u>JANEWAY</u>: Along the same lines, what fraction of the radio iodinated class I actually binds to the peptide at saturation?

<u>GOTCH</u>: Between 10-30%.

<u>JANEWAY</u>: And how do you prepare the class I after you have radiolabelled? Its radiolabelled on cell surface isn't it?

<u>GOTCH</u>: No, its prepared first.

<u>JANEWAY</u>: Is it affinity purified?

<u>GOTCH</u>: Its affinity purified on affinity columns.

<u>JANEWAY</u>: And eluted with what?

<u>GOTCH</u>: Its eluted at very high pH around pH11. I didn't actually prepare the A2 myself, there is also some detergent at that point.

<u>JANEWAY</u>: And then it is radiolabelled?

<u>GOTCH</u>: No then its thawed, we made a very large batch of it and we store it at -170 C and then we radiolabel once a week

<u>JANEWAY</u>: With chloramine?

<u>GOTCH</u>: Yes.

H A ERLICH - SESSION CHAIRMAN'S SUMMING UP- EVOLUTIONARY ANALYSIS OF HLA CLASS II POLYMORPHISMS

As I said earlier this morning, rather than use this time for summary of the very interesting talks we have heard, I thought I would very briefly go through some of the evolutionary analysis and just discuss how that might elucidate some aspects of the functional properties of the polymorphism. The very high degree of polymorphism that is observed in the human population could be due either to recent and rapid mutation of gene conversion selection or the ancestral species that gave rise to the humanoid linaeges might have contained the alleleic diversity that we see and that ancient alleles have simply been maintained. The most straightforward way to look at that is really to construct a phylogenetic tree of all sequences that are available for given class II loci from humans and the non-human species. If speciation predated diversification, that is, if the diversification happened after speciation, obviously the alleles would show limited similarity between species. However, if the divergence preceded speciation then the clustering of sequences would not go by species but simply by allelic similarity. We have done this for DQ alpha. This was all done with a PCR where we used primers to conserve regions of the polymorphic second exon and this is just HLA DQ alpha sequences from humans, chimpanzees, gorillas, some old world monkeys and some new world monkeys and the only point that I will try to make here is that first, these major allelic groups are what we call DQA1, DQA3 DQA2 and DQA4. If you look at a given sequence for instance, the

NATO ASI Series, Vol. H 38
The Molecular Biology of Autoimmune Disease
Edited by A. G. Demaine et al.

DQA3 sequence which is on DR4s and DR9s you find that it is much more similar to a chimpanzee or gorilla sequence than it is to any of the other human sequences. This indicates that the ancestral species that gave rise to the humanoids had these major allelic types so they are in fact very ancient. The one exception to this is the human with a DQA2 allele which we have never seen in any of the non-human primates, and so its possible that this allele arose after speciation. In fact it looks like a recombination between DQA4 and one of the other alleles. The overall conclusion from this kind of analysis is that the alleles are quite ancient. Looking at amino acid changes one could argue that the kind of clustering you get could be due to conversion evolution but, if you have constructed a phylogenetic tree based on silent changes alone, you get essentially the same topology. Again, this indicates that if you look at given groups, the so called alpha 4, you have chimpanzees, gorillas and in fact some of the old world monkeys clustering as well as humans. If you look at the A1 group, you get humans, gorillas, chimpanzees and, some old world monkeys. This suggests that the age of the DQ alpha alleles is very ancient, with the exception of the DQA2 as this particular allele doesn't cluster that well with any group and that's because it is essentially a recombinant between the A4 and the A3 groups. However, if this kind of recombination took place frequently you wouldn't have the maintenance of these allelic types so that gene conversion and recombination does not seem to be a major factor in generating polymorphism at least at the DQ alpha locus. There are a number of different ways of estimating the age of the alleles but, if you base them on known divergence times using the molecular clock, then the DQ alpha alleles with one exception were present before the divergence of the humanoid lineage which occurred more than 5 million years ago. In fact, some of the alleles were present before the split of the humanoids and old world monkeys. I would say that they are more than 20 million years old.

There may be possible selective constraints on evolution so that one can make an estimate as to the rate at which these different allelic types are evolving. If you take one allelic type DQ alpha 1 and you do cross species comparison that is chimp-gorilla, chimp-human, gorilla-chimp and so forth, you can derive a ratio for the extent of replacement to silent substitutions. This ratio is a measure of the extent of the rate of evolution. In other words, it normalises for the time difference and for the number of functional changes that have occurred. For instance, with respect to the DX alpha locus which is presumably a non-expressed locus, this has a ratio of about 3 which is the theoretical expectation for neutral gene or a gene under very weak functional constraints. Therefore, some of the DQ alpha alleles are evolving at about the same rate as the non-expressed gene. This suggests that these genes are evolving slowly at about the neutral rates. However, many of them are much more constrained and are evolving much more slowly than the neutral gene (DX alpha). For instance, DQA4 is evolving much more slowly than is DQA1. A possible explanation is that it is related to some of the issues that were discussed earlier this morning. In our hypothesis that the rate of evolution for DQ alpha reflects constraints on alpha beta pairing then from the hypothesis an alpha chain which is capable of pairing with many different kind of beta chains evolves more slowly than a more permissive alpha chain. That is, an alpha chain which has to pair with many different kind of beta chains is really under more stringent selective constraints. In fact, the alpha 4 which was the most slowly evolving, pairs with the most diverse set of beta chains. Now I should point out that this is based on haplotypes in humans. Even so, you still only get alpha A1 pairing on a haplotype with beta 1, which probably reflects functional pairing differences. Nepom pointed out this morning that an alpha 1 does not pair with a beta 2 or 3 but it does pair with beta 1 and in fact some of these haplotypes are conserved within chimpanzees and gorillas. This may account for why DQ alpha is polymorphic and DR alpha isn't, the DR alpha is non-polymorphic and has to pair with very many different kind of beta chains. We would predict, that DR alpha would have a R/S ratio suggesting that it has to pair with many different beta chains. I would just like to discuss briefly the beta chain evolution. Now the conclusion from the studies of the DQ alpha seem to be that the allelic types were ancient with the exception of alpha 2 which may have arisen after speciation in the human lineage. We have done the same kind of analysis of DQ beta from human, chimps, gorillas, old world monkeys, new world monkeys and bird and whale. The phylogenetic tree, shows that the DX beta split off a long time ago and you have these major groups beta-3, beta-2 beta-1 is split into actually beta 1A and 1B, and you have evolutionary conservation of these groups so that if you look in a given group such as beta 3 or B3, that pigmy chimps humans gorillas but anyway you have chimpanzees and humans in the same, and you have humans and gorillas so that again the ancestral species that gave rise to the humanoid lineages all had these major allelic types which are in fact ancient. However, when we look within these major types - at the twigs of the branches you can see that you get species clustering. For instance, even though in DQ beta 1A you have gorillas and humans showing that the 1A type is ancient, you can see that the humans cluster and the gorillas cluster. In fact, in pigmy chimps there are clustering showing that within these major allelic branches species clustering occurs showing that there is significant allelic diversification within the groups after speciation. One of the things we are interested in using this kind of analysis for is to look at individual residues. As you heard earlier this morning position 57 has been implicated in a number of disease studies as a critical residue. I think the clearest example of that is pemphigus vulgaris where there are two alleles, one of which has a relative risk of 100 and one has a relative risk of 1 or less than 1 and they differ only by a valine to an aspartic acid substitution suggesting that it is a critical residue. In pemphigus, as well as in diabetes, you cannot predict the susceptibility of an allele by their residue at 57. However, we are very interested in looking at the pattern of evolution, particularly the valine to aspartic acid changes or the neutral alanine, valine, serine or aspartic acid substitutions at that position. If you look at beta 2 you find that human and gorilla are very similar. But this is a balanced polymorphism that has been maintained in all of the class II beta chains that we have looked at in humans and non-human primates, in which all species have either aspartic acid or a neutral residue at that position 57. In the disease susceptibility studies, for instance, pemphigus which changes from a valine to aspartic acid, whilst in diabetes its an aspartic acid versus a valine, alanine or serine, this kind of balanced polymorphism is true of all the class II beta chains and these include both humanoids as well as the new and old world monkeys. Therefore, this is a very ancient balanced polymorphism and one of the things that the phylogenetic analysis has allowed us to do is look at individual residues in a quantitative way - this is a phyllogenetic tree again using the method maximum parsimony which, just for those of you who are not familiar with it, is a method of looking at a gene sequences in which one looks at individual positions in the sequence and then tries to generate an ancestral type. From an ancestral type in a particular branch structure you minimise the number of changes that are required to diverge, thats why its called maximum parsimony. This method unlike others of phylogenetic tree construction, allows one to look at the evolutionary history of a single position. For example, there appears to be balanced selection that results in a polymorphism between aspartic acid on the one hand and alanine, valine or serine at residue 57 of all the class II beta chains. Therefore, from the humanoid DQ beta sequence you follow a particular branch, say beta 1A - the ancestral sequence has aspartic acid whilst the 'twigs of the branch' have either valine, serine or aspartic acid or alanine. In fact there are two aspartic acid codons and two valine codons. Similarly you can go into a branch and start out with aspartic acid but at the twigs you diversify so you have a balanced polymorphism within the group of aspartic acid versus valine. So there seems to be selective pressure to generate a balanced polymorphism at this position and this kind of change in a branch structure can be quantitated, that is, you can quantitate the number of changes a given residue goes through within a phylogenetic tree. Finally, in the quantitation of the number of phylogenetically and inferred changes in a given phylogenetic tree you can deduce the residues, positions which are polymorphic and the number of amino acids that are tolerated in the second exon based on the humanoid sequences. Position 57 is quite striking, the only residues allowed are those that we see in humans - valine, aspartic acid alanine and serine and the number of changes for any one residue is greatest for 57. Now 57 is the residue which has gone through the highest number of these changes and we can infer that it is the one under strongest selective pressure and balancing selection. Obviously those residues which are invarient are also under selection in a sense that they are under negative or purifying selection as they are not allowed to diverge. The one that shows the most selection is in the alpha helix, there are other positions that are selected and this is interesting, particularly with respect to some of the points that Gerry Nepom was making - that position 26 in the beta pleated sheets shows this kind of selection. Nonetheless position 57 shows the highest degree, and it is interesting that this phylogenetic analysis can implicate a particular residue as being critical for function in much the same way that the disease susceptibility studies have implicated an individual residue as being critical. Again, the evolutionary studies suggest that its important to have both kinds, that is, an aspartic acid DQ beta and a DQ beta allele which codes for either alanine, valine or serine. In fact, the evolutionary mechanism that can best explain the maintenance of polymorphic alleles over 20 millions years is a model known as over dominant or heterozygote advantage, and it may be that there is a selective advantage to have class II beta chain alleles that have both aspartic acid and a neutral residue at this position as this position may be critical in determining the overall complementation as in the original Brown et al paper in 'Nature' which first presented the HLA-A2 disguised as a class II molecule. They suggested the possibility that there is in fact a salt bridge formed between aspartic acid at 57 and I think arginine at 86 over on the alpha chain.

<ins>TROWSDALE</ins>: I don't know if you have looked at this yet Henry, but is it possible to go through the different species and correlate a particular residue at position 57 of the DQ beta with a particular residue in DQ alpha, or is that not possible with your data?

ERLICH: Well yes

TROWSDALE: A particular one, but a group residue, they should correlate if there is association between the alpha and beta of course?

ERLICH: We haven't done that but I don't think that one would expect that because clearly in humans you can get both kinds of beta chains pairing with the same alpha. For instance, on the DR4 haplotype the DQA3 combines with beta 3.1 which has aspartic acid, 3.2 which has alanine, and 3.3 which has aspartic acid so I don't think position 57 necessarily influences the potential to make an alpha beta pair. However, if you believe the salt bridge model you might speculate that the cleft or the peptide binding groove is somewhat different depending on whether you have an aspartic acid or alanine, valine or serine and therefore to maximise the potential for an immune response an individual with both kind of grooves may have the highest chance of responding, or the largest repertoire of possible responses. What we have done in the primates is to try and evaluate whether the human haplotypes, that is, the observed non random associations of DQ alpha and DQ beta which we see in humans are maintained. Only one of these is maintained, and that is in non- human primates, it is a case of DQ alpha 1 which goes almost invariably with DQ beta 1 so that is conserved. As Gerry pointed out earlier, alpha 1 apparently cannot pair with beta 2 or beta 3, but some of the other DQ alpha and DQ beta haplotypes in humans are not conserved, you don't see the restriction on cis combinations.

<u>TROWSDALE</u>: If you look again at an individual species, do you have any evidence that an individual species has less alleles than another one?

<u>ERLICH</u>: That's a very interesting question - I don't know if we can really address that rigorously because you would have to look at 40 or 50 chimps instead of 9 or 10. However if you look at the human beta alleles beta 1, beta 2, beta 3 and beta 4, we have not found beta 4 in the chimps or gorillas, but we have found it in old world monkeys. May be we just haven't looked at enough chimps and gorillas but one possibility is just as the alpha 2 may have arisen after speciation, it may be that the ancestral species that gave rise to the humanoids have beta 1, beta 2, beta 3 and beta 4, but it was lost in the chimps and gorillas. In contrast, in pigmy chimps we only found beta 3, we did not find any beta 1, beta 2 or beta 4, however, we found six different alleles. Since we only sampled 9 individuals it doesn't seem to have a restricted diversity of alleles, but it does seem to be restricted in the allelic types so that there are a number of alleles but they are all of a particular type. For the data we have, the numbers are too small to make any generalisations but I think it is possible that some species will have a different distribution of possible allelic types.

<u>TROWSDALE</u>: In certain species it appears that DP seems more important than DR. For example, in the mole rat and various rat species there appears to be duplication of DP genes and in one species, I don't know if it is the mole rat or the rat, the DR has gone altogether so it might be a little bit

dangerous to compare varied species without looking at the whole range of different loci because it could be that the DQ job is taken over by DP in some species?

ERLICH: That's an important point within the primates. We are analysing DR, DQ and DP and they all have them. In the case of the non human primates they all had DR, DQ and DP and they also have the same beta 1 and beta 3. One of the things that has been striking and somewhat puzzling to us, we identified this gene which unfortunately we also called DR beta 2 just to confuse things for us and we were discussing with Lars Rask this morning that in humans it is just on DR1 DR2 and DR10 but in the non human primates it is on all haplotypes so that the restriction of expression seemed to have come after speciation.

MOLECULAR GENETICS OF TWO MAJOR THYROID AUTO-ANTIGENS : THYROGLOBULIN AND THYROPEROXIDASE

M. Ludgate and G. Vassart
Institut de Recherche Interdisciplinaire and
Service de Génétique Médicale
Faculté de Médecine
Université Libre de Bruxelles
Campus Erasme
Route de Lennik 808
B - 1070 BRUSSELS
Belgium

NATO ASI Series, Vol. H 38
The Molecular Biology of Autoimmune Disease
Edited by A. G. Demaine et al.

1. INTRODUCTION

The biochemical pathway leading to the synthesis of thyroid hormones involves two thyroid-specific proteins : thyroglobulin and thyroperoxidase. Thyroglobulin is the biosynthetic precursor of iodothyronines which result from the iodination and coupling of selected tyrosine residues in thyroglobulin (Nunez & Pommier, 1982). Thyroperoxidase, in the presence of H_2O_2 provided by a still to be defined enzymatic system, is the enzyme responsible for both the iodination and the coupling hormonogenic reactions. These two proteins are the main differentiation markers of the thyrocyte and, as such, they have been extensively studied from structural, regulatory and pathological viewpoints.

A significant proportion of thyroid diseases are due to -, or, at least, accompanied by - autoimmune manifestations. Depending on the target and the intensity of the autoimmune reaction, the disease leads to hyper - (Grave's disease) or hypothyroidism (idiopathic myxoedema), to destruction of the thyroid gland (Hashimoto's thyroiditis) or is compatible with normal thyroid function (Weetman & McGregor, 1984). The three major autoantigens implicated in these diseases have been identified as the thyrotropin (TSH receptor, thyroglobulin and thyroperoxidase (formerly known as the "microsomal antigen"). While the TSH receptor still resists analysis by cloning techniques, thyroglobulin and thyroperoxidase have yielded to the recombinant DNA methodology so that their structure, the regulation of their production and their antigenic characteristics are now amenable to direct study at the molecular level.

2. THYROGLOBULIN

2.1. Primary structure

Thyroglobulin is the homodimeric (2x330,000Da) glycosylated

iodoprotein of sedimentation 19S that accumulates in the follicular lumen of thyroid follicles. Its abundance and degree of iodination vary greatly depending on the activity of the gland. Immunoreactive thyroglobulin is also found in the plasma where its role, if any, remains unknown.

Thyroglobulin protomer is translated from an 8.4 kb mRNA encoded by a large (> 250,000 bp) transcription unit on the long arm of chromosome 8 (Baas et al., 1985). The coding information is scattered amongst 42 exons (Musti et al., 1986). Cloning and sequencing of human, and bovine thyroglobulin cDNA have provided a detailed picture of the primary structure of the protein (Malthiery and Lissitzky, 1987; Mercken et al., 1985). Following a 19-amino acid signal peptide, the polypeptide chain is composed of 2748 residues. Analysis of the protein sequence for internal homology led to its subdivision into four regions from amino to carboxy terminus as follows : domain A is composed of 10 type I repeats containing about 60 amino acids including 24 highly conserved residues, six of which are cysteines. Sequences of variable length, unrelated to the motif, interrupt the repeats at fixed positions (see Fig. 2 in ref. Mercken et al 1985). Domain B (from positions 1439 to 1486) contains three type II repeats of a shorter motif (17 residues). Domain C is composed of the repetition of a type III motif existing as two subtypes (IIIa, IIIb) sharing a similar pattern of cysteine residues. Both subtypes are repeated twice in tandem, between positions 1586 and 2111. A third copy of motif IIIa is found further downstream. Domain D, constituting the last 600 residues of thyroglobulin, shows no internal homology, is poor in cysteine compared to the other regions, and contains a cluster of tyrosine residues.

Structure-function relationships of thyroglobulin have emerged from the comparison of its primary structure with that of iodothyronine-containing peptides.

Four tryptic peptides containing thyroid hormones have been isolated from thyroglobulin of various species and sequenced.

The corresponding tyrosine residues have been identified in the primary structure of the protein. Two of them map at subterminal positions (residues 5 and 2748 in the bovine sequence) (see fig. 4 in ref. Mercken et al., 1985). They correspond to sites involved preferentially in the synthesis of T4 and T3, respectively. The two other sites are closely linked around position 2560. The amino-terminal hormonogenic domain (around Tyr 5) occurs just before the first type I motif and may share sequence characteristics with it. The three other hormonogenic tyrosines map in domain D.

Comparison of the primary structure of thyroglobulin to available polypeptide sequences revealed a significant sequence similarity (28 percent) between domain D and the whole sequence of acetylcholinesterase from Torpedo Californica (Schumacher et al., 1986). The similarity and the identical location of some introns within the corresponding gene portions indicate that these proteins share a common ancestor and that they exhibit conserved tridimensional characteristics (Swillens et al, 1986). The functional significance, if any, of this homology is unclear, as the residues involved in the enzymatic activity of acetylcholinesterase and in thyroid hormonogenesis are not conserved. The similarity could have pathophysiological implications in thyroid autoimmunity since immunologic cross-reactions between the two proteins could be demonstrated (see below). Sequence similarity between the type I motif of domain A and an exon found in certain transcripts of the invariant chain of class II antigens (Koch et al., 1987) and GA773, a major gastrointestinal tumor associated antigen (Linnenbach) et al, 1989) have been reported. Again, the sequence similarity is suggestive of a common ancestor but does not reveal functional relationships. As the invariant chains are apparently involved in antigen processing and presentation on the surface of macrophages, it was proposed that this segment in thyroglobulin could play a role in addressing the molecule to specific subcellular compartments.

2.2. Microheterogeneity

Apart from the heterogeneity related to glycosylation and to iodine and hormone content, analysis of thyrogloblulin cDNA has revealed a heterogeneity in primary structure originating from the alternative splicing of thyroglobulin primary transcripts. Minor transcripts in which one or two exons are missing have been sequenced in bovine and human species (Mercken et al, 1989, Malthiery, 1987). Except for the case of the hereditary goiter of the Afrikander cattle (which relies on thyroglobulin molecules lacking exon 9 to achieve euthyroidism) nothing is known about the possible function of these minor thyroglobulins. The possibility that they play a role in the triggering of autoimmune processes is conjectural.

2.3. Epitope mapping

A lambda gt11 cDNA library was constructed containing cDNA inserts from human thyroid (Libert et al, 1987a). Screening of recombinant phages was performed with heteroantibodies (rabbit anti-human Tg) and the border of the inserts encoding immunoreactive peptides was sequenced. As most of the clones corresponded to relatively short inserts, individual epitope-containing segments of thyroglobulin could be readily identified. This approach lead to the identification of ten non-overlapping hetero epitope-bearing fragments (see figure 1 in Dong et al, 1989). It demonstrated that the 22 amino-acids at the c-terminus of the protein contain a highly reactive hetero epitope. When the same approach was used with autoantibodies from patients with Hashimoto thyroiditis, not a single recombinant phage could be identified out of $2x10^6$ plaques which were screened. This strongly suggests that autoantibodies are directed to conformation-dependent epitopes and/or structures containing iodine.

The sequence similarity between domain D of thyroglobulin and acetylcholinesterase lead us to propose that immunological cross reaction between thyroglobulin and acetylcholinesterase of eye muscles could play a role in the etiopathogeny of Graves' ophthalmopathy (Ludgate et al., 1985). While definite proof for such a role is still lacking, the existence of shared epitopes between both molecules has been demonstrated by the isolation of two thyroglobulin clones from the lambda gt11 library with rabbit antiacetylcholinesterase antibody (see M7, M9 in fig. 1 in Ludgate et al, 1989a). This Tg/ACHE shared epitope has been shown to be an autoepitope by testing sera from patients with autoimmune thyroid diseases in an ELISA in which recombinant peptides corresponding to M7 and M9 were used as an antigen to coat microtitre plates.

3. THYROPEROXIDASE

Thyroperoxidase is a glycosylated hemoprotein bound to the apical plasma membrane of thyroid follicular cells with its catalytic domain facing the colloid space. It seems to exist in two molecular forms, 105 kDa and 110 kDa, and was identified as the major antigenic component of the thyroid "microsomal antigen" involved in thyroid autoimmunity (Czarnocka et al., 1985, Portman et al, 1985). The primary structure of human thyroperoxidase has been deduced from cloned cDNA (Libert et al, 1987b). Two cDNAs differing by 171 nucleotides were obtained resulting from alternative splicing (Kimura et al, 1987), which accounts most probably for the 105- and 110-kDa protein species observed on western blots. Analysis of hydropathy profiles of the encoded polypeptides indicates that the protein is anchored in the membrane by a segment close to its carboxy terminus. The extracellular domain has similarities with myeloperoxidase (42 percent over 745 residues (Libert et al, 1987a) indicating a common evolutionary origin. Screening of a lambda gt11 cDNA library with hetero- (rabbit anti TPO) and auto-antibodies (from Hashimoto patients with high titres of anti microsomal antibodies) demonstrated unequivocally that TPO and the microsomal antigen are one and the same molecule (Libert et al, 1987a). Interestingly, a single peptide (containing 85 amino acid residues of TPO, was shown to bear (an) epitope(s) recognized by 65% of patients with AITD and antibodies to the intact TPO molecule (see figure 3 in Ludgate et al, 1989b).

4. CONCLUSION

The analysis of the primary structure of thyroglobulin and thyroperoxidase obtained from the sequencing of cDNAs has provided information on structure-function and evolutionary relationships of these proteins. The availability of recombinant molecules provided the tools allowing direct investigation of their antigenic properties. Important differences in antigenicity were found between the two proteins. In thyroperoxidase, sequential epitopes were found to be recognized by auto- and hetero- antibodies. In particular, a short segment of the protein behaves as a major autoepitope recognized by antibodies from patients with autoimmune thyroid diseases. On the contrary, sequential epitopes of thyroglobulin seem to be recognized only by heteroantibodies. Out of an estimated number of 40 heteroepitopes of thyroglobulin (Heidelberger, 1938), a minimum of 10 have been localized and shown to belong to the category of sequential epitopes. Autoantibodies must be mainly directed towards conformational or iodine containing epitopes since they do not react with the vast majority of recombinant thyroglobulin polypeptides.

An interesting exception to this observation is found in the recognition by autoantibodies of thyroglobulin peptides identified on the basis of their cross-reaction with anti acetylcholinesterase antibodies (Ludgate et al, 1989a). Although this immunoreactivity is definitely weaker than that displayed by the thyroperoxidase peptide, it is clearly demonstrable in Hashimoto thyroiditis and, more interestingly, in Graves'disease. Preliminary observations show that these acetylcholinesterase-like thyroglobulin segments are recognized even by serum from patients with Graves'disease showing no antithyroglobulin autoantibodies as measured by standard assays. Future studies are required to explore possible relationships between this observation and a role for these antibodies in the etiopathogenesis of Graves'ophthalmopathy.

ACKNOWLEDGMENTS

The continuous support and critical interest of J.E. Dumont is deeply acknowledged. Amongst the many individuals who participated actively to this study, we want to thank C. Dinsart, Q. Dong, F. Libert and S. Mariotti. Supported by grants from Ministère de la Politique Scientifique (Sciences de la Vie), NIH, Wellcome Foundation and ARBD.

REFERENCES

Baas F, Bikker H, Geurts Van Kessel A, Melsert R, Pearson PL, De Vijlder JJM, Van Ommen GJ (1985) The human thyroglobulin gene: a polymorphic marker localized distal to c-myc on chromosome 8 band q24. Human Genet 69:138-142

Czarnocka B, Ruf J, Fernand M, Carayon P, Lissitzky S (1985) Purification of the human thyroid peroxidase and its identification as the microsomal antigen involved in autoimmune thyroid diseases. FEBS Lett 190:147-152

Dong Q, Ludgate M, Vassart G (1989) Towards an antigenic map of thyroglobulin : identification of ten epitope bearing sequences within the primary structure of thyroglobulin. J Endocr in press

Heidelberger M (1938) The molecular composition of immune precipitates from rabbit sera. J Am Chem Soc 60:242-251

Kimura S, Kotani T, Bride OW, Umeki K, Hirai K, Nakayama T, Ohtaki S (1987) Human thyroid peroxidase: complete cDNA and protein sequence, chromosome mapping and identification of two alternatively spliced mRNAs. Proc Natl Acad Sci USA 86:5555-5559

Koch N, Lauer W, Hibichi J, Dobberstein B (1987) Primary structure of the gene for the murine IA antigen associated invariant chain. An alternatively spliced exon encodes a cysteine rich domain homologous to a repetitive sequence of thyroglobulin. EMBO J 6:1677-1683

Libert F, Ruel J, Ludgate M, Swillens S, Alexander S, Vassart, G, Dinsart C (1987a) Thyroperoxidase : an autoantigen with a mosaic structure made of nuclear and mitochondrial gene modules. EMBO J 6:4193-4196

Libert F, Ruel J, Ludgate M, Swillens S, Alexander S, Vassart, G, Dinsart C (1987b) Complete nucleic acid sequence of the human thyroperoxidase - microsomal antigen cDNA. Nucleic Acids Res 15:6735.
Linnenbach AJ, Wojcierowski J, Wu S, Pyre JJ, Ross AH, Dietzschold B, Speicher D, Koprowski H (1989) Sequence investigation of the major gastro intestinal tumor-associated antigen gene family, GA 733. Proc Natl Acad Sci USA 86:27-31
Ludgate M, Swillens S, Mercken L, Vassart G (1986) Homology between thyroglobulin and acetylcholinesterase : an explanation for pathogenesis in Graves'ophthalmopathy. Lancet ii:219-220.
Ludgate M, Dong Q, Dreyfus PA, Zakut H, Taylor P, Vassart G, Soreq H (1989a) Definition, at the molecular level, of a thyroglobulin-acetylcholinesterase shared epitope : study of its pathophysiological significance in patients with Graves'ophthalmopathy. Autoimmunity, in press
Ludgate M, Mariotti S, Libert F, Dinsart C, Piccolo P, Santini F, Ruf J, Pinchera A, Vassart G (1989) Antibodies to human thyroid peroxidase in autoimmune thyroid disease : Study with a cloned recombinant cDNA epitope. J Clin Endocrinol Metab, in press
Malthiéry Y (1987) Structure primaire de la thyroglobuline humaine. Thèse d'Etat Université d'Aix-Marseille
Malthiéry Y, Lissitzky S (1987) Primary structure of human thyroglobulin deduced from the sequence of its 8448 base complementary DNA. Eur J Biochem 165:491-498
Mercken L, Simons MJ, Brocas H, Vassart G (1989) Alternative splicing may be responsible for heterogeneity of thyroglobulin structure. Biochimie 71:223-226
Mercken L, Simons MJ, Swillens S, Massaer M, Vassart G (1985) Primary structure of bovine thyroglobulin deduced from the sequence of its 8431 base complementary DNA. Nature 316:647-651
Musti AM, Avvedimento E, Polistina V, Ursini VM, Obici S, Nitsch L, Coccoza S, Di Lauro R (1986) The complete structure of the rat thyroglobulin gene. Proc Natl Acad Sci USA 83:323-327
Nunez J, Pommier J (1982) Formation of thyroid hormones. Vitam Horm 39:175-182
Portmann L, Hamada N, Heinrich G, DeGroot LJ (1985) Anti-thyroid peroxidase antibody in patients with autoimmune thyroid disease: Possible identity with anti-microsomal antibody. J Clin Endocrinol Metab 61:1001-1003
Schumacher M, Camp S, Maulet Y, Newton M, McPhee-Quigley K, Taylor S, Friedman T, Taylor P (1986) Primary structure of Torpedo Californica acetylcholinesterase deduced from its cDNA sequence. Nature 319:407-409
Swillens S, Ludgate M, Mercken L, Dumont J, Vassart G (1986) Analysis of sequence and structure homologies between thyroglobulin and acetylcholinesterase : possible functional and clinical significance. Biochem Biophys Res Commun 137:142-148
Weetman AP, McGregor AM (1984) Autoimmune thyroid diseases : developments in our understanding. Endocr Rev 5:309-355

DISCUSSION

CHARREIRE: How can you explain the discrepancies in identifying autoantigenic epitopes on recombinant Tg and TPO segments from your library? For example, it is well known that Tg is the autoantigen in thyroiditis but when you screen your library with autoantibodies, you were unable to identify a single positive clone. On the other hand, at present the role of TPO in mediating thyroiditis is not certain, but when you screen your library with autoantibodies you found a super epitope on one of your clones.

VASSART: I think that the answer probably comes through the weak point of the whole story which is that we study B cell epitopes and not T cell responses or those triggering epitopes. We are studying the antibodies present in patients and apparently these antibodies need the native structure of thyroglobulin containing iodine, which are not present in recombinant portions. Hence, Tg autoantibodies fail to show reactivity with recombinant Tg.

WILKIN: Do you have any estimate at all of the frequency of cross-reaction between the thyroglobulin autoantibody and Acetylcholinesterase?

VASSART: I wish to make two kinds of comments. First, a note of caution about the methodology for people using lambda gt11 libraries. It is quite surprising to note the difference in antibody recognition when you take segments from a protein which is fused to another protein and for which you get antibodies against it. For example, you get a segment of 100 amino acids which shows a positive reaction with its antibody.

You can then find a segment of 400 amino acids containing the sequence of 100 amino acids which I alluded to earlier and you find that it is negative for that same antibody. This brings us to your question; clearly screening a thyroid cDNA library with anti cholinesterase antibodies picks clones and when you sequence these clones the majority are thyroglobulin within the acetylcholinesterase-like domain. When these clones showing reactivity with rabbit anti-acetyl-cholinesterase sera are examined for reactivity against sera from a whole variety of patients, surprisingly it is not the Hashimoto patient's which give the best response although they have highest titre against thyroglobulin; it is the Graves' patient which give the best response. Furthermore, Graves' patients which are negative in classical Tg autoantibody tests still show reactivity with these recombinant clones. I think this tells us something very important about the kind of structure of the epitope involved and might open the way to define new epitopes on Tg which are missed by classical autoantibody tests.

KOHN: Is the active site of the acetylcholinesterase present in the region showing homology to thyroglobulin?

VASSART: This is an interesting question although I think in terms of evolution it is probably not directly relevant. If you examine the sequences, only 30% of the thyroglobulin sequence is homologous with acetylcholinesterase. However, the specific active serine residue involved in the active site of acetylcholinesterase is not present in the homologous region in thyroglobulin. Conversely, the important hormonogenic tyrosine residue of thyroglobulin is not present in acetylcholinsterase.

DEMAINE: When you were looking at the sequence homology between thyroglobulin and acetylcholinesterase, did you also examine the exon intron boundaries and were they conserved?

VASSART: That is not our work. I should quote from Lockridge's work. The intron exon junction in that region of the gene have been mapped to seven exons by Roberto De Lauro. Lockridge has mapped the exons of acetylcholinesterase and I don't remember the exact numbers, but about 3 out of the total exons are exactly at the same place, so I think these signs point to the evolutionary relationship between two proteins despite the relatively low (30% level) of amino acid homology.

ANALYSIS OF AUTOANTIGENIC DETERMINANTS OF THYROID PEROXIDASE ANTIGEN, GENERATED USING POLYMERASE CHAIN REACTION

J Paul Banga, Philip S Barnett, David L Ewins, Martin J Page* and Alan M McGregor

Department of Medicine, King's College School of Medicine & Dentistry, Denmark Hill, LONDON SE5 8RX, UK

* Wellcome Research Laboratories, Department of Molecular Biology, Langley Park Road, Beckenham, KENT BR3 3BS, UK

NATO ASI Series, Vol. H 38
The Molecular Biology of Autoimmune Disease
Edited by A. G. Demaine et al.

INTRODUCTION

Immune reactivity manifests itself in the form of B cell, that is antibody and T cell reactivity. In autoimmune disease, immune reactivity is directed towards particular target antigens (Weetman & McGregor, 1984). It has been difficult to experimentally study a large proportion of autoimmune disease due to the lack of knowledge on the nature of the autoantigen or, in cases where the autoantigen is known, the lack of available purified antigen. This lack of antigen may be due to the difficulty in purifying the material or difficulty in obtaining sufficient human tissue for biochemical purifications.

We have approached this problem by generating recombinant preparations of human autoantigen, the thyroid microsomal/thyroid peroxidase antigen (TMA/TPO) involved in destructive autoimmune thyroid disease (AITD). We have previously shown that the TMA is a 105kd protein (Banga et al, 1985) on which several autoantigenic sites have been delineated to which the pathogenetic autoantibodies (aAb) are directed (Doble et al, 1988; Banga et al, 1989). By using the recently introduced technique of amplifying DNA by the Polymerase Chain Reaction (PCR) (Saiki et al, 1985), we have been able to express selected segments of the TMA/TPO polypeptide as recombinant fusion proteins. This has allowed us to delineate some of the aAb binding sites to different segments of the TMA/TPO. The availability of discrete segments of the TMA/TPO protein will now allow studies on the accurate localization of autoantigenic epitopes recognized by aAbs and the T cell populations involved in AITD.

METHODS

Recombinant DNA techniques

i. Human thyroid cDNA library: mRNA from a Graves' thyroid gland was isolated, poly A^+ purified and used for cDNA synthesis using standard procedures (Davis et al, 1987). The amplified, lambda gt10 library was screened with a ^{32}P labelled, 40 mer synthetic oligonucleotide complementary to the 3' end of the TPO gene using hybridization conditions already described (Collison et al, 1989). Positive plaques were picked and plaque purified through two or three successive rounds of screening, phage preparations made using the plate lysate method and then EcoR1 digested (Maniatis et al 1983). The largest insert was gel purified and subcloned into M13 for sequence analysis using several synthetic 20 mer oligonucleotides as primers. The TPO clones were subcloned in PUC 18.

ii. Polymerase Chain Reaction (PCR): This was performed on cloned TPO cDNA templates of TPO 18 and TPO 32. Gel purified cDNA insert (10ng) was mixed with 45 pmol of each oligonucleotide primer (oligo 3B and 3E for Reg 3 and oligo 2bB and 2bE for Reg 2b) using Gene Amp DNA amplification reagent kit and 2.5U Taq polymerase (Perkin Elmer Cetus) in a total volume of 100ul. The samples were subjected to PCR in a Perkin Elmer Cetus DNA thermal cycler. Each cycle consisted of 1 minute denaturation at 95°C, 2 minutes annealing at 37°C and three minutes of chain extension at 72°C. Following PCR, the overlaying oil was removed, 10ul sample was electrophoresed in 1% agarose gel in EtBr to visualize the PCR products. The remainder of the amplified DNA was extracted with phenol/chloroform, ethanol precipitated and following suspension in 100ul TE8, digested with BamH1 and EcoR1.

iii. Expression in pGEX-2T: The amplified BamH1/EcoR1 digested DNA was ligated into BamH1/EcoR1 digested pGEX-2T plasmid and used to transform TG1 cells. Expression with recombinant or non-recombinant TG1 cultures and purification of fusion polypeptides was performed as described by Smith and Johnson (1988).

Immunoblotting: SDS-PAGE and immunoblotting with human sera was performed as already described (Banga et al, 1989) using 1:100 diluted sera and ^{125}I-Protein A followed by autoradiography.

RESULTS AND DISCUSSION

Isolation of TPO cDNA: A human Graves' thyroid cDNA library was constructed in lambda gt10. The library was screened with ^{32}P-labelled 40 mer synthetic oligonucleotide complementary to the human TPO nucleotide sequence 2600-2640 (Kimura et al, 1987). The 40 mer oligonucleotide corresponds to the 3' end of the TPO gene and identifies both species of TPO mRNA transcript reported by Kimura and colleagues (Kimura et al, 1987). The specificity of the oligonucleotide probe for TPO mRNA was confirmed by Northern blotting using mRNA from Graves' thyroid glands. Using the optimised hybridization conditions, the 40 mer probe recognized an approximately 3.0kb mRNA from human thyroid glands which was absent in human or bovine retina mRNA preparations, confirming the specificity of the probe under our hybridization conditions (Collison et al, 1989).

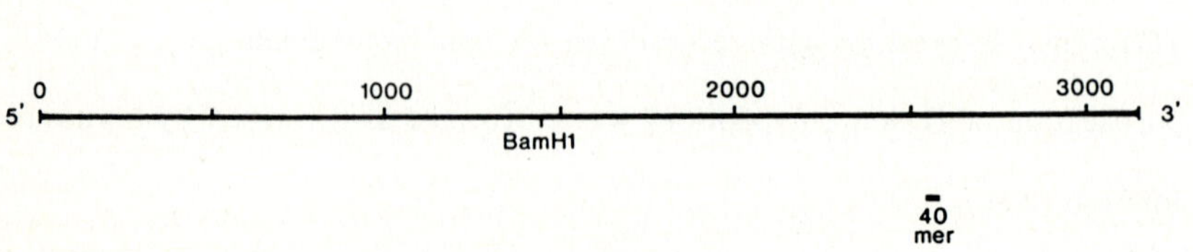

Figure 1. Strategy for cloning TPO cDNA
(see text for details)

Screening of 10^5 recombinant plaques from the lambda gt10 library in duplicate filters with the 40 mer TPO oligonucleotide probe identified twenty positive plaques containing cDNA inserts ranging from 0.6kb - 2.0kb. The largest insert (TPO 18) was fully sequenced in M13 using synthetic oligonucleotides as primers and corresponded to the TPO-1 species starting at nucleotide 1011 (Kimura et al, 1987). A 5' TPO probe (430bp) from TPO 18 was generated by BamH1/EcoR1 digestion of TPO 18 phage DNA and used to rescreen the thyroid cDNA library to identify a full length TPO cDNA (TPO 32) (Fig. 1). Both TPO18 and TPO32 cDNA were purified following subcloning in pUC18.

Polymerase Chain Reaction: This was used to amplify the selected regions of TPO cDNA for expression as fusion polypeptides with glutathione S-transferase (GST). The oligonucleotide primers used in these experiments were designed with BamH1 and EcoR1 restriction sites on their 5' and 3' ends respectively for directional subcloning. Furthermore, the restriction sites on the ends were placed in a way that allowed the generation of, in frame, amplified cDNA product for the purposes of ligation and expression in the plasmid pGEX-2T. In this report, the amplification and expression of region 3 (R3) and Region 2b (R2b) of TPO cDNA are reported (Fig. 2). Using TPO 18 cDNA insert and the respective pairs of oligonucleotide primers for amplification, bands of 807 and 399 base pairs of R3 and R2b respectively were amplified, as shown in Fig. 3.

Expression and purification of TPO polypeptide segments of GST-TPO fusion proteins: The gel purified, amplified segments of TPO DNA were ligated into BamH1/EcoR1 digested expression plasmid pGEX-2T. The plasmid directs the expression of C-terminal fusion polypeptides based on the glutathione S-transferase enzyme, a 26kd molecular weight soluble protein. Besides the relatively small molecular weight of GST, an added advantage is the ease of purification of the GST enzyme or fusion polypeptides of GST under non-denaturing conditions by affinity chromotography

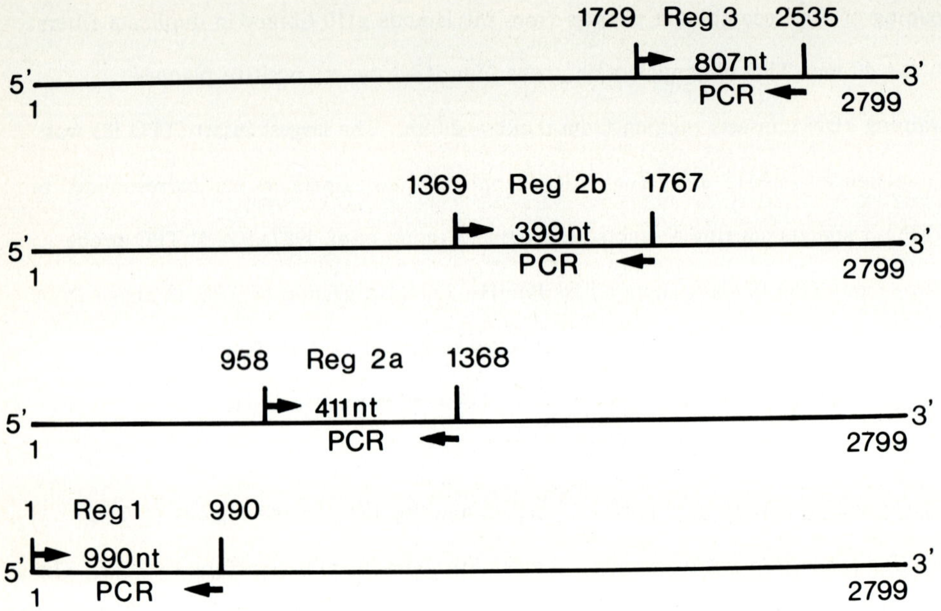

Figure 2: Location of oligonucleotide primers for amplification by PCR of selected regions of TPO cDNA. The polypeptide coding region comprises of 2799 nucleotides (933 amino acids). The 5' and 3' ends are indicated. The arrows on each line indicate the position of the primers and the direction of chain elongation during the PCR reaction; the numbers indicate the location of the nucleotides from which priming is initiated. The TPO molecule was divided into four segments for amplification and expression; these were Reg. 3 (269 amino acids), Reg. 2b (133 amino acids), Reg. 2a (137 amino acids) and Reg. 1 (330 amino acids). Data for Reg. 3 and Reg. 2b is reported in this communication.

using glutathione-agarose followed by elution of the bound material with glutathione or urea extraction of the inclusion body (Smith et al, 1988).

Non-recombinant pGEX-2T cultures induced with 0.1mM IPTG synthesize abundant GST protein which after the affinity chromatography purification step is recoverable in virtually 100% purity (Fig. 4). Recombinant pGEX-2T constructed with PCR amplified, in frame DNA of Reg 3 and Reg2b of TPO synthesize GST-fusion polypeptides of approximately 56kd and 39kd respectively (Fig. 5 and Fig. 6 respectively). Extraction of the proteins in 6M urea yields recombinant TPO as fusion

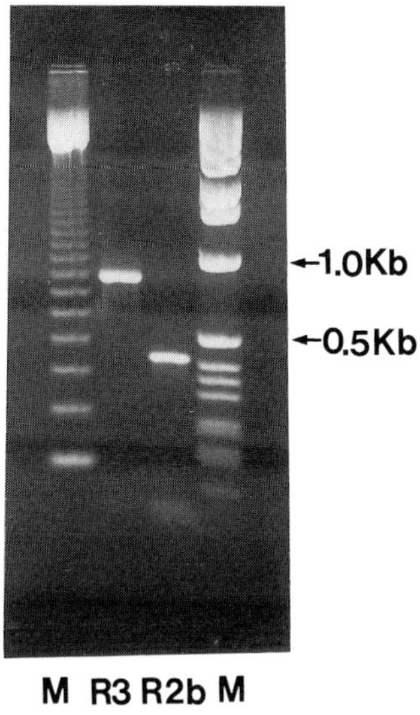

Figure 3. EtBr-stained agarose gel to show the PCR products derived from TPO cDNA. R3 and R2b refer to Reg. 3 and Reg. 2b amplification products of 807 and 399 base pairs respectively. M refers to the 123kb (left) and 1kb (right) base pair ladder.

proteins of 50-60% purity (Fig 5, lane 5; Fig 6, Lane 5). The enriched recombinant GST-TPO fusion polypeptides were analysed for aAb binding using sera from AITD patients.

Immunoblotting: Recombinant fusion polypeptides of TPO encompassing R3 and R2b segments were assessed for the presence of autoantigenic epitopes by immunoblotting. Non-induced and induced total bacterial extracts carrying the recombinant plasmid together with purified inclusion bodies and 6M urea extracts were utilized. In addition, inclusion bodies from bacteria containing non-recombinant plasmid together with affinity purified GST polypeptide from the IPTG induced cells were also electrophoresed.

Immunoblotting with normal human sera shows non-specific reactivity with several bands, the strongest band at approximately 55kd and others at 50kd, 44kd, 32kd and

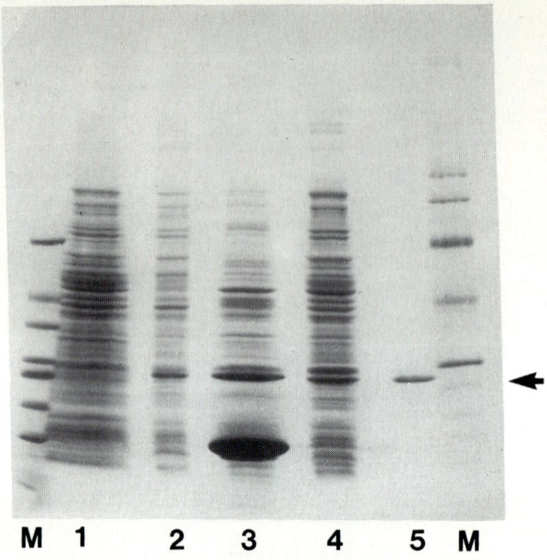

Figure 4. SDS-PAGE analysis of the parental, non-recombinant plasmid products expressing the glutathione-S-transferase (GST) protein. Lane 1 = total extract of non-induced bacteria. Lane 2 = total extract of IPTG-induced bacteria, expressing the GST protein at 26kd (arrowed). Lane 3 = total soluble protein extract of induced bacteria applied to glutathione-agarose affinity column. Lane 4 = flow through the affinity column. Lane 5 = pure GST eluted with reduced glutathione from the affinity column. M refer to the low mol. wt. (left) and high mol. wt. markers

28kd (Fig. 7, panel A, Lanes 1-12). However, no binding to the thyroid microsome was observed (Fig. 7, Panel A, Lane 12). Immunoblotting with a patient's sera containing aAbs to TMA/TPO, identified the TMA/TPO polypeptide in thyroid microsomes together with the TMA band (Fig. 7, Panel B, Lane 12). In addition, this sera also reacts with the R3 TPO polypeptide co-migrating at 56kd (Fig. 7, Panel B, Lanes 2, 3 and 4); no visible specific bands at 56kd were observed in non-induced R3 plasmid containing bacterial extract (Fig. 7, Panel B, Lane 1) confirming the specificity of the aAbs for the R3 fusion polypeptide. No specific binding was observed to R2b fusion polypeptide (Fig. 7, Panel B, Lanes 5-8) or, as expected, to the purified GST protein (Fig. 7, Panel B, Lane 11).

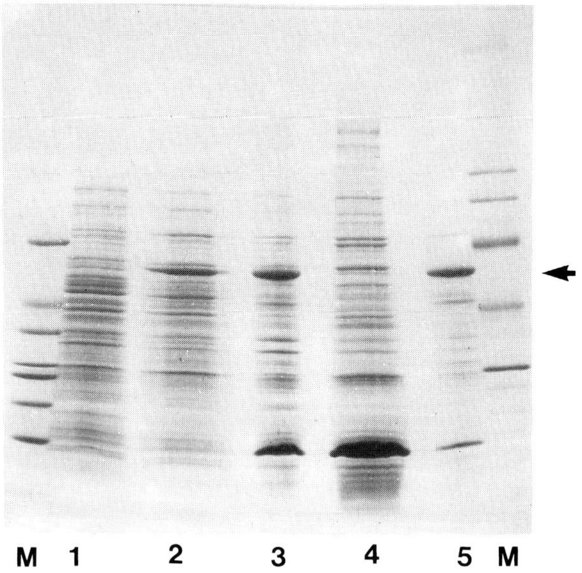

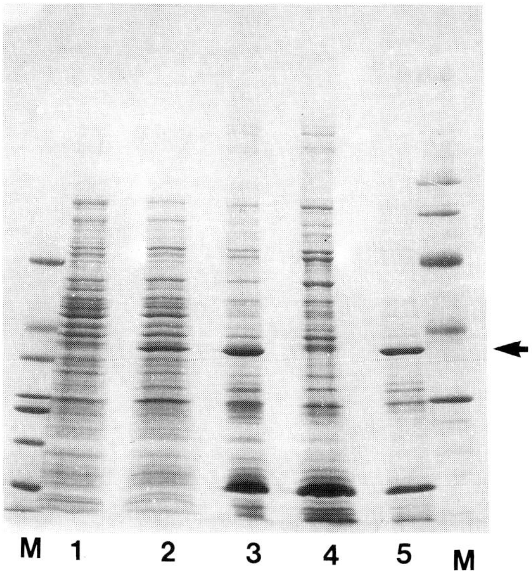

Figure 5 and Figure 6. SDS-PAGE analysis of recombinant TPO-GST fusion polypeptides derived from Reg. 3 (Fig. 5) and Reg. 2b (Fig. 6) segments of the TPO molecule. The arrow shows the position of the Reg. 3 fusion polypeptide at 56kd (Fig. 5) and Reg. 2b fusion polypeptide at 39kd (Fig. 6). Lane 1 = total extract of non-induced bacteria. Lane 2 = total extract of IPTG-induced bacteria expressing the fusion polypeptide. Lane 3 = purified total inclusion bodies. Lane 4 = 2M urea extract of inclusion body showing absence of recombinant fusion protein. Lane 5 = 6M urea extract showing the enrichment of recombinant fusion protein.

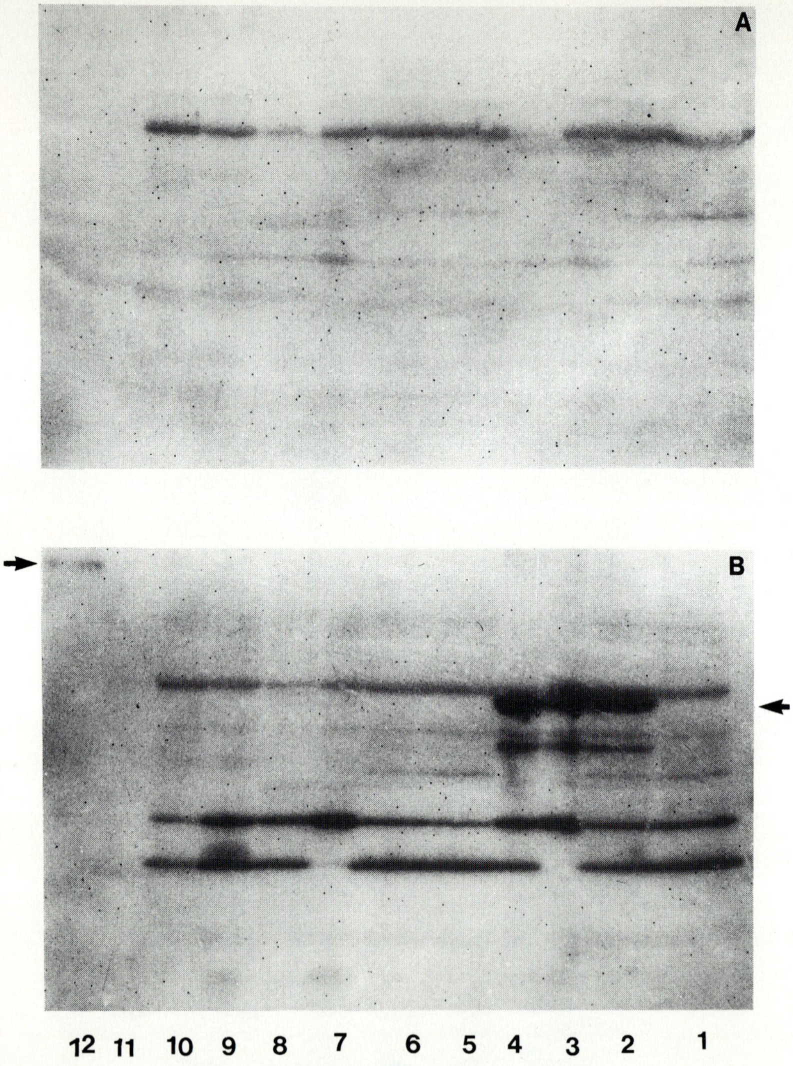

Figure 7. Immunoblotting with normal human serum (Panel A) and serum from an AITD patient containing aAbs and TMA/TPO (Panel B). Lane 1-4 are R3 TPO-GST proteins. Lane 4-8 are R2b TPO-GST proteins. Lane 9-11 are the parental non-recombinant GST protein. Lane 1 and 5 are non-induced bacterial total cell lysate. Lane 2 and 6 are IPTG-induced bacterial total cell lysate. Lane 3, 7 and 9 are the total purified inclusion bodies. Lane 4, 8 and 10 are 6M urea enriched proteins whilst Lane 11 contains affinity purified GST protein. Lane 12 contains thyroid microsomes run as a positive control. Within the spectrum of bacterial binding proteins by antibodies to *E.coli* present in the normal human serum (Panel A) and the patient's serum (Panel B), a binding of microsome aAbs can be seen to the TMA polypeptide in thyroid microsomes (Lane 12, arrowed) and to the R3 fusion proteins (Lanes 2, 3 and 4, arrowed) (Panel B).

CONCLUSIONS

i. Selected segments of TPO cDNA can be amplified by PCR. Using oligonucleotide primers containing BamH1 and EcoR1 restriction sites allows in frame cloning and expression of the amplified DNA as GST-TPO fusion polypeptide in the expression vector pGEX-2T.

ii. The GST-TPO recombinant proteins have been purified to > 50% purity by 6M urea extraction. By immunoblotting, using aAbs from sera of patients with AITD autoantigenic sites have been mapped to the C-terminal (Reg 3) segment of the recombinant TPO protein.

ACKNOWLEDGEMENTS

We wish to thank Dr David Snary for valuable comments throughout the study, Dr Kevin Johnson for advice on cloning with pGEX vectors and Mr Hugh Spence for synthesis and purification of the oligonucleotides.

REFERENCES

Banga, J.P., Pryce, G., Hammond, L. & Roitt, I.M. (1985). Structural features of the autoantigens involved in thyroid autoimmunity: The thyroid microsomal/microvillar antigen. Mol. Immunol. 22; 629-642

Banga, J.P., Tomlinson, R.W.S., Doble, N., Odell, E. & McGregor, A.M. (1989). Thyroid microsomal/thyroid peroxidase autoantibodies show discrete patterns of cross-reactivity to myeloperoxidase, lactoperoxidase and horseradish peroxidase. Immunol. 67; 197-204

Collison, K.S., Banga, J.P., Barnett, P.S., Kung, A.W.C. & McGregor, A.M. (1989). Activation of the thyroid peroxidase gene in human thyroid cells: Effect of thyrotropin, forskolin and phorbol ester. J. Mol. Endocrinol. 3; 1-5

Davis, L.G., Dibner, M.D. & Battey, J.F. (1986). Basic Methods in Molecular Biology. Elsevier; New York, Amsterdam, London

Doble, N., Banga, J.P., Pope, R., Lalor, E., Kilduff, P. & McGregor, A.M. (1988). Autoantibodies to the thyroid microsomal/thyroid peroxidase antigen are polyclonal and directed to several distinct antigenic sites. Immunol. 64; 23-29

Kimura, S., Kotani, T., McBride, O.W., Umeki, K., Hirai, K., Nakayama, T. & Ohtaki, S. (1987). Human thyroid peroxidase: Complete cDNA and protein sequence, chromosome mapping and identification of two alternately spliced mRNA's. Proc. Natl. Acad. Sci. 84; 5555-5559

Maniatis, T., Fritsch, E.F. & Sambrook, J. (1982). Molecular cloning: A Laboratory Manual. Cold Spring Harbor Laboratory, New York

Saiki, R.K., Bugawau, T.L., Horn, G.T., Mullis, K.B. & Erlich, H.A. (1986). Analysis of enzymatically amplified B-globin and HLA-DQ DNA with allele specific oligonucleotide probes. Nature, 324; 163-166

Smith, D.B. & Johnson, K.S. (1988). Single step purification of polypeptides expressed in *Escherichia coli* as fusions with glutathione S-transferase. Gene 67; 31-40

Weetman, A.P. & McGregor, A.M. (1984). Autoimmune thyroid disease: developments in our understanding. Endocrine Revs. 5; 309-361

DISCUSSION

KOHN: Do you have any information on the upstream regulatory elements of the TPO gene?

BANGA: We have not looked at the promoter regions of the TPO gene. Our main interest has been to focus on the expression of the TPO as a recombinant protein. In this context, we are expressing the 5' region of TPO cDNA which codes for the N-terminal of the protein to examine whether any autoantigenic sites reside in that region of the molecule.

PUJOL-BORRELL: How certain are we that the autoantibodies to the thyroid microsomal antigen (TMA) and the TMA/TPO protein are the pathogenetic elements in destructive thyroid disease. By immunofluorescence studies, it is clear that the TMA is found exclusively on the apical pole of the thyroid follicular cells and thus not easily accessible to the elements of the immune system.

BANGA: The evidence that autoantibodies to TMA maybe involved in the pathogenesis of destructive thyroid disease resides in the fact that these autoantibodies fix complement whilst, in contrast, the anti-thyroglobulin autoantibodies do not fix complement. The cytotoxic potential of the microsomal autoantibodies and, indeed, some monoclonal antibodies have been demonstrated in vitro on primary cultures of human thyroid cells. Furthermore, I believe that the autoantigenic epitopes on the TMA to which these autoantibodies are directed may well be important and relevant to pathogenesis. We recently demonstrated the multiplicity of the autoantibody response to TMA, with at least several distinct autoantigenic sites discernible including the active enzyme site (Doble et al, Immunol. 64; 23 1988). A number of thyroid autoimmune disease patients have high titres of autoantibody to TMA but no destructive thyroid disease. It is possible that differences in TMA epitope specificity of these autoantibodies may explain these differnces and using our PCR generated, recombinant TPO we can begin to answer these questions.

CHARREIRE: Have you injected mice with your recombinant TPO preparations to induce an experimental model of thyroid disease? This would also demonstrate that this protein is pathogenetic.

BANGA: These experiments are currently in progress and I do not have any preliminary data as yet. However, Kotani has recently demonstrated that biochemically purified porcine TPO is pathogenetic and will induce thyroid lesions in certain strains of mice. (Kotani et al, 8th Int. Cong. Endocrinol., Kyoto, Japan, 1988).

GLYCOLIPID ANTIGENS IN TYPE I DIABETES MELLITUS AND ITS LONG TERM COMPLICATIONS

Ramesh C. Nayak, Ph.D.
Joslin Diabetes Center
One Joslin Place
Boston, Massachusetts 02215 U.S.A.

Address for Correspondence:

Immunology Section
Research Division

Joslin Diabetes Center
One Joslin Place

Boston, Massachusetts 02215
U.S.A.

NATO ASI Series, Vol. H 38
The Molecular Biology of Autoimmune Disease
Edited by A. G. Demaine et al.

A. Introduction

The accumulated evidence of the past two decades is overwhelmingly in favour of an autoimmune mechanism of beta cell destruction leading to insulin dependent (Type I diabetes mellitus. This evidence includes the association of insulin dependent diabetes with certain alleles of major histocompatibility complex genes, elevated levels of circulating activated T-cells, recapitulation of the beta cell destructive process in pancreas grafts in the absence of graft rejection, and the presence of anti-islet cell autoantibodies (Bottazzo GF, et al. 1974; MacCuish AC, et al. 1974) in the circulation of the majority of patients. It is this latter feature, anti-islet cell autoantibodies, that can be considered to be a hallmark of autoimmune diabees. While these autoantibodies have been extensively studied and have been shown to be present in individuals up to 10 years prior to development of overt diabetes. The biochemical nature of the target autoantigen(s) with which these autoantibodies react still remains to be elucidated.

Antibodies to a 64 KD protein have been found in diabetic humans, rats, and mice (Baekkeskov S, et al. 1982; Baekkeskov S, et al. 1984; Atkinson MA, and MacLaren NK. 1988); however, autoantibodies to a ganglioside antigen may represent the majority of islet cell autoantibody binding to frozen pancreas sections in immunofluorescence assays (Nayak RC, et al. 1985; Colman PG, et al. 1988; Bright GM, 1989; Nayak RC and Eisenbarth GS, 1989).

B. What Are Gangliosides?

Gangliosides are a series of structurally related glycosphingolipids (glycolipids) that contain acidic sugars known as sialic acids. These molecules are amphipathic, i.e., they contain hydrophobic domains due to the oligosaccheride components and they bear a strong negative charge due to the presence of sialic acid.

Gangliosides are primarily membrane components and are predominantly found in plasma membranes, where they represent a minor component of the total membrane but can represent up to 60% of the lipid content of the outer membrane leaflet. The lipid moiety of glycosphingolipids is known as ceramide and it consists of a long chain fatty acid linked through an amide bond to the nitrogen atom on carbon-2 of the long chain amino-alcohol sphingosine or the related molecule, sphinganene. The oligo-saccheride chain consists of sialic acid, hexoses and N-acetylated hexosamines, and is linked through a glycosidic bond to carbon-1 of the sphingosine portion of ceramide gangliosides were first identified in the brain more than a half century ago and have since been found in all tissues. The amounts and types of gangliosides found vary from tissue to tissue with the central nervous system containing the largest amounts.

A systematic nomelature for gangliosides has been developed (IUPAC-IUB commission on biochemical nomenclature, 1976) by the International Union of Pure and Applied Chemistry (IUPAC), but it is still common to find the nomenclature of Svennerholm (Svennerholm L., 1963) used in the current literature. In this system, gangliosides are given an alpha-numeric designation such that G represents ganglio-series glycolipids, M(mono), D(di), T(tri), etc., represents the number of sialic acid moieties in the molecule, and a number 1, 1 a, 1b, 2, 3, etc., represents the molecules migration position on thin layer chromatography (TLC) plates under the conditions of the initial description (Svennerholm L. 1963). Therefore, GM3 was the third monosialoganglioside migrating up the TLC plate.

C. <u>The Islet Cell Autoantigens in Frozen Pancreatic Sections has the Biochemical Properties of a Sialoglycoconjugate</u>

In order to shed some light on the immunochemical nature of the autoantigen to which islet cell autoantibodies bind to in frozen sections of pancreata, a series of biochemical perturbations were performed on these sections (Nayak RC, et al. 1985). The rationale behind this approach being that any ablation or enhancement of islet cell autoantibody (ICA) binding to these perturbed sections would yield information on the nature of the antigen due to the biochemical specificity of the perturbations (see Table I). It was found that pre-oxidation of pancreatic sections with sodium meta-periodate ablated the ability of ICA to bind to these islets in these sections, however, if these oxidised sections were then reduced with a solution of sodium borohydride, the ability of ICA to bind to the islets was restored. This result suggested that sialic acid was involved in the antibody binding site as (under the conditions used) periodate specifically oxidises the extra-cyclic glyceryl side chain of sialic acids. The involvement of sialic acid was confirmed by neruaminidase digestion of sections which removes sialic acids and irreversibly ablates antibody binding to such treated islets. As sialic acids are found as components of glycoconjugates such as glycoproteins and glycolipids, efforts were made to discern whether the sialic acid moiety of the autoantigen was linked to protein or lipid. It appeared unlikely that the autoantigen was a glycoprotein as it was insensitive to Pronase digestion, in fact, it appeared more likely that the autoantigen was a lipid as it could be extracted with organic solvents (Table I and Nayak RC, et al. 1985; Colman PG et al. 1988). Furthermore, the autoantigen(s) had identical properties to the ganglioside antigen reacting with the monoclonal antibody 3G5 and was distinct from the binding properties of monoclonal antibody to an islet cell protein antigen (Table I and Nayak RC, et al. 1985), which tends to support the conclusion that the autoantigen is a ganglioside.

TABLE I

Effect of Various Biochemical Treatments of Sections on Antibody Binding to Human Islet Cells

	Patient 1,	2,	3	3G5 Monoclonal Anti-Ganglioside
No treatment	+	+	+	+
Periodate	-	-	-	-
Periodate/Borohydride	+	+	+	+
Neuraminidase	-	-	-	-
Pronase	+	+	+	+
Chloroform:methanol	-	-	-	-
Methanol	-	-	-	-

Reproduced from Nayak RC, et al 1985 with permission from the American Diabetes Association.

D. The Islet Cell Autoantigen(s) has the Properties of a Monosialoganglioside

As it was apparent that pretreatment of frozen sections of pancreas with organic solvents ablated ICA bidning to the islets in these sections, organic solvents were used to extract the autoantigen(s) from pancrea tissue. The crude glycolipid extracts produced were shown to be able to block ICA binding to pancreas sections in a dose-dependent manner (Colman PG, et al. 1988; Bright GM, 1989; Nayak RC and Eisenbarth GS, 1989). This extract was also able to block the binding of monoclonal antibody 3G5 to islets in pancreatic sections but could not block the islet cell binding of monoclonal antibodies to islet proteins. This extract has been subfractionated by preparative thin layer chromatography, and a subfraction containing a number of monosialogangliosides was found to block ICA binding to sections. A similar fraction from a human liver extract did not exhibit any blocking activity (Colman PG, et al. 1988). Subfractionation of pancreatic glycolipids into mono-, di-, tri-, and poly-sialogangliosides by ion exchange chromawas also performed.

Only the monosialogangliosides were able to block ICA binding to islets, confirming the results obtained by preparative TLC (Nayak RC, et al. 1988b); Bleich D, et al. 1989). Furthermore, the abundant monosialogangliosides GM3, GM2 and GM1 were not able to block ICA binding to sections of pancreas and neither were the di-sialogangliosides GD1a and GD1b nor the tri-sialoganglioside GT1b, suggesting that the autoantigen may be a novel monosialoganglioside.

E. The Ganglioside Antigen Reacting with the 3G5 Monoclonal Antibody is Distinct from the Islet Cell Ganglioside Autoantigens

In all of the above studies, the islet cell ganglioside antigen's properties were essentially indistinguishable from that of the 3G5 antigen. Furthermore, the 3G5 antigen was found to migrate as a monosialoganglioside between GM1 and GM2 on TLC. On ion exchange chromatography, however, the 3G5 antigen eluted in the disialoganglioside fraction but was still found to migrate between GM1 and GM2 on TLC. This paradoxical behaviour is reminiscent of gangliosides containing O-acetylated sialic acids, and such O-acetyl groups are labile in the presence of base. It was found that monoclonal antibody 3G5 binding to its antigen is indeed ablated by pre-exposure of the antigen to base suggesting that the 3G5 antigen is a disialoganglioside containing an O-acetylated sialic acid moiety and, therefore, id distinct from the islet cell autoantigen (Nayak RC, et al. 1987a).

F. Islet Cell Antigens are Expressed in Tissues Involved in Diabetic Complications

The long-term complications of diabetes include microvascular disease, macrovascular disease (atherosclerosis) and peripheral neuropathy. The microvascular disease of diabetes is manifested as diabetic retinopathy and diabetic nephropathy. One of the earliest events in diabetic retinopathy is the loss of pericytes from the capillary wall, termed pericyte drop out. The functions of the pericyte have not been definitively described but appears to include regulation of vascular perfusion through contractility and pericytes have recently been shown to inhibit endothelial cell proliferation *in vitro* (Orlidge A and D'Amore P, 1987). The development of proliferative retinopathy is characterised by the presence of an abundance of leaky vessels, which (one might speculate) may arise due to pericyte loss and hence control of endothelial cell proliferation. The cause of pericyte drop out is still elusive, however, an association of of retinopathy with HLA B15 and DR4 has been reported (McCann VJ, et al., 1983) and even higher relative risks for retinopathy have been found with HLA-DR3/0, DR4/0, DR4/0 and X/X haplotypes in the absence of myopia (Rand LI, et al, 1985; Baker RS, et al. 1986). While a preponderance of literature on biochemical and rheological mechanisms of microvascular disease exists, the literature on immunological mechanisms in diabetic complications has been sporadic and inconclusive. Consequently, monoclonal antibodies to islet cell antigens were screened for reactivity with bovine pericytes in vitro (Table II and Eisenbarth GS, et al. 1988). Of the antibodies tested, only 3G5 and HISL-8 were found to react with pericytes. Additional studies with the 3G5 antibody showed that this antibody also reacted with pericytes in baboon retinal capillaries in vivo, and that the antigen was a ganglioside migrating between the GM1 and GM2 markers on TLC similar to the islet antigen (Nayak RC, et al. 1988a). The 3G5 antigen has also been found in glomeruli in frozen sections of human, bovine, and rat kidneys, and also on rat glomeruli isolated by sieving. Staining on tissue cultured glomerular cells indicated that neither endothelial no mesangial cells expressed the 3G5 antigen, but this antigen was expressed on glomerular epithelial cells (podocytes) which form the filtration slit pore structure (Nayak RC et al. 1988c). Similarly, the 3G5 antigen has been found in atherosclerotic smooth muscle (Nayak RC, et al. 1989) and in brain (Nayak RC, et al. 1987). The presence of islet type antigens in the tissues affected by diabetic complications tempts one to suppose that this might be a basis for immunological mediation of complications. However, the cross reactions of these monoclonal antibodies cannot support any contention of autoimmunity as they are not autoantibodies.

TABLE II

Indirect Immunofluorescence of Bovine Retinal Pericytes Using A Panel of Monoclonal Anti-Pancreatic Islet Cell Antibodies

Antibodies	Binding*
3G5	+
HISL-1	-
HISL-5	-
HISL-8	+
HISL-9	-
HISL-14	-
HISL-19	-
4F2	-
LC7/2	-
P3X63.Ag8	-

* + = the observation of stained cells; - = that stained cells were not observed. Reproduced with premission from Eisenbarth GS, et al. 1988.

G. Are Autoantibodies Involved in Diabetic Complications?

To date, I an mot aware of the existence of any literature describing autoantibodies to microvascular pericytes, and I have not yet looked for these myself. It has, however, been reported that some diabetics have circulating antibodies to vascular endothelial cells (Cerilli J, et al. 1985), but no attempts to correlate these antibodies with complications has been made. I have recently found that ICA positive sera react with glomeruli in frozen sections of rat kidney (Nayak RC, et al. 1988c), however, it is unclear whether this represents reactivity with endogenous immunoglobulin as it has been shown that Type I diabetics have circulating anti-immunoglobulin (DiMario U, et al. 1988). In atherosclerosis, immunoglobulin deposition in the vascular wall has been observed, and may represent immune complex deposition and insudative processes. In diabetic subjects, it has been suggested that antibodies may bind to a neoantigen in the vascular wall. It is suggested that the neoantigen arises over a long period of time by non-enzymatic glycation of proteins due to the hyperglycaemic environment caused by diabetes (Brownlee M and Cerami A, 1981). Antibodies reacting with intrinsic antigens of the vessel walls have thus far not been described in atherosclerosis, however, the anti-endothelial cell antibodies described above could potentially be involved in atherosclerosis as an endothelial injury is thought to initiate the process (Ross R and Glomset JA, 1976). With regard to diabetic neuropathy, autoantibodies reacting with sympathetic nerves have been recently described (Brown FM, et al. 1989) and the presence of these antibodies has been found to correlate with clinical measures of neuropathy such as aberations in control of postual variation in blood pressure (Rabinowe SL, et al. 1989). The antigens with which these autantibodies react in peripheral nerves are under study and preliminary results suggest that they may be glycolipids (Nayak RC, Rabinowe SL, unpublished results).

H. Final Remarks

In recent years, it has become apparent that the genetic susceptibility to Type I diabetes mellitus may be encoded by genes within and outside of the major histocompatibility complex (Hattori M, et al. 1986; Todd JA, et al, 1988; Hattori M, et al. 1989). The MHC serves to restrict antigen specific immune responses and is a restriction element in the molecular recognition process. The "diabetogenic" MHC haplotype in the context of pathogenesis can be cnsidered to be a permissive element in that it allows recognition of self antigens and permits consequent autoreactivity. While the immunogenetics of Type I diabetes in man and animals share fundamentally similar concepts of permissive roles of MHC antigens in autoreactivity, the pathogenic mechanisms of islet cell destruction in human diabetes remains unclear. Although islet cell autoantibodies have been demonstrated in the circulation of patients having Type I diabetes, and have been shown to precede the clinical onset of diabetes by as much as a decade, there is still no definitive evidence to indicate a role of these autoantibodies in beta-cell destruction. In animal models such as the BB rat and the NOD mouse, it appears that the disease is primarily T-cell mediated (Mordes JP and Rossini AA. 1987). A pathogenic role for T-cells in human diabetes also remains largely unproven, although activated T-lymphocytes have been found to present in elevated amounts in the peripheral blood of Type I diabetic patients. It seems, at least to me, that there is a pressing need to identify and characterise autoantigens of the islets of Langerhans to enable the identification of antigen specific effectors of autoimmunity, be they antibodies or T-lymphocytes.

I. Acknowledgements

This work was supported by fellowship grants to Dr. Nayak from the Juvenile Diabetes Foundation International and is currently funded by a National Institutes of Health Grant (DK39783). This project also received support from the Glycoconjugate, Tissue Culture and Flow Cytometry Cores of the Diabetes and Endocrinology Research Center Grant (DK36836) awarded to the Joslin Diabetes Center.

J. Literature Cited

Atkinson MA, MacLaren N (1988) Autoantibodies in non-obese diabetic mice immunoprecipitate 64,000 M_r islet antigen. Diabetes 37:1587-1590.

Baekkeskov S, Nielse JH, Marner B, Bilde T, Ludvigsson J, Lernmark A. (1982) Autoantibodies in newly diagnosed diabetic children immunoprecipitate human pancreatic islet cell proteins. Nature 298:167-169.

Baekkeskov S, Dyrberg T, Lernmark A (1984) Antibodies to 64 kilodalton islet cell protein precede the onset of spontaneous diabetes in the BB rat. Science 224:1348-1350.

Baker RS, Rand LI, Krolewski AS, Maki T, Warram JH, Aiello LM (1986) Influence of HLA-DR phenotype and myopia on the risk of non-proliferative and proliferative diabetic retinopathy. Am. J. Ophth. 102:693-700.

Bleich D, Dotta F, Eisenbarth GS, Nayak RC (1989) Isolation of an autoantigenic monosialoganglioside from human pancreas. Clin. Res. 37:446A.

Bottazzo GF, Florin-Christensen A, Doniach D (1974) Islet cell antibodies in diabetes mellitus with autoimmune polyendocrine diseases. Lancet ii:1279-1283.
Bright GM (1989) Inhibition of islet cell antibody binding by organic solvent extracts of whole human pancreas. Diabetes 38:(Suppl. 2)187A.
Brown FM, Brink SJ, Freeman R, Rabinowe SL (1989) Anti-sympathetic nervous system autoantibodies: Diminished catecholamines with orthostasis. Diabetes 38:938-941.
Brownlee M, Cerami A (1981) The biochemistry of the complications of diabetes mellitus. Ann. Rev. Biochem. 50:385-432.
Cerilli J, Brasile L, Karmody A (1985) Role of vascular endothelial cell antigen system in the etiology of atherosclerosis. Ann. Surg. 202:329-334.
Colman PG, Nayak RC, Campbell IL, Eisenbarth GS (1988) Binding of cytoplasmic islet cell antibodies is blocked by human pancreatic glycolipid extracts. Diabetes 37:645-652.
DiMario U, Dotta F, Crisa L, Anatasi E, Andreani D, Dib SA, Eisenbarth GS (1988) Circulating anti-immunoglobulin antibodies in recent onset Type I diabetic patients. Diabetes 37:462-466.
Eisenbarth GS, Nayak RC, Rabinowe SL (1988) Type I diabetes as a chronic autoimmune disease. J. Diabetic Complications 2:54-58.
Hattori M, Buse JB, Jackson RA, Glincher L, Dorf ME, Minami M, Makino S, Moriwaki K, Kuzuya H, Imura H, Strauss WM, Seidman JG, Eisenbarth GS (1986) The NOD mouse: Recessive diabetogenic gene in the major histocomplex. Science 231:733-735.
Hattori M, Fukuda M, Horio F, Kato H, Makino S (1989) A single non MHC linked recessive gene determines the development of insulitis in NOD mice. Diabetes 38(Suppl. 2):90A.
IUPAC-IUB Commison on Biochemical Nomenclature (CBN) (1976). Nomenclature of lipids recommendations. Eur. J. Biochem. 79:11-21.
MacCuish AC, Barnes EW, Irvine WJ, Duncan LJP (1974) Antibodies to pancreatic islet cells in insulin dependent diabetes with co-existant autoimmune disease. Lancet ii:1529-1531.
McCann VS, McCluskey J, Kay PH, Zilko PJ, Christiansen FT, Dawkins RL (1983) HLA and complement gentic markers in diabetic retinopathy (letter). Diabetologia 24:221.
Mordes JP, Rossini AA (1987) Keys to understanding autoimmune diabetes mellitus. IN: Doniach D, Bottazzo GF. Endocrine and other organ-oriented autoimmune disorders. Bailliere's Clinical Immunology and Allergy. Vol. 1 pp. 29-52.
Nayak RC, Eisenbarth GS (1989) The humoral anti-islet immune response: Immunochemical studies of glycoconjugate antigens. IN: Ginsberg-Fellner F, McEvoy R (eds). Autoimmunity in the pathogenesis of diabetes. Springer, New York, in press.
Nayak RC, Omar MAK, Rabizadeh A, Srikanta S, Eisenbarth GS (1985) "Cytoplasmic" islet cell antibodies: Evidence that the target antigen is a sialoglycoconjugate. Diabetes 34:617-619.
Nayak RC, Colman PG, Eisenbarth GS (1987) How are monoclonal antibodies related to autoimmune serology? IN: Doniach D, Bottazzo GF (eds). Endocrine and other organ-oriented autoimmune disorders. Baillere's Clinical Immunology and Allergy. Vol. 1 pp. 81-99.
Nayak RC, Berman AB, George KL, Eisenbarth GS, King GL (1988) A monoclonal antibody (3G5)-defined ganglioside antigen is expressed on the cell surface of microvascular pericytes. J. Exp. Med. 167:1003-1015.

Nayak RC, Colman PG, Eisenbarth GS (1988b) Characterization of islet cell gangliosides reacting with islet cell autoantibodies and anti-islet cell monoclonal antibody 3G5. Diabetes Res. Clin. Practic. 5(Suppl 1):554.

Nayak RC, Attawia MA, Eisenbarth GS, King GL (1988c) Are anti-glomerular antibodies associated with diabetic nephropathy? XIIIth International Workshop on the Immunology of Diabetes. Melbourne Australia, November 27-29, 1988. J. Autoimmunity, in press.

Nayak RC, Colman PG, Spitalnik S, King GL, Eisenbarth GS (1988d) Identification and characterisation of ganglioside antigens defined by anti-islet cell monoclonal antibody 3G5. Diabetes 37(Suppl. 5):29A.

Nayak RC, Attawia MA, King GL (1989) Monoclonal antibody 3G5 is a marker of proliferating smooth muscle cells in atherosclerosis. International Research Symposium on Diabetes, Lipoproteins and Atherosclerosis, Hilton Head, South Carolina, March 6-8, 1989.

Orlidge A, D'Amore P (1987) Inhibition of capillary endothelial cell growth by pericytes and smooth muscle cells. J. Cell. Biol. 105:1455-1462.

Rabinowe SL, Brown FM, Watts M, Kardofske MM, Vinik AI (1989) Anti-sympathetic ganglia antibodies and postural blood pressure in IDDM subjects of varying duration and patients at high risk of developing IDDM. Diabetes Care 12:1-6.

Rand LI, Krolewski AS, Aiello LM, Warram JH, Baker RS, Maki T (1985) Multiple factors in the prediction of risk of proliferative diabetic retinopathy. N. Engl. J. Med. 313:1433-1438.

Ross R, Glomset JA (1976) The pathogenesis of atherosclerosis. N. Engl. J. Med. 295:420-425.

Svennerholm L (1963) Chromatographic separation of human brain gangliosides. J. Neurochem. 10:613.

Todd JA, Acha-Orbea H, Bell JI, Chao N, Fronek Z, Jacob CO, McDermott M, Sinha AA, Timmerman L, Steinman L, McDevitt HO (1988) A molecular basis for MHC class II-associated autoimmunity. Science 240:1003-1008.

DISCUSSION

JANEWAY: You have shown us the tissues that stain positive with 3G5; how many tissues are negative for 3G5?

NAYAK: Skeletal and cardiac muscle are totally negative for 3G5. However, some cells in the liver are positive whilst other liver cells are negative. Subpopulations of lymphocytes are also negative for 3G5.

JANEWAY: Is the antigen recognized by the islet cell autoantibodies like the antigen recognized by 3G5?

NAYAK: They are both distinct gangliosides. The islet cell autoantibody binding antigen is a monoganglioside whilst 3G5 binds to a disialo ganglioside.

JANEWAY: Does binding of 3G5 block the binding of islet cell autoantibodies?

NAYAK: These are difficult experiments to interpret due to differences in the affinity of the monoclonal 3G5 antibody and the autoantibodies.

PAPADOPOLOUS: Would it be possible to replace the islet cell immunofluorescence assay with a simple ELISA using your purified pancreatic glycolipid extract?

NAYAK: We have tried this using glycolipid extracts to coat microtitre wells. However, the backgrounds obtained with normal human sera are very high, probably due to neutral glycolipid binding antibodies normally found in human sera.

ON THE MAIN IMMUNOGENIC REGION OF THE ACETYLCHOLINE RECEPTOR. STRUCTURE AND ROLE IN MYASTHENIA GRAVIS

S.J. Tzartos, D. Sophianos, A. Kordossi, I. Papadouli,
I. Hadjidakis*, C. Sakarellos*, M.T. Cung+ and M. Marraud+.

Hellenic Pasteur Institute, Athens, Greece;
*University of Ioannina, Ioannina, Greece; and
+CNRS-UA-494, ENSIC-INPL, Nancy, France.

INTRODUCTION

The nicotinic acetylcholine receptor (AChR) from mammalian muscle and fish electric organ consists of four homologous subunits with the stoichiometry $\alpha_2\beta\gamma\delta$. Each subunit transverses the membrane at least four times (Changeux and Revan, 1987; Numa et al., 1983). The AChR molecule is the major autoantigen in the human autoimmune disease, myasthenia gravis (MG) (Willcox and Vincent, 1988). Anti-AChR antibodies result in loss of AChRs and also directly block the function of the remaining AChR molecules, thereby causing a defect in neuromuscular transmission.

Two-thirds of the anti-AChR antibodies in MG patients and rats immunized with intact AChR are directed against an extracellular area of the α-subunit, named the main immunogenic region (MIR) (Tzartos and Lindstrom, 1980; Tzartos et al., 1982). In a series of recent studies, the binding sites of some anti-MIR mAbs were gradually localized (Ratnam et al., 1986a; Barkas et al., 1987; 1988) and finally were found between residues 67-76 of the α-subunit (Tzartos et al., 1988).

Anti-MIR mAbs injected in rats cause experimental autoimmune MG (Tzartos and Lindstrom, 1980; Tzartos et al., 1987) and when added to mouse muscle cell cultures cause antigenic modulation, i.e. AChR loss due to antibody-mediated AChR crosslinking (Tzartos et al., 1985). More

NATO ASI Series, Vol. H 38
The Molecular Biology of Autoimmune Disease
Edited by A. G. Demaine et al.

importantly, the anti-MIR antibody fraction of human MG, when tested on mouse muscle cells, was found to be the principle etiologic agent in the capacity of the sera to cause AChR loss (Tzartos et al., 1985). Therefore the MIR seems to play a critical role in the pathogenesis of MG. Furthermore, anti-MIR mAbs have been used extensively in the elucidation of various aspects of AChR research (Merlie et al. 1986, Lindstrom et al. 1988; Zhang et al. 1988). Clearly, a better understanding of this region is valuable for the study of the AChR and the disease.

A brief description of some of our recent studies on both the pathogenic role and the fine structural characterization of the MIR will be given below.

RESULTS AND DISCUSSION

A. FUNCTION OF THE ANTI-MIR ANTIBODIES

As was mentioned above, the anti-MIR antibodies of MG sera were found to be the major contributors in causing AChR loss in mouse cell cultures (Tzartos et al., 1985). However, since only 5-10% of the human anti-AChR antibodies bind to the mouse AChR, the significance of the above results was limited. In order to study the whole anti-AChR repertoire of the human sera we subsequently used a human cell line, the TE671. This cell line was initially thought to be a medulloblastoma one (McAllister et al. 1977) but has recently been shown to be rather a rhabdomyosarcoma one (Stratton et al. 1989). TE671 produce an AChR apparently identical with that of human muscle (Luther et al. 1989).

We first established that the TE671 cell culture system is appropriate for studies on AChR antigenic modulation. This was inferred

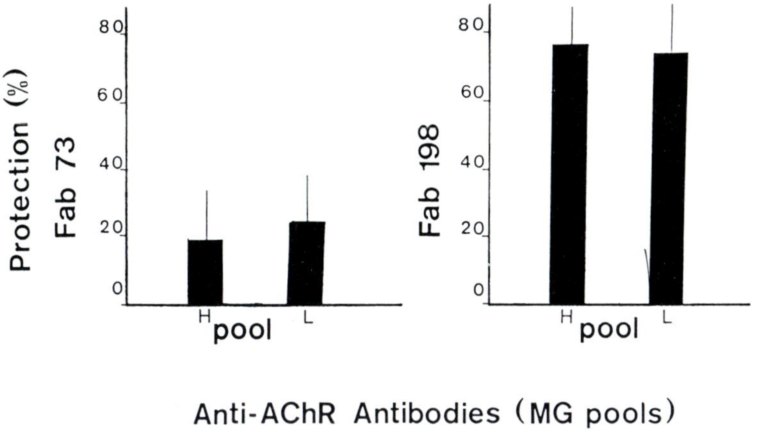

Figure 1. Protection of TE671 cell-bound AChR against antigenic modulation caused by two pools of MG sera. Protection was achieved by preincubation of the cells with excess of Fab.mAbs directed to the MIR (mAb 198) or to a region of the AChR β-subunit (mAb 73). H and L, pools of subsequently added high and low titer MG sera, respectively.

from the observation that the normal half life and the antigenic modulation of the TE671 AChR (Sophianos and Tzartos, 1989) was similar to that of the AChR on normal human muscle cell cultures (Tzartos et al., 1986). Consequently, the TE671 cells were subsequently used to study the functional role of distinct anti-AChR specificities and especially of the MIR. Any of 10 MG sera studied, when added to these cell cultures, dramatically accelerated AChR degradation. Similar activity was exhibited by four anti-MIR mAbs or a mAb to the β-subunit (mAb 73). However, as expected, univalent Fab fragments of the same mAbs (Fab.mAbs) bound but did not accelerate AChR degradation, apparently because they could not crosslink the AChR molecules. High excess of these Fab.mAbs were used in order to shield the corresponding AChR regions against binding of subsequently added antibodies. The Fabs totally inhibited the activity of the subsequently added homologous intact mAbs (Sophianos and Tzartos, 1989).

Protection of the AChR, by the above Fab.mAbs, against the activity of the human MG sera was finally tested. Two pools of a total of 38 human MG sera were used. Fig. 1 shows that the anti-MIR mAb 198 (like two other not shown anti-MIR mAbs) protected by about 80% the AChR against MG serum mediated antigenic modulation. On the contrary, Fabs of the anti-β mAb 73 had little only protecting effect. These results show that the anti-MIR antibody fraction from MG sera is mainly responsible for the antigenic modulation capacity of these sera. Furthermore, the ability of anti-MIR Fab.mAbs to protect the AChR against antigenic modulation in this system might be of therapeutic interest.

B. LOCALIZATION OF THE MIR ON THE INTACT AChR.

Although the epitopes for some anti-MIR mAbs were mapped to the α67-76 decapeptide, two major points remained unclear: a. Since the MIR epitope(s) are quite conformation-dependent, most anti-MIR mAbs (30 of the 41) could not be mapped by using synthetic peptides. Therefore it cannot be excluded that the majority of these mAbs bind to AChR segments different from the α67-76. b. Even those anti-MIR mAbs which bind to the α67-76, do so, with an affinity lower by several orders of magnitude than to the intact AChR (Tzartos et al., 1988; 1989). Thus, it could be argued that their primary epitopes are located in various irrelevant discontinuous sites. Therefore, studies on the intact AChR were also needed to clarify the above uncertainties. We show below that all anti-MIR mAbs compete with each other for binding on the intact AChR, and we identify antigenic regions neighboring to the MIR.

Twenty-one anti-AChR mAbs, were used in the competition experiments for binding to the Torpedo AChR. These included all available anti-MIR mAbs which bind well to the Torpedo AChR. Fig. 2A shows that all the 16

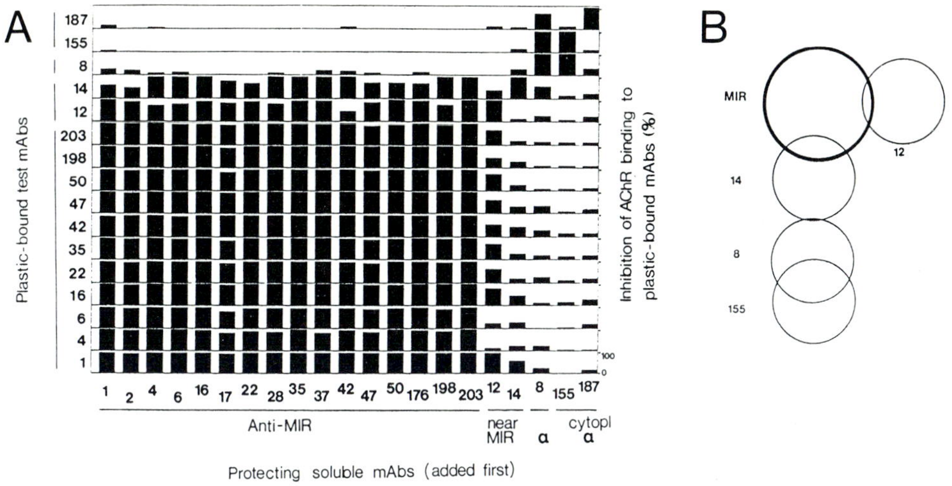

Fig. 2. A. Mapping the binding sites of anti-AChR mAbs by competition experiments between mAb pairs for binding to intact 125-I-α-bungarotoxin labelled *Torpedo* AChR. 125-I-toxin-AChR was preincubated with a soluble protecting mAb and the complex was added to microwells coated with a test mAb. The specifically bound radioactivity on the microwells was measured and the percentage inhibition of binding due to the protecting soluble mAb was estimated. Numbers denote mAb codes. B. Model for the possible arrangement of the binding sites of anti-AChR mAbs, relative to the MIR, on the intact AChR. Circles represent the traces of the mAbs bound on the AChR. Overlapping circles represent effective competition between the corresponding mAbs whereas non-overlapping cycles denote that the corresponding mAbs do not compete against each other. Numbers denote mAb codes (from Kordossi and Tzartos, 1989).

anti-MIR mAbs effectively competed against each other for binding to the same region of the intact *Torpedo* AChR, the MIR. Complete competition was also obtained among the anti-human MIR mAbs for binding to the human AChR (not shown, Kordossi and Tzartos, 1989).

Fig. 2B shows a model for the possible arrangement of the binding sites of some mAbs relative to the MIR as deduced from the results of Fig. 2A. The epitope for mAb 8 overlaps with the epitopes for mAbs known to bind to the cytoplasmic side (like mAb 155) (Ratnam et al., 1986b; Tzartos et al., 1988). It was earlier proposed that this epitope is located within the lipid binding area of the AChR (Gullick et al. 1981).

Since the MIR seems to be located on the side of the AChR molecule (Kubaleck et al. 1987) we suggest that the overlapping mAb 14 also binds on the side but nearer the intramembranous portion of the AChR, thus partially competing with mAb 8. In turn, the epitope for the cytoplasmic mAb 155 should be located very near the membrane.

It has been shown earlier that the mAb-competition technique is capable of distinguishing between epitopes a few amino acids apart (Kordossi and Tzartos, 1987). Therefore, the complete competition observed among the anti-MIR mAbs for binding to the AChR, in any of the combinations tested, strongly suggests that the MIR is a single and small area with rather distinct limits. This information lends support to the peptide mapping experiments (Barkas et al., 1988; Tzartos et al., 1988; 1989) which localized the MIR between α67-76.

C. ANTIGENIC ROLE OF SINGLE RESIDUES WITHIN THE MIR DECAPEPTIDE α67-76

In order to evaluate the contribution of each residue to the antigenicity of the MIR, we synthesized peptides corresponding to Torpedo (WNPADYGGIK) and human (WNPDDYGGVK) α67-76 together with 13 peptide analogs. Nine analogs had one residue of the Torpedo decapeptide replaced by L-Alanine, three had a structure intermediate between the Torpedo and human α67-76, and one had D-Alanine in position 73. Using one-and two-dimensional NMR spectroscopy, the conformation of these peptides in DMSO was recently studied. Both the presence of strong and multiple short-and long-range NOEs in the Torpedo peptide and the temperature dependence measurements argue in favor of a rigid folded conformation. This is stabilized by three interactions involving the Asp^{71}, Gly^{74} and Lys^{76} amide protons (Cung et al. 1989).

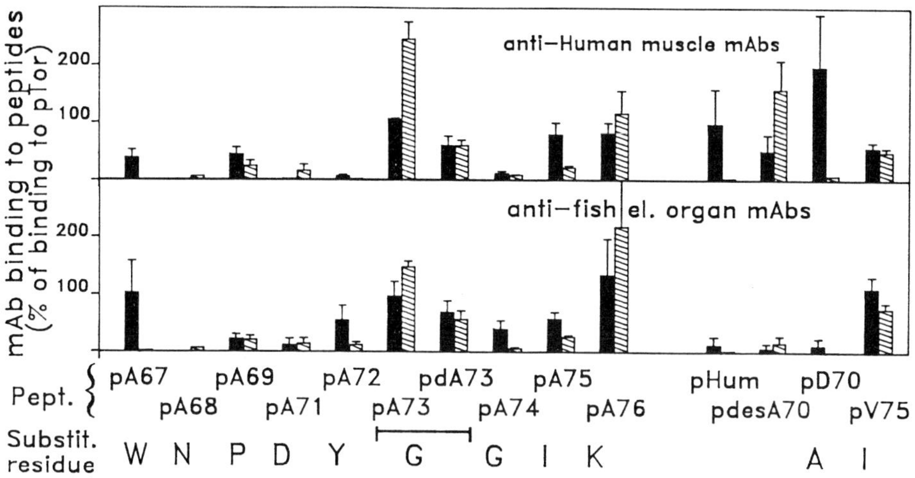

Fig. 3. Summary of anti-MIR mAb binding to synthetic peptide analogs of the Torpedo AChR α67-76 peptide. Each bar represents the average binding of four anti-fish (lower part) or two anti-human (higher part) mAbs to a peptide analog as a percentage of binding to the Torpedo α67-76, under conditions of either direct peptide plating (black bars) or plating via poly-A-K/ glutaraldehyde (hatched bars). SD bars show the variations between the different mAbs. pA67, pA68 etc. denote alanine substitutions of the Torpedo α67-76 residues W67, N68 etc. pdA73: D-alanine, instead of L, was used. pHum: human α67-76. pdesA70: residue 70 was eliminated. pD70 and pV75: intermediate analogs between Torpedo and human decamers which differ at residues 70 and 75.

A direct solid phase RIA was used for testing binding of anti-MIR mAbs to the above peptides. Peptides were attached to 96 well plates, a. by using poly-Ala-Lys and the test peptide was bound covalently to the poly-Ala-Lys via glutaraldehyde; or b. the peptides were adsorbed directly to the plate. Binding of the subsequently added mAb was detected by the use of ^{125}I-protein A (Papadouli et al. 1989).

Fig. 3 shows the average binding patterns of two anti-human muscle and four anti-fish electric organ AChR anti-MIR mAbs using all 15 peptides. Use of the poly-Ala-Lys/glutaraldehyde technique, although in most cases produced similar with the direct peptide plating results, dramatically inhibited mAb binding to some peptides and enhanced binding to a few others.

Monoclonal antibody binding specificity was very high. Single conservative substitutions (peptides pA69, pA74) or simple stereochemical changes within a single amino acid (pdA73 versus pA73) were sufficient for dramatic alterations in the binding capacity of the mAbs. At least two "key positions", i.e. residues essential for binding by any tested anti-MIR mAb, were identified. These were Asn68 and Asp71. Other residues are important only for binding by some mAbs. Overall, antibody binding was mainly restricted to α68-74, the most critical part being α68-71. Residue α70, rather than α75, plays the major role in the difference between human and fish AChR MIR. Fish electric organ and human MIR seem to form two distinct groups of strongly overlapping epitopes. Finally, some peptide analogs (pA73 and pA76) enhanced mAb binding, suggesting that the construction of a very antigenic MIR is feasible.

CONCLUSIONS

The presented experiments show that:

a. The anti-MIR antibodies of human patients play a major role in causing human AChR loss.

b. The MIR, at least as far as it concerns all available anti-MIR mAbs, is a small region with defined limits, apparently located within or including residues α67-76.

c. Within α67-76, some residues are indispensable for antibody binding (especially Asn68 and Asp71) while others play little if any role. Residue α70 plays the critical role in the differences observed between human and fish AChR MIR.

ACKNOWLEDGMENTS

We thank Mr. S. Potamianos, Miss A. Kokla and Mr. A. Efthimiadis for excellent technical assistance. We also thank Dr. the. Barkas and Dr. R. Matsas for valuable discussions. Supported by grants from the Greek General Secretariat of Research and Technology, the Muscular Dystrophy Association of America and the Association des Myopathes de France.

REFERENCES

Barkas T, Mauron A, Roth B, Alliod C, Tzartos SJ, Ballivet M (1987) Mapping the main immunogenic region and toxin binding site of the nicotinic acetylcholine receptor. Science 235:77-80

Barkas T, Gabriel J-M, Mauron A, Hughes GJ, Roth B, Alliod C, Tzartos SJ, Ballivet M (1988) Fine localisation of the main immunogenic region of the nicotinic acetylcholine receptor to residues 61-76 of the α-subunit. J Biol Chem 263:5916-5920

Changeux JP, Revah F (1987) The acetylcholine receptor molecule: allosteric sites and the ion channel. TINS 10:245-250

Cung M T, Marraud M, Hadjidakis I, Bairaktari H Sakarellos C, Kokla A, Tzartos S (1989) 2D-1H NMR study of a synthetic peptide containing the main immunogenic region of the Torpedo acetylcholine receptor. Biopolymers 28,465-478

Gullick WJ, Tzartos SJ, Lindstrom J (1981) Monoclonal antibodies as probes of acetylcholine receptor structure. I. Peptide mapping. Biochemistry 20:2173-2180

Kordossi A, Tzartos SJ (1987) Conformation of cytoplasmic segments of acetylcholine receptor α and β subunits probed by monoclonal antibodies. Sensitivity of the antibody competition approach. EMBO J 6:1605-1610

Kordossi A A, Tzartos SJ (1989) Monoclonal antibodies against the main immunogenic region of the acetylcholine receptor. Mapping on the intact molecule. J Neuroimmunol In press

Kubalek E, Ralston S, Lindstrom J and Unwin N (1987) Location of subunits within the acetylcholine receptor by electron image analysis of tubular crystals from Torpedo marmorata. J Cell Biol 105:9-18

Lindstrom J, Schoepfer R, Whiting P (1987) Molecular studies of the neuronal nicotinic AchR family. Molecular Neurobiology 1:281-337

Luther M A, Schoepfer R, Whiting P, Casey B, Blatt, Montal M S, Montal M, Lindstrom J (1989) A muscle acetylcholine receptor is expressed in the human cerebellar meduloblastoma cell line TE671. J Neurosci In press

McAllister R M, Isaacs H, Rongey R, Peer M, Ann W, Soukup S W, Gardner M B (1977) Establishment of a human meduloblastoma cell line. Int J Cancer 20:206-212

Merlie JP, Smith MM (1986) Synthesis and assembly of acetylcholine receptor, a multisubunit membrane glycoprotein. J Membr Biol 91:1-10

Numa S et al. (1983) Molecular structure of the acetylcholine receptor. Cold Spring Harb Symp Quant Biol 48:57-69

Papadouli I, Potamianos S, Hadjidakis I, Bairaktari H, Tsikaris V, Sakarellos C, Cung MT, Marraud M, Tzartos ST (1989) Antigenic role of single residues within the main immunogenic region of the nicotinic acetylcholine receptor. Submitted

Ratnam M, Le Nguyen D, Rivier J, Sargent P, Lindstrom J (1986a) Transmembrane topography of the nicotinic acetylcholine receptor: immunochemical tests contradict theoretical predictions based on hydrophobicity profile. Biochemistry 25:2633-2643

Ratnam M, Sargent P, Sarin V, Fox JL, Le Nguyen D, Rivier J, Criado M, Lindstrom J (1986b) Location of antigenic determinants on primary sequences of the subunits of the nicotinic acetylcholine receptor by peptide mapping. Biochemistry 25:2621-2632

Sophianos D, Tzartos SJ (1989) Fab fragments of monoclonal antibodies protect the human acetylcholine receptor against antigenic modulation caused by myasthenic sera. Submitted

Stratton MR et al. (1989) Characterization of the human cell line TE671. Carcinogenesis In press

Tzartos SJ, Lindstrom JL (1980) MAbs to probe acetylcholine receptor structure: Localization of the main immunogenic region and detection of similarities between subunits. Proc Natl Acad Sci USA 77:755-759

Tzartos SJ, Seybold M, Lindstrom J (1982) Specificities of antibodies to acetylcholine receptors in sera from myasthenia gravis patients measured by monoclonal antibodies. Proc Natl Acad Sci USA 79:188-192

Tzartos SJ, Sophianos D, Efthimiadis A (1985) Role of the main immunogenic region of acetylcholine receptor in myasthenia gravis. An Fab monoclonal antibodies protects against antigenic modulation by human sera. J Immunol 134:2343-2349

Tzartos SJ, Sophianos D, Zimmermann K, Starzinski-Powitz A (1986) Antigenic modulation of human muscle acetylcholine receptor by myasthenic sera. Serum titer determines receptor internalization. J Immunol 136:3231-3237

Tzartos SJ, Hochschwender S, Vasquez P, Lindstrom J (1987) Passive transfer of experimental autoimmune myasthenia gravis by monoclonal antibodies to the main immunogenic region of the acetylcholine receptor. J Neuroimmunol 15:185-194

Tzartos SJ, Kokla A, Walgrave S, Conti-Tronconi B (1988) Localization of the main immunogenic region of human muscle acetylcholine receptor to residues 67-76 of the α-subunit. Proc Natl Acad Sci USA 85:2800-2903

Tzartos SJ, Loutrari H, Tang F, Kokla A, Walgrave S, Milius R P, Conti-Tronconi B (1989) The main immunogenic region of Torpedo electroplax and human muscle acetylcholine receptor. Localization and micro-heterogeneity reveiled by the use of synthetic peptides. J Neurochem In press

Willcox N, Vincent A (1988) Myasthenia gravis as an example of organ-specific autoimmune disease. In "B lymphocytes in human disease" A.G. Bird and J. Calvert, eds. Blackwells, Oxford, pp469-506.

Zhang Y, Tzartos SJ, Wekerle H (1988) B-T lymphocyte interactions in experimental autoimmune myasthenia gravis: antigen presentation by rat/mouse hybridoma lines secreting mAbs against the nicotinic acetylcholine receptor. Eur J Immunol 18:211-218

DISCUSSION

NEWSOM-DAVIS: Would you like to speculate on what is special about the MIR that might be provoking antibodies preferentially in the disease? Do you think it lies in the structure of the segments you have been talking about, the fact that the alpha subunit is duplicated or do you think it lies, for example, in the immunoglobulin genes of the respondents?

TZARTOS: I believe it is the structure. The special features of the structure of this region are the two alpha subunits. The paper by Nigel Unwin (Kubalet et al, 1987 J. Cell Biol. 105, 9) reported the arrangement of the subunits of the receptor and showed the MIR on the periphery of the receptor. I think the close arrangement of the two alpha subunits allows it to be easily crosslinked by the antibody to the receptor.

SCHWEIBER: I want to refer to the experimental autoimmune myasthenia gravis (EAMG) model using Torpedo acetylcholine receptor. We have good evidence that the Torpedo receptor is not the appropriate model to induce EAMG. We have therefore tried very hard to purify mammalian acetylcholine receptor to induce experimental disease. We find that the immunogenic region in the experimental model is different with Torpedo receptor from that of mammalian acetylcholine receptor.

LOHSE: What is the relationship between the main immunogenic region and functional site of the alpha chain of the acetylcholine receptor? Perhaps this will provide a clue to this region being the immunogenic region. We know from other autoantibodies that they are often directed against the functional site of a protein. What is the functional site of the alpha chain of the acetylcholine receptor and what is its relation to the main immunogenetic region?

TZARTOS: The main immunogenic region, as far as we know, does not have an effect on the function of the receptor. It is away from the toxin binding site since we know that the toxin binding site is near the acetylcholine binding site between residues 170 and 190. Furthermore, antibodies to the main immunogenic region do not block the channel.

ACETYLCHOLINE RECEPTOR-EXPRESSING FIBROBLASTS

Toni Claudio
Department of Cellular & Molecular Physiology
Yale University School of Medicine
333 Cedar Street
New Haven CT 06510
USA

INTRODUCTION

Two key and as yet unresolved questions concerning the autoimmune disease myasthenia gravis (MG) are: 1) what initiates the autoimmune response, and 2) what sustains it. It is known that autoantibodies to the acetylcholine receptor (AChR) can be detected in MG patient sera, that the disease symptoms can be passively transferred from humans to mice with the IgG fraction from MG patient sera (Drachman et al. 1976), that the AChR can induce experimental autoimmune myasthenia gravis (EAMG) in test animals (reviewed in Lindstrom 1985; Newsom-Davis 1986; Engel 1987), and that the AChR is the only protein at endplates which is capable of inducing EAMG (Claudio & Raftery 1980). The importance of the AChR in this disease cannot be disputed, but what role does it play in the initiation and/or maintenance of the disease. Are there specific epitopes on the AChR that are required for induction? It has been suggested that alterations of AChRs on myoid cells in the thymus might serve to break tolerance and initiate the autoimmune response directed against AChRs. Penicillamine has been shown to react with AChRs and to enhance EAMG (Bever et al. 1984). If alterations in the AChR can cause MG, do they occur by an exogenous or an endogenous mechanism? An endogenous mechanism acting directly on AChRs could have several sites of action. Various posttranslational modifications of the AChR are known to occur naturally, including disulfide-bond formation, glycosylation, phosphorylation, and fatty acylation. If such modifications are not executed faithfully, the expression or the chemical or structural nature of the molecule could be slightly or severely affected. The expression of a chemically or structurally altered AChR could easily lead to the expression of new or altered immunogenic determinants.

NATO ASI Series, Vol. H 38
The Molecular Biology of Autoimmune Disease
Edited by A. G. Demaine et al.

Our interest has been in expressing the AChR in an artificial system which readily lends itself to various experimental manipulations. Some of these manipulations include antigenic modulation, nerve-induced AChR clustering, and the effects of posttranslational modifications on subunit assembly, AChR structure, and function. For these types of studies, we require an expression system in which large numbers of identical cells express receptors on their surface for long periods of time. These requirements are not readily attained with transient systems, and thus we have chosen to establish a stable expression system in cultured cell lines.

The muscle-like AChR is a heterologous multisubunit complex composed of four different subunits in the stoichiometry $\alpha_2\beta\gamma\delta$. In addition to the complex subunit composition, each subunit undergoes several posttranslational modifications and spans the membrane a multiple number of times. In order to reconstitute all of the functional properties of this AChR, the four subunits must be present and at least some of the posttranslational modifications must be executed correctly. Thus, whatever system one uses to express AChRs, the ability to introduce all four subunits into the same cell and to express them in a cell type that is capable of performing the necessary modifications is of considerable importance. Although muscle-like and neuronal AChR subunit genes and cDNAS have been isolated from a number of species (reviewed in Claudio 1989), we have chosen to work with the AChR isolated from *Torpedo californica* electric organ (Claudio 1987). *Torpedo* AChR is the most extensively studied and best characterized AChR and the one for which the most structural information is available (reviewed in Karlin 1980; Conti-Tronconi & Raftery 1982; Popot & Changeux 1984). In addition, several monoclonal antibody libraries are available which are directed against *Torpedo* AChR providing us with subunit-specific and conformation-specific antibodies.

ESTABLISHING THE EXPRESSION SYSTEM

We have established several cell lines which express functional cell surface *Torpedo* AChRs. These have been established by two different gene transfer methods: calcium phosphate-DNA-mediated cotransfection and viral infection using packaged retroviral recombinants. Using a calcium phosphate precipitation method (Graham & van der Eb 1973; Wigler et al. 1977) we recently showed that the cotransfection efficiency of introducing four different cDNAs plus a selectable marker gene into the same cell was 80% (Claudio, 1987). In that study, we described the introduction of the four *Torpedo* subunit cDNAs plus the adenine phosphoribosyltransferase gene (aprt) into mouse fibroblast L cells deficient in thymidine kinase (tk) and aprt (Ltk^-aprt^-). We found (by genome blotting) that nine of eleven clonal isolates had incorporated the four cDNAs plus aprt and that the majority of the material had been integrated correctly into the genome. In addition, of the nine positive cell lines, half had picked up approximately equal copy numbers (10 to 20) of each of the four cDNAs. In that particular study, the cDNAs were not engineered into vectors that would express efficiently in mammalian cells and thus no information was available on the efficiency of protein expression.

In a subsequent study (Claudio et al. 1987), the four AChR subunit cDNAs engineered into SV40 expression vectors (pSV2, Subramani et al. 1981) and the tk gene were cotransfected into Ltk^-aprt^- cells. Analysis of two clonal isolates revealed that one line (all-11) had integrated copies of all four subunit cDNAs (4:2:2:8 copies per cell for α, β, γ, δ, respectively) and the other line (all-6) had integrated three of the four subunit cDNAs (0:1:8:4 for α, β, γ, δ, respectively). The all-11 cell line was analyzed pharmacologically, biochemically, and electrophysiologically at the single channel level and it was shown to express fully functional cell surface *Torpedo* AChRs (Claudio et al. 1987).

In the previous studies, selectable marker genes were used that complimented cellular mutations (tk^- or $aprt^-$). We have also established AChR-expressing fibroblast cell lines after cotransfection using a dominant selectable marker gene (Claudio et al. 1989b). The marker gene used was the neomycin resistance gene (neo^r) which encodes G418 (a neomycin analog) resistance in mammalian cells (Davies & Jimenez 1980) and the recipient cell line was mouse fibroblast NIH3T3. As in the other studies, the DNAs were introduced into cells using a calcium phosphate precipitation procedure, the cells were put into selective medium, individual colonies were isolated using cloning cylinders and grown into stable cell lines. Of twenty-three clonal isolates, seventeen were analyzed at the protein level for expression of subunits. Four of the cell lines expressed all four subunits, four cell lines expressed three subunits, five lines expressed two subunits, two lines expressed one subunit, and two lines expressed no subunits. Approximately one-fourth of the transfected cells that had incorporated the selectable marker gene, expressed all four subunits. We have not yet performed genome blots on these lines and thus do not know whether our cotransfection efficiency was lower than in previous studies, or whether it remained high (~80%) but the efficiency of protein expression of all four subunits was low (25%).

One other method of introducing DNA into host cell genomes was to use helper-free recombinant retroviruses. AChR subunit cDNAs were engineered into direct orientation murine leukemia virus vectors (kindly provided by RC Mulligan or J Morgenstern), DNA was transfected into the retrovirus NIH3T3 packaging cell line φ2 (Mann et al. 1983), helper-free infectious viral particles containing the recombinant were harvested, and used to infect various cell lines. Cell lines we have successfully infected include mouse fibroblast L and NIH3T3 cells and three muscle cell lines: rat L6 (Yaffe 1968), mouse C2 (Yaffe & Saxel 1977; Blau et al. 1983), and mouse BC_3H-1 (Schubert et al. 1974). Two types of AChR-expressing cell lines were established using retroviruses: all-*Torpedo* AChR-expressing fibroblast cell lines and *Torpedo*-endogenous rat hybrid AChR-expressing L6 cell lines. When the all-6 cell line (Ltk^-aprt^- cells containing integrated copies of pSV2-β, -γ, -δ cDNAs and the tk gene) was infected with packaged retroviral α-recombinants, fully functional receptors were expressed on the surface of the cells (Claudio et al 1989c). When rat L6 muscle cells were infected with the recombinant, three types of AChRs were expressed on the surface: AChRs containing two rat α subunits (normal endogenous AChRs), hybrid AChRs containing two *Torpedo* α subunits, and hybrid AChRs containing one rat and one *Torpedo* α subunit (Paulson & Claudio 1988).

PROPERTIES OF ACHRS EXPRESSED IN FIBROBLASTS

The maximum level of surface expression in all-11 cells that we have obtained thus far is ~40,000 AChR molecules per cell, giving a site density of ~50/μm^2. This quantity is sufficient for biochemical and pharmacological analyses, as well as electrophysiological analyses using single channel recording techniques (Claudio et al. 1987). We have shown that only a single population of AChRs is expressed on the surface of these cells in terms of structural composition and function. Surface receptors are composed of all four subunits, they are assembled into proper $\alpha_2\beta\gamma\delta$ pentamers (Hartman et al 1989), and they migrate on sucrse gradients with a sedimentation coefficient of 9*S* (Claudio et al 1987). Amplitude and kinetic analyses of single channel recordings made from AChR-fibroblasts also support the observation that only a single population of cell surface AChRs is expressed in these cell lines (Claudio et al 1987). The receptors display proper physiological properties (similar desensitization kinetics, mean channel open time, single channel conductance) and they display all of the pharmacological properties of *Torpedo* AChRs isolated from *Torpedo* membranes [same rank order of affinities for agonists and antagonists, dissociation constant for α-bungarotoxin (a competitive antagonist) of 7.8×10^{-11} M, reversible antagonists exhibit different affinities for the two binding sites on the AChR]. The cell surface distribution of AChRs on AChR-fibroblasts was also investigated using rhodamine conjugated α-bungarotoxin and fluorescence microscopy (Hartman et al 1989). The results indicated that every cell was expressing AChRs, the level of expression was essentially the same in each cell, and the receptors were fairly evenly distributed over the surfaces of cells.

All of the above characterizations have been made on the all-11 cell line (L cells expressing AChRs). Analysis at the single channel level of AChRs expressed in 3T3 cells (all-15) has revealed that they have properties identical to those expressed in all-11 cells (Sine, Claudio, Sigworth, manuscript in preparation). These two AChR-expressing cell lines were established using a calcium phosphate-DNA-mediated cotransfection procedure, however, different selectable marker genes were employed for the two cell lines: the tk gene was cotransfected into Ltk$^-$aprt$^-$ cells (recessive drug resistance) and the neomycin resistance gene was cotransfected into NIH3T3 cells (dominant drug resistance). The observation that functional AChRs are expressed in non-muscle cells after stably introducing the cDNAs by cotransfection using a dominant or a recessive marker gene, greatly broadens the range of recipient cell types that can be used for studying heterologous multisubunit protein complexes. Although we have not established AChR-expressing cell lines by introducing each subunit cDNA into cells with recombinant retrovirus vectors, we have introduced one subunt cDNA into cells using this method (Claudio et al 1989a,b). In those cell lines expressing just three of the *Torpedo* subunits, functional cell surface AChRs were formed after introduction of the missing subunit by viral infection (Claudio et al 1989c). In addition, if one *Torpedo* AChR subunit was introduced into a muscle cell line by infection, hybrid AChRs capable of binding α-bungarotoxin with high affinity were produced (Paulson & Claudio 1988). These results would suggest that proper AChR molecules can be expressed in several cell types after introducton of subunit cDNAs into cells by transfection or viral infection.

MANIPULATIONS OF ACHRS EXPRESSED IN FIBROBLASTS

The availability of large quantities of identical cells stably expressing functional AChRs, individual AChR subunits, or combinations of subunits has enabled us to investigate several aspects of AChR biology. Individual uncomplexed subunits have now been characterized in terms of their molecular mass, antigenicity, posttranslational processing, cell surface expression, stability in fibroblasts, stability in differentiated and undifferentiated muscle cells, and ability (of α) to bind α-bungarotoxin (Claudio et al 1989c).

One posttranslational modification long thought to play a role in AChR function, is phosphorylation (reviewed in Schuetze & Role 1987; Huganir & Greengard 1987). Phosphorylation of other membrane-bound receptors has been shown to cause diverse effects including a decrease in agonist binding, an increase in the rate of receptor internalization, or an increase in desensitization. The AChR-fibroblast system has allowed us to correlate direct measurements of AChR phosphorylation with *in vivo* measurements of AChRs. The cell lines readily take up ^{32}P, they respond to stimulators and inhibitors of various protein kinases, large quantities of modified AChR complexes and individual subunits can be isolated, and the cells are amenable to pharmacological, immunological, biochemical, and electrophysiological analyses before and after treatments. After treatment with ^{32}P, three classes of labeled AChR subunits can be isolated: 1) unassembled, cytoplasmic subunits, 2) assembled, cytoplasmic AChR complexes, and 3) assembled, cell surface AChR complexes. The degree and pattern of AChR phosphorylation was found to be different among these three pools suggesting a possible role of phosphorylation in assembly of AChR subunits (Green & Claudio 1988).

One other goal of establishing this system was to be able to investigate some of the early events of synaptogenesis. There is ample evidence demonstrating that nerves exert a profound influence (directly and/or indirectly) over AChRs in muscle cells. It is known that nerves markedly affect receptor cluster formation (reviewed in Rubin & Barald 1983) and that cluster formation may influence the state of phosphorylation of the AChR (Ross et al 1988). AChR synthesis, insertion into the plasma membrane, and possibly selective activation of synaptic nuclei may also be under the control of neurons (see Schuetze & Role 1987). The question is, are any of these specific interactions between nerves (or nerve trophic factors) and AChRs. The AChR-fibroblast cells are ideal for investigating the specificity question because the only muscle-specific proteins expressed in these cells are AChRs. Thus far, it has been possible to coculture AChR-fibroblasts with 1-day old *Xenopus laevis* embyronal neurons and maintain expression of cell surface AChRs. In such cocultures, it appeared that *Xenopus* neurons made physical contact and formed stable associations with AChR-fibroblasts. Recordings from AChR-fibroblasts that had been contacted by neurons displayed miniature end-plate currents with amplitudes consistent with the site density of surface AChRs (Hartman et al 1989). In another study, agents known to induce AChR clusters in muscle cells (reviewed in Rubin & McMahan, 1982) were shown to induce clusters in AChR-fibroblasts (Claudio et al 1989b). The results from both studies would suggest that our AChR-fibroblasts are an appropriate "simplified muscle cell system" with which to investigate early events of synaptogenesis.

CONCLUSIONS

Using cotransfection, viral infection, or a combination of the two techniques, we have established cell lines expressing one, two, three, or four different AChR subunits. In those cell lines expressing all four subunits, fully functional, cell surface AChRs are expressed. The system is easily manipulated allowing for analyses at many levels, including biochemical, pharmacological, immunological, and electrophysiological. The system also appears to be ideally suited for investigations of heterologous multisubunit protein complexes. Questions we are now able to address concerning the biology of the AChR include, where does subunit assembly occur, what effects do posttranslational modifications have on AChR structure, function, and modulation, and, what role does the AChR play in some of the early events of synaptogenesis.

ACKNOWLEDGEMENTS

This work was supported by National Institutes of Health grants NS21714 and HL38156.

REFERENCES

Bever CT, Dretchen KL, Blake GJ, Chang HW, Asofsky R (1984) Augmented anti-acetylcholine receptor response following long-term penicillamine admisistration. *Ann Neurol* **16**:9-13

Blau HM, Chiu C-P, Webster C (1983) Cytoplasmic activation of human nuclear genes in stable heterocaryons. *Cell* **32**:1171-1180

Claudio T (1987) Stable expression of transfected *Torpedo* acetylcholine receptor α-subunits in mouse fibroblast L cells. *Proc Natl Acad Sci USA* **84**:5967-5971

Claudio T (1989) Molecular genetics of acetylcholine receptor-channels. In: Glover DM, Hames D (eds) *Frontiers in Molecular Biology*. IRL Press, London (in press)

Claudio T, Raftery MA (1980) Is experimental autoimmune myasthenia gravis induced only by acetylcoline receptors? *J Immunol* **124**:1130-1140

Claudio T, Green WN, Hartman D, Hayden D, Paulson HL, Sigworth FJ, Sine SM, Swedlund A (1987) Genetic reconstitution of functional acetylcholine receptor-channels in mouse fibroblasts. *Science* **238**:1688-1694

Claudio T, Paulson HL, Hartman D, Sine S, and Sigworth FJ (1989a) Establishing a stable expression system for studies of acetylcholine receptors. In: Hoffman JF, Giebisch G (eds) *Current Topics in Membranes and Transport*, Molecular Biology of Ion Channels, vol **33**. Academic Press, New York, p 219-247

Claudio T, Hartman DS, Green WN, Ross AF, Paulson HL, Hayden D (1989b) Stable expression of multisubunit protein complexes in mammalian cells. In: Maelicke A (ed) *NATO ASI Series H, Cell Biology,* Molecular Biology of Neuroreceptors and Ion Channels, vol **32**. Springer-Verlag, Berlin, p 469-480

Claudio T, Paulson HL, Green WN, Ross AF, Hartman DS, Hayden D (1989c) Fibroblasts transfected with *Torpedo* acetylcholine receptor β, γ, and δ subunit cDNAs express functional AChRs when infected with a retroviral α-recombinant. *J Cell Biol* **108** (in press)

Conti-Tronconi, BM, Raftcry MA (1982) The nicotinic cholinergic receptor: correlation of molecular structure with functional properties. *Ann Rev Biochem* **51**:491-530

Davies J, Jimenez A (1980) A new selective agent for eukaryotic cloning vectors. *Am J Trop Med Hyg* (Suppl) **29**:1089-1092

Drachman D, Kao J, Pestronk A,Toyka K (1976) Myasthenia gravis as a receptor disorder. Ann NY Acad Sci 274:226-234

Engel, AG (1987) Molecular biology of endplate diseases. In: Salpetyer, MM (ed) *The Vertebrate Neuromuscular Junction.* Alan R Liss, Inc., New York, p 361-424

Graham R, van der Eb A (1973) A new technique for the assay of infectivity of human adenovirus 5 virus. *Virol* **52**:456-467

Green WN, Claudio T (1988) Differences in the phosphorylation of unassembled, assembled but cytoplasmic, and surface acetylcholine receptors. *Soc Neurosci Abstr* **14**:1045 (419.3)

Hartman DS, Poo M-m, Green WN, Ross AF, Claudio T (1989) Synaptic contact between embryonic neurons and acetylcholine receptor-fibroblasts *J Physiol Paris* (in press)

Huganir RL, Greengard P (1987) Regulation of receptor function by protein phosphorylation. *Trends in Pharm Sci* **8**:472-477

Karlin A (1980) Molecular properties of nicotinic acetylcholine receptors. In: Cotman CW, Poste G, Nicolson GL (eds) *The Cell Surface and Neuronal Function,* vol **6**. Elsevier/North-Holland Biomedical Press, Amsterdam, p 191-260

Lindstrom J (1985) Immunobiology of myasthenia gravis, experimental autoimmune myasthenia gravis, and lambert-eaton syndrome. *Ann Rev Immunol* **3**:109-131

Mann R, Mulligan RC, Baltimore D (1983) Construction of a retrovirus packaging mutant and its use to produce helper-free defective retrovirus. *Cell* **33**:153-159

Newsom-Davis, J (1986) Diseases of the neuromuscular junction. In: Asbury RK, Guy M, McKhann W, McDonald I (eds) *Diseases of the Nervous System, Clinical Neurobiology*, vol **I**. Ardmore Medical Books, Philadelphia, p 269-282

Paulson HL, Claudio T (1988) Temperature-sensitive expression of all-*Torpedo* and *Torpedo*-rat hybrid AChRs in mammalian cells. *Soc Neurosci Abstr* **14**:1045 (419.4)

Popot J-L, Changeux P-J (1984) Nicotinic receptor of acetylcholine: structure of an oligomeric integral membrane protein. *Physiol Rev* **64**:1162-1239

Ross AF, Rapuano M, Prives JM (1988) Induction of phosphorylation and cell surface redistribution of acetylcholine receptors by phorbol ester and carbamylcholine in cultured chick myotubes *J Cell Biol* **107**:1139-1145

Rubin LL, Barald KF (1983) Neuromuscular development in tissue culture. In: Burnstock G, Vrbova G, O'Brien R (eds) *Somatic and Autonomic Nerve-Muscle Interactions*. Elsevier Science Publisher, BV, Amsterdam, New York, p 109-151

Rubin LL, McMahan UJ (1982) Regeneration of the neuromuscular junction: steps toward defining the molecular basis of the interaction between nerve and muscle. In: Schotland DL (ed) *Disorders of the Motor Unit.* John Wiley & Sons, p 187-196

Schubert D, Harris AJ, Devine CE, Heinemann S (1974) Characterization of a unique muscle cell line. *J Cell Biol* **61**:398-413
Schuetze SM, Role L (1987) Developmental regulation of nicotinic acetylcholine receptors. *Ann Rev Neurosci* **10**:403-457
Subramani S, Mulligan RC, Berg P (1981) Expression of the mouse dihydrofolate reductase cDNA in simian virus 40 vectors. *Mol Cell Biol* **1**:854-864
Wigler M, Silverstein S, Lee L-S, Pellicer A, Cheng Y-c, Axel R (1977) Transfer of purified herpes virus thymidine kinase gene to cultured mouse cells. *Cell* **11**:223-232
Yaffe D (1968) Retention of differentiation potentialities during prolonged cultivation of myogenic cells. *Proc Natl Acad Sci USA* **61**:477-483
Yaffe D, Saxel O (1977) Serial passaging and differentiation of myogenic cells isolated from dystrophic mouse muscle. *Nature* **270**:725-727

DISCUSSION

NEWSOM-DAVIS: One of the features about innervation and synaptogenesis is that where there is an epsilon chain present, at least in some species, that gets put in place of the gamma chain and perhaps as a consequence the open time shortens. Do you have any evidence of that. You don't have an epsilon chain but do you have any evidence about the open time?

CLAUDIO: We have not done any single channel recordings on those patched receptors. We have looked hard for an epsilon chain in Torpedo and there does not appear to be one.

RAKOVITZ: On that question about epsilon, if the mammalian muscle is denervated do you get the converse process where instead of clustering, as in the Torpedo receptor, you get non-clustering and the diffuse distribution of the receptor as in the mammalian foetal calf muscle system. Is the epsilon subunit found in the foetal calf muscle AchR? Are they differently expressed in inervated or non-inervated muscle tissue??

CLAUDIO: The epsilon subunit is not found in AchR from Torpedo or the mammalian foetal AchR. It should not have been given a new Greek symbol but simply been called foetal or adult mammalian subunit since in mammalian AchR, this subunit is termed epsilon in adult and gamma in foetal tissues. Its expression varies in muscle tissue depending on the degree of innervation.

<u>RAKOVITZ</u>: Can your data on clustering of the AchR in fibroblasts be reconciled by different receptor subunits being expressed under different conditions?

<u>CLAUDIO</u>: The AchR receptor on mammalian muscle cells can cluster without going through an epsilon and gamma switch.

<u>KOHN</u>: Do you know the effect of AchR antibodies on your transfected fibroblasts?

<u>CLAUDIO</u>: This is being done in collaboration with S Tzartos. An advantage of our system is that a large variety of well characterized epitope specific monoclonal antibodies to the Torpedo AchR are available allowing us to answer important questions on modulation and down-regulation of the receptor induced by crosslinking with the appropriate monoclonal antibodies.

THE INTERACTION BETWEEN MHC CLASS II MOLECULES AND IMMUNOGENIC PEPTIDES

S. Buus , A. Sette [*], E. B. Shaeffer [°], and H. M. Grey [*]
Institute for Experimental Immunology
Nørre Allé 71
DK-2100 Copenhagen Ø
Denmark

Our immune system performs the crucial task of defending us against attack from microorganisms such as bacteria, parasites, and viruses. To this end the immune system has been endowed with very powerful weapons against foreign, and, to avoid unwanted destruction of the body itself, with the ability to distinguish between "self" and "non-self". The main players of the immune system are the blood borne lymphocytes, the so-called B and T cells, the only cells known sofar with the capacity to examine and respond to molecules (antigens) in their surroundings. Especially the T cells appear to occupy a central role in regulating the immune system and in distinguishing between self and non-self. Antigen recognition by T cells is unusually complicated. T cells on their own seem to be blind; they require the presence of another cell type, the so-called accessory cell. Among other requirements, the accessory cell must be able to take up and alter antigens (in a function called antigen processing), and subsequently display processed antigen in association with accessory cell synthesized proteins, the major histocompatibility gene complex (MHC) molecules. The MHC genes which encodes for these membrane glycoproteins are the most polymorphic loci known ie. many different alleles exist in the population, however each individual only possesses a few of these.

Here, we will deal with some recently gained insights into how T cells recognize antigens. The main emphasis will be on the interaction between MHC class II molecules and immunogenic peptides, however, we will first introduce antigen processing.

[*] Cytel, 11099 North Torrey Pines Road, La Jolla, CA 92037, USA
[°] National Jewish Center, 1400 Jackson Street, Denver, CO 80220, USA

NATO ASI Series, Vol. H 38
The Molecular Biology of Autoimmune Disease
Edited by A. G. Demaine et al.

ANTIGEN PROCESSING

In general, T cells only recognize proteins. Prior to recognition by T cells protein antigens need to be physically altered or "processed" by accessory cells (Reviewed Unanue 1984, Buus et al. 1987b). The exact nature of antigen processing is still poorly understood despite almost two decades of intense research. Thus, the molecules and cellular compartments of the accessory cell involved in antigen processing have not been identified. It is believed that protein antigens are non-specifically taken up by the accessory cell and partially degraded by proteolysis. The fragments thus generated are specifically bound to MHC molecules, and the resulting peptide/MHC complexes are presented at the accessory cell surface to T cells. It has been demonstrated that proteolytic degradation of the native antigen in the test tube can substitute for whatever processing event(s) that take place within an accessory cell (Shimonkevitz et al. 1983). In recent years, several antigen derived peptides have been identified that without further alteration, can be presented to T cells. Data have also been obtained to suggest that naturally processed antigens are peptides commonly of the MW size 2,000 - 12,000 with a mean MW of approximately 3,000 (Buus et al. 1988).

PRESENTATION TO T CELLS OF PROCESSED ANTIGEN IN THE CONTEXT OF MHC MOLECULES.

T cells do not recognize soluble protein antigens, but only antigens presented in association with MHC molecules (Rosenthal and Shevach, 1973; Zinkernagel and Doherty,1974). Thus, antigen recognition by T cells is heavily influenced by the MHC haplotype of the individual. One important immune phenomenon is known as *MHC-restriction* which means that the specificities of T cells are restricted since they must co-recognize antigen and MHC. Another phenomenon is known as *responder/non-responder status* which means that an animal, when immunized with a simple antigen, will give a high or low response depending on its MHC haplotype. Any theory dealing with the nature of MHC control of T cell responses must explain these two different MHC related immune phenomena. One theory, the so-called *hole in the T cell repertoire* hypothesis explains low-responder status, as well as MHC restriction, as the result of defects in the T cell repertoire against certain antigen/MHC combinations. In contrast, the so-called *determinant selection* hypothesis proposes that the function of the MHC molecule is to specifically bind some, but not all, peptides created during antigen processing, and that T cells only recognize peptides that can be bound by the MHC. In any event, the final antigen-specific step in T cell activation is thought to be the creation of a tri-molecular complex consisting of MHC, processed antigen, and the

T cell receptor.

Two classes of MHC molecules, class I and II, are known to function as T cell restriction elements. Though distinctly different, they are closely related to one another structurally. Both are glycoprotein dimers with similar domain structures and intramolecular S-S bridges. The X-ray crystallographic structure of a human MHC class I molecule, HLA-A2, has recently been described (Björkman et al, 1987), and based on these findings a model describing the structure of MHC class II molecules has been proposed (Brown et al, 1988). It is thought that the two outer domains of the MHC molecule form a rectangular antigen binding groove between a floor of β-pleated strands and two α-helical walls.

DEMONSTRATION OF PEPTIDE-MHC COMPLEXES

That processed antigen and MHC interact specifically prior to T cell recognition was supported by the observation that antigens could compete with one another for presentation apparently at the level of the accessory cell (Werdelin, 1982). Direct biochemical evidence of the existence of peptide-MHC complexes has recently been obtained. Using equilibrium dialysis Babbitt et al. demonstrated that the affinity purified mouse MHC molecule, I-A^k, was capable of binding an immunogenic peptide derived from hen egg lysozyme (HEL 46-61). The binding of this peptide to I-A^k was specific and had a dissociation constant of 2-4 μM (Babbitt et al., 1985).

We have for some time been investigating the I-A^d restricted T cell response to an immunodominant peptide from chicken ovalbumin (Ova 323-339). Using equilibrium dialysis we were also able to show a specific binding between ^{125} I-labeled Ova 323-339 and affinity purified I-A^d. During the course of these investigations we noted that the peptide-MHC complexes, once formed, were very stable. We reasoned that it should be possible to assay the binding between Ova 323-339 and I-A^d by separating peptide-MHC complexes from uncomplexed peptide by size exclusion chromatography. Indeed, this turned out to be possible ,and we have subsequently used gel filtration to assess peptide-MHC binding (Buus et al, 1986). The peptide-MHC complexes assayed by this method could be isolated and used to stimulate T cells thus demonstrating their immunological relevancy.

The gel filtration method also allowed us to examine the thermodynamics of peptide-MHC complex formation (Buus et al, 1986). The overall equilibrium dissociation constants for peptide-MHC interactions were found to be approximately 10^{-5}M. In comparison, the affinity of antigen-antibody interactions is typically 10^{-9}M to 10^{-11}M. This difference is mainly explained by the slow on-rate. Assuming pseudo-first order kinetics, the rate of association was calculated to be approximately 1 $s^{-1}M^{-1}$ which is about 5 orders of magnitude less than the known rate of association for most antigen-antibody interactions. Dissociation of peptide-MHC complexes followed a first order reaction with a rate of dissociation which, in contrast, was similar to the one found for most antigen-antibody interactions, about 10^{-5} s^{-1}.

THE IMMUNOLOGICAL RELEVANCY OF PEPTIDE-MHC INTERACTIONS

In order to correlate the capacity of a given MHC molecule to bind a peptide with its capacity to serve as a T cell restriction element we examined the ability of four different MHC molecules to bind twelve peptides already known to be immunogenic (Buus et al, 1987a) A very good correlation was found between immunogenicity and binding to MHC; the binding appeared specific and saturable; and peptides restricted to the same restriction element inhibited the binding of one another to the MHC suggesting the existence of only one peptide binding site per MHC molecule. This strongly suggested that binding of a peptide to MHC is a prerequisite for presentation ie. that determinant selection is operative in defining T cell immune responses. In one instance, however, T cell responses directed against a peptide/MHC combination were very difficult to demonstrate even though the peptide could clearly be shown to bind to the MHC molecule. This would argue that peptide binding in itself is insufficient to assure immunogenicity, and that additional factors, such as holes in the T cell repertoire, would have to exist superimposed on determinant selection. This would make biological sense since, as mentioned below, MHC molecules are unable to distinguish between self and non-self. This function belongs entirely with the T cells which must be able to override the potential responses directed against self peptides that inevitably will be presented in the context of MHC.

To analyze the relative distribution of determinant selection and and potential holes in the T cell repertoire, we examined the immune response to the 149 amino acid protein antigen, Staphylococcal Nuclease (Nase) (Schaeffer et al, submitted). Fourteen overlapping peptides representing the entire antigen were synthezised, and tested both for their binding to four different MHC molecules and for their usage of these restriction elements in T cell responses. A total of 54 independent peptide-MHC combinations were examined. T cell responses (ie. immunogenicity) were found in 24% of these events, and binding to MHC could be detected in all, but one, case (12/13). Conversely, binding was detected in 31% of the 54 events many, but not all, of which led to a T cell response (12/17). Thus, the specific binding of processed antigen to MHC (ie.determinant selection) appears to be an absolute requirement for immunogenicity, and, in addition, holes in the T cell repertoire may act in concert with determinant selection to define T cell immune responses. In these experiments about 70% of the binding events led to an immune response leaving the remaining 30% of the binding events as potential examples of hole in the T cell repertoire.

THE SPECIFICITY OF PEPTIDE-MHC INTERACTIONS

Animals with only one MHC class II molecule are known to exist. If binding of processed antigen to MHC is a prerequisite for T cell immunogenicity, then how can one MHC molecule present the sizable part of the universe of peptides that would be needed to fulfill this task? To address this question we first defined the residues within the I-A^d restricted Ova peptide 323-339 involved in binding to I-A^d. A "core-region" consisting of the residues 327-332 was identified by C- and N terminal truncations of the original peptide. Subsequently, a total of 55 single substituted analogs of the Ova peptide 323-336 were made and tested both for their I-A^d binding and for their capacity to stimulate two Ova 323-336 specific/ I-A^d-restricted hybridomas. This approach also implicated the region 327-332, and in particular the residues 327 and 332, as critical for the binding of Ova 323-336 to I-A^d. Overall, it was found that the peptide-MHC interaction was very permissive since about 85% of the analogs had MHC binding capacity equivalent to that of the native peptide. In contrast, T cell recognition was found to be much more specific since only about 30% of the analogs could be recognized by T cell specific for the native antigen (Sette et al., 1987). Similar observations have now been made in a system using the MHC molecule, I-E^d, as the T cell restriction element (Sette et al.,submitted).

The data from the Nase experiments and from the single substituted analog experiments both described above, clearly demonstrate that, whereas the final T cell response is quite specific, the interaction between processed antigen and MHC is very permissive. Thus, it is feasible that binding of processed antigens to MHC is a prerequisite for the ability of T cells to recognize a sufficient part of the universe of antigens - that is, it is difficult to envision that any microorganism could escape the immune system by being made up of proteins that could not be presented due to a lack of MHC binding peptides upon processing. How is this broad "MHC repertoire" created? In looking through the sequences of peptides known to be very good I-A^d or I-E^d binders we noted certain sequence similarities (motifs). The I-A^d binding motif was largely hydrophobic (Sette et al. 1987), whereas the I-E^d binding motif was mostly positively charged (Sette et al, submitted). With very few exceptions, good I-A^d or I-E^d binders contained the appropriate motif, and the actual usage of these motifs were confirmed by truncation analysis. The MHC recognition of a large repertoire of seemingly unrelated peptides is therefore likely to be accomplished by the recognition of broad structural motifs. It is noteworthy, that the two motifs identified so far are very dissimilar. This would argue against algorithms that claim to identify general T cell epitope motifs.

MHC MOLECULES CONSTITUTIVELY BIND PEPTIDES DERIVED FROM SELF PROTEINS

We have previously found that only a minor proportion, approximately 5%, of the MHC molecules were available for peptide binding and suggested that endogenously derived peptides might constitutively occupy the peptide binding site on the majority of MHC molecules (Buus et al, 1987b). This was later supported by X-ray crystallographic data showing radiodense material in the putative peptide binding site of a MHC molecule (Björkman et al, 1987). Importantly, it has been shown that MHC molecules can bind self-peptides (Babbitt et al 1986, Lorenz et al, 1988), and it has been possible to elute off peptide-like material, supposedly derived from self proteins, from affinity purified MHC molecules (Buus et al 1988). Thus, MHC molecules do not distinguish between self and non-self.

REFERENCES

Babbitt BP, Allen PM, Matsueda GR, Haber E, Unanue ER (1985) The binding of immunogenic peptides to Ia histocompatibility molecules. NAture 317:359

Babbitt BP, Matsueda GR, Haber E, Unanue ER, Allen PM (1986) Antigenic competition at the level of peptide-Ia binding. Proc Natl Acad Sci USA 83:4509

Björkman PJ, Saper MA, Samraoui B, Bennett WS, Strominger JL, Wiley DC (1988) Structure of the human class I histocompatibility antigen, HLA-A2. Nature 329:506

Brown JH, Jardetzky T, Saper MA, Samraoui B, Björkman PJ, Wiley DC (1988) A hypothetical model of the foreign antigen binding site of class II histocompatibility molecules. Nature 332:845

Buus S, Sette A, Colon SM, Jenis DM, Grey HM (1986) Isolation and characterization of antigen-Ia complexes involved in T cell recognition. Cell 47:1071

Buus S, Sette A, Colon SM, Miles C, Grey HM (1987a) The relation between major histocompatibility complex (MHC) restriction and the capacity of Ia to bind immunogenic peptides. Science 235:1353

Buus S, Sette A, Grey HM (1987b) The interaction between protein derived immunogenic peptides and Ia. Immun Rev 98:115

Buus S, Sette A, Colon SM, Grey HM (1988) Autologous peptides constitutively occupy the antigen binding site on Ia. Science 242:1045

Lorenz RG, Tyler AN, Allen PM (1988) T cell recognition of bovine ribonuclease. Self/non-self discrimination at the level of binding to the I-A^k molecule. J Immunol 141:4124

Rosenthal AS, Schevach EM (1973) Function of macrophages in antigen recognition by guinea pig lymphocytes. I Requirement for histocompatible macrophages and lymphocytes. J exp Med 138:1194

Sette A, Buus S, Colon SM, Smith JA, Miles C, Grey HM (1987) Structural characteristics of an antigen required for its interaction with Ia and recognition by T cells. Nature 328:395

Shimonkevitz R, Kappler J, Marrack P, Grey HM (1983) Antigen recognition by H-2 restricted T cells. I Cell-free processing. J exp Med 158:303

Unanue ER (1984) Antigen presenting function of macrophages. Annu Rev Immunol 2:395

Werdelin O (1982) Chemically related antigens compete for presentation by accessory cells to T cells. J Immunol 129:1883

Zinkernagel RM, Doherty PC (1974) Restriction of in vitro T cell-mediated cytotoxicity in lymphocytic choriomeningitis within a syngeneic or allogeneic system. Nature 248:701

DISCUSSION

ALLEN: The ability of a peptide to bind to MHC and the failure to generate a T cell response suggests that 'holes in the repertoire' at the T cell receptor level may be operating. Have you looked at F1 animals?

BUUS: No we have not.

JANEWAY: It is worth pointing out that 'determinant selection' has also been experimentally observed by Bersofsky. They can identify an immunogenic peptide but when native protein is used, no immunogenicity is apparent in the peptide presumably because it cannot be processed.

BUUS: Malissen too has shown that some of their transfectants can present a peptide, but fail to present the native protein due to a failure of processing.

DEMAINE: How many MHC molecules bind to one antigen?

BUUS: There is one peptide binding site per MHC molecule.

DEMAINE: The majority of MHC molecules that you find in your experiments would be complexed to an antigen. Is this the same in all MHC backgrounds between different strains of animals?

BUUS: It is the same in all four MHC elements that we have examined. However, like Paul Allen, we get some inhibition of binding of the peptides to MHC by mouse serum.

ALLEN: This leads to the question of whether there are free Ia molecules that are functional *in vitro* that are bound to foreign peptides in most cases, or otherwise to self peptides. In general, most of all the Ia molecules (> 90%) on the cell surface will have their binding site occupied. As this is not covalent binding, there is an equilibrium with an extremely slow rate which, at present, makes it very difficult to perform precise quantitation sites.

MOLECULAR MIMICRY BETWEEN VIRUS PROTEINS AND AUTOANTIGENS IN AUTOIMMUNITY

Thomas Dyrberg
Hagedorn Research Laboratory
Niels Steensensvej 6
DK-2820 Gentofte
Denmark

Viruses have been implicated in the etiopathogenesis of many diseases of unknown origin, and in particular diseases where autoimmunity has been speculated to play a role (Mims, 1985). Several of the characteristic features of a virus infection have been proposed to enable the virus to precipitate an autoimmune response or to turn a protective immune response into a, potentially harmful, self reactive immune response. Virus may infect cells of the immune system thereby perturbing their function (McChesney and Oldstone, 1987). Thus, examples from spontaneous and experimental diseases have demonstrated that virus infection of T and/or B cells interfere with the function of these cells, in vitro and in vivo, e.g., following infection with measle and human immunodeficiency virus (HIV) and in mice lactic dehydrogenase virus infects macrophages through their Ia molecules (Inada and Mims, 1984) and may thus interfere with these cells' antigen presenting function.

Another mechanism by which virus could cause a spurious immune response is through the induction of crossreactive antibodies or lymphocytes (Mims, 1985). Potential ways this could take place include immunogenic presentation of self antigens in the context of viral proteins, destruction of cells with release of immunologic silent cell proteins, induction of crossreactive antiidiotypic immune responses to virus antibodies or through non-specific, polyclonal B cell activation, e.g., following Epstein-Barr virus infection (EBV).

One variation on this theme is the presence of homologous epitopes on virus and host cell proteins, a phenomenon which has

NATO ASI Series, Vol. H 38
The Molecular Biology of Autoimmune Disease
Edited by A. G. Demaine et al.

been termed molecular mimicry (Oldstone, 1987). An autoimmune response could be initiated by a mimicking epitope if the microbial and host cell determinants are similar enough to crossreact, but different enough to break immunologic tolerance. The immune response to the crossreactive self determinant may thereafter continue stimulated by the host antigen. At the time of clinical onset of the ensuing disease, the infectious agent may have been cleared leaving only the autoimmune response behind. That pathogenic microbes share antigenic determinants with the host cell proteins have been known for a long time, e.g., the development of cardiac myosin crossreactive antibodies following infection with hemolytic streptococci (Dale and Beachey, 1985). The concept of molecular mimicry originated from studies on parasites, although the phenomenon then was proposed as a mechanism whereby parasites could evade immune attack through antigen similarity to the host (Damian, 1988). Subsequent work has focused more on the possible pathogenic role that mimicking epitopes may have induction of autoimmunity. Crossreactive epitopes have been identified between parasites, bacteria and virus proteins and potential human autoantigens, often by analysis of antibody crossreactivities. With the rapid advances in molecular cloning of virus and cell proteins it has become possible to directly search for shared sequences between virus and host proteins. This approach at present only allows for analysis of linear sequence homologies. In humoral immunity the antigen epitopes are primarily conformational, however, there is ample evidence that linear epitopes may elicit antibody responses. The T cell recognizes peptide fragments presented by MHC class II molecules (Buus et al., 1987). The initial recognition of an antigen by T cells has a pivotal role in induction of an (auto)immune response and analysis at the T cell level of the implications of mimicking epitopes on virus and host cell proteins, require further studies.

What is the evidence that molecular mimicry can play a role in the pathogenesis of autoimmune diseases. The encephalotigenic site of myelin basic protein (MBP) for rabbits was found to share a sequence of six consecutive amino acids with the hepatitis B virus polymerase (Fujinami and Oldstone, 1985). Rabbits, immunized with a peptide containing the shared sequence, contained antibodies and peripheral blood lymphocytes that recognized intact MBP. In addition, central nervous system tissue from rabbits immunized with the peptide by the peripheral route showed histologic lesions resembling those found in experimental allergic encephalitis. These results, in an experimental model system, suggest that virus infection may tricker the production of antibodies and lymphocytes with the potential of crossreacting with biologically important self proteins in vivo.

Antibodies against the acetylcholine receptor (AChR) play an important role in the pathogenesis of autoimmune myasthenia gravis (MG). By using synthetic peptides representing regions of the immunodominant AChR α chain, it has been demonstrated that some MG patients have autoantibodies recognizing residues 160 to 167 (Schwimmbeck et al., 1989). When such antibodies were affinity purified from MG patient serum on a column coupled with the AchR peptide, it was shown that they bound the native AChR and inhibited the binding of α-ungaro toxin to the receptor. The AChR α-chain sequence in addition demonstrated specific immunological crossreactivity with a shared homologous determinant on a herpes simplex virus protein both at the peptide and at the protein level (Schwimmbeck et al., 1989). The immunological crossreactivity of AChR and herpes simplex virus indicate that this virus may be associated with the initiation of some cases of myasthenia, and provides an example of a potentially significant pathogenic molecular mimicry between an autoantigen and virus protein in a human autoimmune disease.

Molecular mimicry between a microbial antigen and an autoantigen may, however, represent only one mechanism for initiation of autoimmunity. An alternative hypothesis is that a crossreactive autoimmune response to a determinant on an immune regulatory cell mimicking a microbial antigen could interfere with a function of the particular cell. One candidate for such regulatory cell proteins is the HLA antigens.

Several reports have demonstrated crossreactivities or amino acid homologies between HLA class I molecules and bacterial proteins, e.g., between HLA B27 associated with ankylosing spondylytis and a Klebsiella pneumonia protein (Schwimmbeck et al., 1987). More pertinent to this discussion may be the findings of mimicking epitopes between virus proteins and HLA class II antigens. The presence of a shared epitope between the HIV gp41 envelope protein and a conserved N-terminal region of HLA class II β-chain molecules was thus speculated to contribute to the functional impairment of $CD4^+$ T cells and development of autoimmune phenomena in AIDS patients (Golding et al., 1988). Serum from AIDS patients contained antibodies reacting with synthetic peptides representing the shared epitope as well as with native class II molecules. In vitro, the proliferative response of normal $CD4^+$ T cells to Tetanus toxoid and allogenic stimulation was significantly decreased after incubation with class II crossreactive rare patient sera but not control sera (Golding et al., 1989). Further, such patient sera could destroy class II bearing cells by antibody dependent cellular cytotoxicity. Other examples of sequence homologies and immunologic crossreactivity have been reported between virus and HLA class II proteins, e.g. between cytomegalo virus and HLA-DR β-chain proteins (Fujinami et al., 1988) and between EBV and HLA-DQ β-chain molecules associated with autoimmune type 1 diabetes (Horn et al., 1988; Dyrberg and Michelsen, 1988).

In conclusion, one of the mechanisms whereby virus infection may precipitate an autoimmune response could be through molecular mimicry between a microbial protein and an autoantigen or an immune regulatory protein. Further studies on molecular mimicry as a cause of autoimmunity are, however, required with particular emphasis on the importance of conformational epitopes and of T cell crossreactivities.

REFERENCES

Buus S, Sette A, Colon S, Miles C, Grey HM (1987) The relationship between major histocompatibility complex (MHC) restriction and the capacity of Ia to bind immunogenic peptides. Science 235: 1353-1358

Dale JB, Beachey EH (1985) Epitopes of streptococcal M proteins shared with cardiac myosin. J Exp Med 162: 583-591
Damian RT (1988) Parasites and molecular mimicry. In: Lernmark Å, Dyrberg T, Terenius L, Hökfelt B (eds) Molecular mimicry in health and disease. Excerpta Medica, Amsterdam, New York, Oxford, p 211
Dyrberg T, Michelsen B, Oldstone M (1988) Virus and host cell antigen sharing in myasthenia gravis and autoimmune diabetes. In: Lernmark Å, Dyrberg T, Terenius L, Hökfelt B (eds) Molecular mimicry in health and disease. Excerpta Medica, Amsterdam, New York, Oxford, p 245
Fujinami RS, Nelson JA, Walker L, Oldstone MBA (1988) Sequence homology and immunologic cross-reactivity of human cytomegalovirus with HLA-DR β chain: a means for graft rejection and immunosuppression. J Virol 62: 100-105
Fujinami RS, Oldstone MBA (1985) Amino acid homology between the encephalitogenic site of myelin basic protein and virus: mechanism for autoimmunity. Science 230: 1043-1045
Golding H, Robey FA, Gates FT III, Linder W, Beining PR, Hoffman T, Golding B (1988) Identification of homologous regions in human immunodeficiency virus I gp41 and human MHC Class II β I domain. J Exp Med 167: 914-923
Golding H, Shearer GM, Hillman K, Lucas P, Manischewitz J, Zajac RA, Clerici M, Gress RE, Boswell RN, Golding B (1989) Common epitope in human immunodeficiency virus (HIV) I-GP41 and HLA class II elicits immunosuppressive autoantibodies capable of contributing to immune dysfunction in HIV I-infected individuals. J Clin Invest 83: 1430-1435
Horn GT, Bugawan TL, Long CM, Erlich HA (1988) Allelic sequence variation of the HLA-DQ loci: relationship to serology and to insulin-dependent diabetes susceptibility. Proc Natl Acad Sci USA 85: 6012-6016
Inada T, Mims C (1984) Mouse Ia antigens are receptor for lactate dehydrogenase virus. Nature 309: 59-61
McChesney MB, Oldstone MBA (1987) Viruses perturb lymphocyte functions: selected principles characterizing virus-induced immunosuppression. Ann Rev Immunol 5: 279-304
Mims CA (1985) Viral aetiology of diseases of obscure origin. Br Med Bull 41: 63-69
Oldstone, MBA (1987) Molecular mimicry and autoimmune disease. Cell 50: 819-820
Schwimmbeck PL, Dyrberg T, Drachman DB, Oldstone MBA (1989) Molecular mimicry and myasthenia gravis: an autoantigenic site of the acetylcholine receptor α subunit that has biologic activity and reacts immunochemically with herpes simplex virus. Submitted for publication
Schwimmbeck PL, Yu DTY, Oldstone MBA (1987) Autoantibodies to HLA B27 in the sera of HLA B27 patients with ankylosing spondylitis and Reiter's syndrome. J Exp Med 166: 173-181

DISCUSSION

ALLEN: Have you looked at cross-reaction at the level of the T cell on any of these, for example, say you have 6 amino acids can you show nice cross reaction in the mouse or some other system?

DYRBERG: No but we are in the process of doing that. This hasn't been thoroughly studied at the level of T cell recognition.

NEWSOM-DAVIES: I was going to follow and really say much the same thing in relation to the myasthenic story because its highly likely that the antibodies depend on T cell help and one can't assume that the epitopes seen by the B cells are going to be the same ones as seen by the T cells so it might really be more relevant to go for the T cell cross reactivity mimicry than the B cell

DYRBERG: That's probably true for a number of autoimmune diseases but particularly with myasthenia gravis I think you could argue that the B cell recognition could be of primary importance because you know the disease is caused by the immune response to the receptor so you could argue that T cell involvement could be brought about by another region leading to antibodies reactive with this sequence on the receptor and that by itself could give the clinical symptoms of the disease.

NEWSOM-DAVIS: To support that argument you would really need to show that there are cross reactive epitopes for T cells.

DYRBERG: My point would be that the clinically important cross reactions would be at the antibody level, at least in myasthenia.

EISENBARTH: I have a general question about the area in terms of the way the hypothesis is tested and what the specificity is of the cross reactions and the sequence homologies that one finds. We have drugs like penicillamine that clearly induce myasthenia gravis perhaps by mimicry. I don't think anyone knows how penicillamine works. The difficulty I have is seeing once one defines a sequence homoolgy as to whether one would be just as likely to define a sequence homology in plant viruses for instance, as the sequence homologies that you've shown, I mean that would be one question. How likely are these sequence homologies when you search your data bank

DYRBERG: Unlikely, but still that doesn't prove anything. They occur and the number of proteins in the databases are increasing. The probability of these kind of homologies coming up is also increasing.

EISENBARTH: I guess my question would be are you just as likely to find homology with plant virus as you are with a human virus?

DYRBERG: Yes, I guess you would be.

EISENBARTH: So then the finding of homology itself is not much of a proof that there is anything pathogenic?

DYRBERG: That was the point I tried to make.

EISENBARTH: If you picked the plant viruses and their homology sequences, would you just as often find an antibody crossreactivity as you do when you pick the human virus and create the peptide sequence?

DYRBERG: If you find the same sequence for instance as some of those shown here in a plant virus and you look at the peptide level then of course you would get the same crossreaction. It is not necessary that you would get the same crossreaction when you look at the protein level

EISENBARTH: The next difficulty is that neither of the tests really tell you that you have a pathogenic mechanism involved so how do you actually test the hypothesis and perhaps epidemiologically get at it that there is some disease relationship with a virus?

DYRBERG: The actual test or the proof that this plays a role will be difficult. One way to go about it would be to look for binding to these regions that we are talking about upon immunisation so as to actually demonstrate that this sequence is immunologically recognized

EISENBARTH: I don't think that would test the hypothesis that would be like creating a peptide immunising with it and seeing a crossreactivity. I think you perhaps have to get to show that the virus is either more common in the disease state.

DYRBERG: That would be difficult with many of these viruses which are so frequent. Another approach would be to look at the effect of these immune reactions be it T cells or antibodies in the intact animal.

WILCOX: I'm really coming to the same question again. Don't you think that if you really believe in these cross reactions you ought to look for epidemiological evidence that a given virus is actually implicated in a given patient group.

DYRBERG: That would be nice but there are a number of problems; one is for instance with EBV infection that in grown up population 70-90% would have had an EBV infection. Now that doesn't show that EBV could not be involved in autoimmunity. In the case of MHC proteins you know that there is a vast excess of persons carrying autoimmune associated MHC type but still you only get the disease in very few persons.

WILCOX: You might be able to use epidemiological approaches because, for example, in the Far East, myasthenia gravis occurs in very young children. There must be some good reason why its so much commoner in very young children than it is in the West.

JANEWAY: I want to return to the issue that both Allen and Newsom-Davis were raising and that is the importance of understanding where the T cells come into the system. One can say if you have an acute infection you can use epitopes on the virus that are non-self for help to drive the B cells that are making these crossreactive autoantibodies but autoimmune diseases when they become established there is persistent production of antibody or persistent T cell activation that at least we imagine (and I think it still has to be proven) is directed at a self antigen and not at the virus and so the virus specific T cells or the virus specific recognition is not autoreactive it can't be called on and so if you are going to invoke this mechanism you have to account for the generation of autoreactive T cells as well as the production of crossreactive antibodies.

McGREGOR: Perhaps I could come to your support and just give you an example of what I think is a very elegant demonstration in vivo of what you have been describing in vitro. John Penhale in Perth, Australia has a beautiful animal model of autoimmune thyroiditis. In 1985 the Australian Government decided to improve the health care of animals in their facilities and moved from having animals maintained under non-sterile conditions in their animal houses to a sterile environment. As soon as that happened he could no longer get thyroiditis in his animals. Luckily for him, the Australian Government moved slowly and they hadn't enforced this legislation in Darwin in the North of Australia where another group working on the same rat animal model still had animals that weren't sterile. If he took the gastrointestinal washings of the animals from Darwin gave them to pregnant rats in his animal house, in other words, recolonised their gut, then the offspring of those animals redeveloped the disease again. Nothing else had changed, the diet was the same, the only thing that was different was that they clearly had been reinfected by normal gut flora and redeveloped the disease. The problem, in a sense, in answer to Nick Wilcox is that you find something and then you follow it but there are so many viruses and bacteria in the gut of these rats now and the question is which one is it that seems to be switching on the disease? I do think, however, this is an example of one of the kinds of mechanisms that you have been describing occurring in vivo and inducing autoimmunity

DYRBERG: Thank you. Just for completeness sake, I would like to suggest the mechanism where crossreactivity indeed could lead and trigger that kind of T cell auto aggression. Virus could activate B cells to produce substantial amounts of a crossreacting antibody. This antibody in the case of myasthenia gravis could bind to the receptor areas and increase the autoimmunogenicity of these by releasing receptors hence T cells would be activated which are really truly autoreactive and would in a way amplify or trigger a completely independent real autoimmune response. I think all the elements for such a potential mechanism have been shown in animal models why shouldn't they occur in real life?

INTRODUCTION BY C A JANEWAY TO SESSION ON THE INTERACTION OF AUTO-ANTIGEN, MHC AND T CELL RECEPTOR

I want to begin by talking about some of the questions I find interesting. What we are talking about is how the T cell receptor, MHC and antigen get together and signal a T cell to become activated. The first question is whether the T cell receptor and MHC bind in a single orientation I don't mean a given T cell and a given MHC antigen but all T cells and all MHC antigens? The receptor and ligand interactions always take place in a certain orientation. Second, what role do the CD4 or CD8 play and how do they play it? Third, what is MLS considered in the broader sense of all of those interesting non-antigens that seem to shape the repertoire by deletion in the thymus? In general and broader terms, how does the T cell receptor repertoire play a role in autoimmunity? I will try and deal with that in my talk. Another question is, are CD4 functional subsets relevant in autoimmunity, in fact do they even exist, and finally, what are the T cell autoantigens - what the T cell recognizes as autoantigens and tissues? I would first like to consider some of the players - TCR alpha beta, MHC class I and II antigen in the form of a peptide, CD8 and CD4 and the products of MLS loci, the question is how do they all fit together? My first consideration is the T cell receptor itself. We don't actually know what it looks like but its similarity to immunoglobulin strongly suggests it will look like an immunoglobulin. In immunoglobulins, the third hypervariable region is located basically in a cleft between the two V domains which are part of the V region determined by V gene segments. The third hypervariable region of the T-cell

NATO ASI Series, Vol. H 38
The Molecular Biology of Autoimmune Disease
Edited by A. G. Demaine et al.

receptor, which is made up of junctions, the V alpha and J junction and the V beta, D beta and J beta junctions and where most diversity occurs, would be predicted to lie in the central region of the T cell receptor. To solve this problem we obviously need soluble T cell receptors so we can do direct binding studies. Now the next question is how the antigenic peptide would lie between the two major helices of the MHC class II, one in the alpha chain and one in the beta chain, lying on the curved beta pleated sheet overlying the two immunoglobulin-like domains of class II on the APC. We have been investigating the response of the T-cell clone D10 to peptide antigens. This clone appears to have a site within V beta but outside of the hypervariable region, with a low affinity contact with class II MHC on the beta chain when recognising the antigenic peptide. I think the following will be of some interest to people who are interested in allo-antigens and autoantigens. This same receptor recognizes auto-antigen, and it recognizes a large group of allo antigens. It can see 5 different class II molecules, but this hybrid class II molecule A alpha K, A beta B, meaning that the beta helix is actually carrying the important information. We say its the helix because all of these 5 haplotypes share a common major change in the top of the helix containing a proline, glutamic acid, isoleucine interchange. That's the only common feature of these 5 haplotypes in sequence, and since we know that its the beta chains from this chain shuffling experiment you see A alpha B, A beta K treated as self by this clone. If you then probe the site that makes a low affinity contact with self Ia, that is, A alpha K, A beta K in the presence of antigen, this is now a site of high affinity in allo recognition, and this T cell receptor may be called a type 3 allo reactor. There is probably direct recognition of MHC independent of what peptides are in the groove. Now there are two other reasons why we think that this orientation is fixed and they have to do with some of my other questions. One of the next players is CD4. CD4 in this case not because the clones we work with are all class II restricted as I think CD8 will do the same, but because there is a lot of data now to suggest that CD4, firstly binds to the same class II molecules in the T cell receptor and then secondly, physically interacts with the T cell receptor and finally, when it does, it brings the cytoplasmic enzyme P56 LCK over to the T cell receptor. P56 LCK then phosphorylates the zeta chain on 4 tyrosines. There is some question as to whether another player that I won't talk much about CD45 or T200, which is a tyrosine specific phosphatase (so it removes phosphates from tyrosines) may also play a key role. It has been shown that inhibiting tyrosine phosphatase activity actually has a very funny effect on zeta phosphorylation. There is clearly going to be a lot of data coming up about CD45 which may well be part of this large collection of molecules. I left the CD3 molecules out because they are somewhat inconvenient but we happen to know that when the TCR visibly associates with CD4 bringing LCK over and that signalling can improve a 100 fold and what I mean by that is you need a 100 times less ligand to get the same amount of activation. We have shown that in several different ways and the fact that this is clearly a signalling molecule has led us to refer to this class of molecules as co-receptors. They are physical parts of the receptor and that's the only known function that they have. They do have a negative signalling function that seems to be important in cell separation when no antigen is present. So because this makes meaningful contacts both with the T cell receptor and class II those are presumably stereo specific and if that's true one would have to think that the complex has to be orientated similarly in all such contacts. I am aware that the group in France has postulated that their peptides derived from this region of class II then interfere with CD4 class II association but we don't see any effect. Now I would like to add one more player to this equation and that's the unknown product of the MLS locus. We got frustrated working with MLS and so a couple of years ago we started exploring MLS analogues and we came across some really good ones which we reported called Staphyloccal enterotoxins. These are proteins produced by Staphylocci which when they go into food they make you sick and nobody knows quite how. But they also turn out to be the worlds most potent T cell mitogens and they are now being worked on by many groups. Now these molecules turn out to bind directly and in intact form to the class II MHC molecule. We don't actually know where they bind on the molecule but I think that information will be forthcoming fairly soon. We do know that they bind to the V beta part of the T cell receptor and they bind to that part which is outside the hyper variable region and hence stimulate the T cells. Everything we have ever done with Staphyloccal enterotoxins gives us exactly the same data that we get when we look at MLS locus polymorphism. Whilst that's not proof it at least says that a protein which binds could easily be the product of the MLS locus. There are a whole series of proteins none of which we have been able to physically identify as being the products of MLS. Finally I would like to point out that MLS differences can alter antigen presenting functions by APC by at least 10 fold. A stimulatory MLS APC can present conventional antigens 10 times better than a non-stimulatory one. The affinities contributed are obviously not sufficient to trigger the cell, you need to have the peptide and the hyper variable contact. We think this may help to move things along.

On a different point, I think it should be borne in mind that we are dealing with the T cell world. Now we are somewhat CD4 eccentric if you will, we think the CD4 T cells sits in the centre of the immunological universe and tells every other cell what to do. They tell bone marrow cells to make more non-specific effector cells, they tell B cells to make antibody, they tell macrophages to become activated and destroy intracellular bacteria and they tell CD8 positive T cells to kill or become activated to kill. The question that comes up is does one T cell do all of this or in fact is there heterogeneity in all T cells and of course there has been a lot of data, at least in the mouse, now in the last 3 or 4 years. There are probably two cells with different functions, they have been called TH1 and TH2 or T helper and T inflammatory, you can take your pick. The TH2 cells turn out to be the major B cell activator and uses interleukins 4,5 and 6 to drive B cells to antibody production. The so-called TH1 cell or what we call T inflammatory cell has as its major lymphokines IL-2 and gamma interferon, which are respectively very good as macrophage activators and CTL activators. In automunity it may make a difference whether you activate TH1 or TH2.

THE ADVANTAGES OF LIMITING THE T CELL REPERTOIRE FOR ANTIGEN & MHC

Ann Pullen, Edward Wakeland*, Wayne Potts*, John Kappler, Philippa Marrack
Department of Medicine
Howard Hughes Medical Institute
1400 Jackson Street
Denver, Colorado 80206

T cell receptors are made up of two polypeptides α and β, which are constructed in each cell by rearrangement of one of a number of V (variable), D (diversity) and J (joining) gene segments. The inclusion of nucleotides not encoded in the germline, or the exclusion of germline nucleotides, at the V-J junction also adds to the number of possible receptors. The tremendous flexibility which this type of construction allows has been well established for immunoglobulins and T cell receptors and many millions of combinations are possible. Besides the well known processes of thymic positive and negative selection, mice use a number of strategies to reduce the enormous T cell receptor repertoire available to them. In this paper these strategies will be outlined and their possible advantages will be discussed.

Three strategies are employed by mice to limit their use of Vβ elements: first, deletion of part of the Vβ locus on chromosome 6, secondly, inactivation of genes by point mutation and thirdly, elimination in the thymus of T cells bearing receptors which have reactivity to self 'super' antigens.

Analysis of the structure of the murine V_β locus in inbred laboratory mice has established that there are two major V_β haplotypes. The majority of common stains carry the V_β^b haplotype which encodes about 20 V_β elements (Behlke et al., 1985, Barth et al., 1985, Patten et al., 1984). A few strains, including SJL, SWR, C57L and C57BR, carry the V_β^a haplotype which has a deletion of 9 of the V_β genes (Behlke et al., 1986).

The few strains which carry the V_β^a haplotype carry a functional $V_\beta17a$ gene (Kappler et al., 1987a) while an inactivated form of this gene ($V_\beta17b$) is present in mice of the V_β^b haplotype. Inactivation of $V_\beta17b$ is due to a point mutation in the coding region which results in a termination codon (Wade et al., 1988).

*Department of Pathology, University of Florida, Gainesville, Florida

NATO ASI Series, Vol. H 38
The Molecular Biology of Autoimmune Disease
Edited by A. G. Demaine et al.

We recently reported that T cells bearing receptors including the $V_{\beta}17a$ element were reactive to IE (Kappler *et al.*, 1987a) and that in mice bearing IE these T cells were eliminated in the thymus (Kappler *et al.*, 1987b). Since this demonstration of tolerance to self antigens by clonal deletion there have been many reports from our lab and others of the elimination of T cells bearing receptors including V_{β} elements with particular reactivities to self antigens (Table 1).

Table 1

V_{β} Recognition of Self 'Super' Antigens

Self Super Antigen	Reactive V_{β} Elements	Reference
Unknown B Cell Product and IE	17a	Kappler, *et al.*, 1987a
Unknown Product and IE	5	Bill, Kanagawa & Palmer, in prep,
	11	Tomonari & Lovering, 1988
		Bill, *et al.*, 1989
	12	Bill, Appel & Palmer, 1988
$Mls\text{-}1^{a}$ (Chromosome 1)	6	MacDonald, *et al.*, 1988,
	8.1	Kappler, *et al.*, 1988
	9	Happ, Woodland & Palmer, 1989
$Mls\text{-}2^{a}$ (Linkage Unknown)	3	Pullen, *et al.*, 1988
$Mls\text{-}3^{a}$ (Linked to Ly-7)	3	Pullen, *et al.*, 1989

We have termed these self antigens 'super' antigens to distinguish them from conventional antigens because they stimulate T cells bearing a particular V_{β} element virtually regardless of the other components of the T cell receptor on these cells. Moreover, recognition of 'super' antigens is not as strictly MHC restricted as that of conventional antigens (Kappler et al., 1988, Pullen et al., 1988). Presentation by class II molecules is required but many different IE or IA molecules are capable of presenting each self 'super' antigen to a particular T cell.

All the above studies on the T cell repertoire have been carried out using inbred mice and we felt it would be informative to examine wild mouse populations to determine whether the phenomena observed in captive inbred mice were reflected in wild mouse populations which are presumably surviving under intense selective pressure.

Using a panel of monoclonal antibodies (Table 2) we examined peripheral T cells and thymocytes from a panel of 27 wild mice for their expression of a number of V_β elements.

Table 2

Antibodies used in these experiments

V_β Target	Antibody	Source
2	B20	Malissen (unpublished)
3	KJ25	Pullen, Marrack & Kappler, 1988
5	MR9-4	Kanagawa (unpublished)
6	RR4-7	Kanagawa, Palmer & Bill, 1988
7	TR130	Okada (unpublished)
8.1, 8.2, 8.3	F23.1	Staerz, et al., 1985
8.1, 8.2	KJ16	Haskins, et al., 1984
8.2	F23.2	Staerz, et al., 1985
11	RR3-15	Bill, et al., 1988
17a	KJ23a	Kappler, et al., 1987a
All	597	Kubo, et al., 1989

When levels of T cells bearing a particular V_β were low in the periphery, analysis of the stained thymocytes was made to determine whether the absence of the cells in the periphery was due to deletion of the gene or elimination of self-reactive cells in the thymus. A summary of the data is shown in Table 3.

Table 3

Elimination of Peripheral T Cells Expressing Particular V_βs is common in Wild Mice

	Strategy for V_β Elimination				
	Homozygous Genetic Deletion	Homozygous Point Mutation	Tolerance to Self Super-Antigens		
			IE	Mls-1[a]	Mls-2[a]
V_β Eliminated	5, 8, 13 12, 11, 9 6, 15	17	5	6, 8.1	3
Number of Wild Mice Showing this Elimination	13/27	27/27	13/14	5/14	22/27

The staining data showed that many of the mice examined bore a homozygous chromosomal deletion which included V_β5, 6, 8 and 11. Southern blot analysis of genomic DNA from these animals showed that the deletion extended over the region from V_β5 - V_β15, and included V_β6 and V_β15 which are not deleted in SJL. None of the wild mice contained any $V_\beta17a^+$ T cells. Southern blot analysis of liver DNA from the wild mice showed a restriction fragment length polymorphism identical with BALB/c V_β17 rather than SJL, suggesting the presence of the V_β17b nonfunctional allele.

All the examples of tolerance to self 'super' antigens which have been reported for inbred strains (Table 1) were also observed in the wild mice analyzed. In fact the extent to which the animals reduced their repertoire by this mechanism was remarkable.

Only one mouse had high levels of V_β5 expression, the others had either deleted the gene or had eliminated the $V_\beta5^+$ T cells in the thymus presumably in response to an unknown product and IE. It should be noted that the picture for $V_\beta11^+$ T cells was less clear, since there were IE^+ wild mice which had not eliminated their $V_\beta11^+$ T cells.

Initially we proposed that the elimination of a large number of self-reactive T cells by self 'super' antigens was advantageous to mice because it would reduce the likelihood of autoimmune disease perhaps by deleting T cell clones with autoimmune potential which might be poorly tolerized by conventional self antigens. The extent of the T cell repertoire in different mice would be determined by a balance between selection for a large repertoire to allow responsiveness to foreign antigens and selection for a small repertoire to limit autoreactivity.

More recently, however, we have realized the significance of another group of 'super' antigens, the Staphylococcal enterotoxins (White et al., 1989, Janeway, et al., 1989). Like self 'super' antigens these proteins are able to stimulate large numbers of T cells bearing particular V_β elements and have degenerate MHC requirements for their presentation. We now think that V_β elimination in mice may have been selected by the deleterious effects of this type of foreign 'super' antigen. Stimulation of large numbers of T cells bearing particular V_β elements by S. aureus may result in massive release of lymphokines with dramatic effects on the physiology of the mouse. We have observed a 17% weight loss in 68 hours after administration of 250 µg SEB ip (unpublished observation) and are currently investigating other lymphokine mediated effects. Moreover, the ability of the mice to respond to other foreign antigens after treatment with SEB is markedly suppressed (unpublished data). This massive T cell activation may be essential to the mechanism of action of some bacterial toxins and perhaps is of some advantage to the micro-organism as a temporary immunosuppressive mechanism.

References

Barth R, Kim S, Lan N, Hunkapillar T, Sobieck N, Winoto A, Gershenfeld H, Okada C, Hansburg D, Weissman I, Hood L (1985) The murine T-cell receptor uses a limited repertoire of expressed V_β gene segments. Nature 316:517.

Behlke M, Chou H, Huppi K, Loh, D (1986) Murine T cell receptor mutants with deletions of β-chain variable region genes. Proc Natl Acad Sci USA 83:767.

Behlke M, Spinella D, Chou H, Sha W, Hartt D, Loh D (1985) T cell receptor β-chain expression: dependence on relatively few variable region genes. Science 229:566.

Bill J, Apple V, Palmer E (1988) An analysis of T-cell receptor V-gene expression in MHC-disparate mice. Proc Natl Acad Sci USA 85:9184.

Bill J, Kanagawa O, Woodland D, Palmer E (1989) The MHC molecule, I-E, is necessary but not different for the clonal deletion of $V_{\beta}11$ bearing T-cells. J Exp Med (in press).

Happ MP, Woodland DL, Palmer E (1989) A third T cell receptor V_{β} gene that encodes reactivity to $Mls\text{-}1^{a}$ gene products. Submitted for publication.

Haskins K, Hannum C, White J, Roehm N, Kubo R, Kappler J, Marrack P (1984) The major histocompatibility complex-restricted antigen receptor on T cells. VI. An antibody to a receptor allotype. J Exp Med 160:452.

Janeway Jr CA, Yagi JY, Conrad PJ, Katz ME, Jones B, Vroegop S, Buxser S (1989) T-cell responses to Mls and to bacterial proteins that mimic its behavior. Immunol Rev107:61-88.

Kanagawa O, Palmer E, Bill J (1989) The T cell receptor $V_{\beta}6$ domain imparts reactivity to $Mls\text{-}1^{a}$. Cell Immunol (in press).

Kappler J, Roehm N, Marrack P (1987b) T cell tolerance by clonal elimination in the thymus. Cell 49:273.

Kappler JW, Staerz U, White J, Marrack PC (1988) Self-tolerance eliminates T cells specific for Mls-modified products of the major histocompatibility complex. Nature 332:35.

Kappler J, Wade T, White J, Kushnir E, Blackman M, Bill J, Roehm R, Marrack P (1987a) A T cell receptor V_{β} segment that imparts reactivity to a class II major histocompatibility complex product. Cell 49:263.

Kubo RT, Born W, Kappler JW, Marrack P, Pigeon M (1989) Characterization of a monoclonal antibody which detects all murine α/β T cell receptors. J Immunol (in press).

MacDonald HR, Scheider R, Lees RK, Howe RC, Acha-Orbea H, Festenstein H, Zinkernagel RM, Hengartner H (1988) T-cell receptor V_{β} use predicts reactivity and tolerance to Mls^{a}-encoded antigens. Nature 332:40.

Patten P, Yokota T, Rothbard J, Chien Y, Arai K, Davis M (1984) Structure, expression and divergence of T-cell receptor β chain variable regions. Nature 314:40.

Pullen AM, Marrack P, Kappler JW (1988) The T cell repertoire is heavily influenced by tolerance to polymorphic self antigens. Nature 335:796.

Pullen AM, Marrack P, Kappler JW (1989) Evidence that Mls-2 antigens which delete $V_{\beta}3^{+}$ T cells are controlled by multiple genes. J Immunol (in press).

Staerz U, Rammansee H, Benedetto J, Bevan M (1985) Characterization of a murine monoclonal antibody specific for an allotypic determinant on T cell antigen receptor. J Immunol 134:3994.

Tomonari K, Lovering E (1988) T-cell receptor-specific monoclonal antibodies against a V_β11-positive mouse T-cell clone. Immunogenetics 28:445-451.

Wade T, Bill J, Marrack PC, Palmer E, Kappler JW (1988) Molecular basis for the nonexpression of V_β17 in some strains of mice. J Immunol 141:2165-2167.

White J, Herman A, Pullen AM, Kubo R, Kappler JW, Marrack P (1989) The V_β-specific superantigen staphylococcal enterotoxin B: stimulation of mature T cells and clonal deletion in neonatal mice. Cell 56:27-35.

DISCUSSION

TROWSDALE: That was very interesting. You slightly glossed over the different IE and IA specificities, could you say anymore about which haplotypes associated with the toxins and which were affecting MLS - that is, is there some specificity in the bindings to IE or IA?

PULLEN: With MLS it certainly binds to IE and IA - some of the data is already published but for example in H2Q the IA of Q does not present, whilst in K and D both IA and IE can bind. With the enterotoxins I'm not familiar with all the haplotypes they have tried.

JANEWAY: Yes, I can add a little bit on that because its not always binding, you have to understand that the enterotoxins have to bind both to the IA and the T cell receptor in such a way that they can be brought together. For instance, strain B10GD which has A of D and E is a very poor responder to staphyloccal enterotoxins whereas B10B2 which has E is also a good responder but if you look at binding the enterotoxin binds equally to A and E so it looks as though the E molecule, and the A molecule are competent to bind but relatively incompetent to stimulate. We have looked at 20 clones that respond to enterotoxin presented by A of D or E of D and none of them respond to it. Also in man, some direct binding studies have been done and I don't recall which of the MHC molecules, enterotoxin binds to, although they bind to different ones and with much higher affinity than they do with the mouse

TROWSDALE: What I am getting at, are there any distinct sequences that you can identify in IA or in IE or in man for example, DQ or DR that might be related to activation with various toxins?

PULLEN: We haven't done those studies.

JANEWAY: I would just like to add a comment. Diane Mathis has shown that none of the amino acids that line the class II cleft and are critical for presentation of peptides are required for presentation of staphyloccal enterotoxins so presumably they bind elsewhere although it hasn't formally been proved.

DEMAINE: Two questions. First, when you look in your wild type mice, do you ever find any duplication and hence selection of the genes which are retained in these mice?

PULLEN: We haven't looked. All we have done is the antibody staining and then gone to check and confirm what we found in the thymus? We haven't looked at the whole chromosome.

DEMAINE: Also, would you expect in the future to find any sort of correlations with V alpha deletions or do you think they will be specific for V beta?

PULLEN: We really don't know, I mean obviously at the moment we can't look at V alpha because there are very few of the alpha monoclonals available but who knows. So far there doesn't seem to be any evidence to suggest its going to be, but we can't exclude it yet.

PUJOL-BORRELL: Just a short question related to the point that was raised this morning by Alan McGregor on the fact that in some spontaneous autoimmune diseases in animals the incidence is dramatically decreased in general if these animals are kept in a germ free environment, do you have any data on the utilisation of V beta genes?

PULLEN: No and I can tell you that every mice that's been fed in our facility is definitely not germ free its probably got every enterotoxin you can imagine.

JANEWAY: Enterotoxins are totally distinct from conventional mitogens on several criteria; first of all you have to have IA or IE to get a response, they have to be bound to an IA bearing cell, whereas T cell mitogens work directly in the T cell. You don't need any class II you need CD4 which generally for T cell mitogens you don't need and the most important and obvious thing is that they work only on certain V betas.

PULLEN: Obviously they result in mitosis but they are not acting directly on the T cell, people get confused about what to call a mitogen but they are not acting directly on the T cell they have this very loose MHC requirement, but they definitely need it.

FUNCTIONAL DISSOCIATION OF T CELL SITES; IMMUNOGENIC, ANTIGENIC AND PATHOGENIC SITES[1]

Dale S. Gregerson*§, Steven P. Fling§ and Wesley F. Obritsch*
Departments of *Ophthalmology and §Microbiology
University of Minnesota
Minneapolis, MN 55455 USA

Carmen F. Merryman
Department of Biochemistry and Molecular Biology
Thomas Jefferson University
Philadelphia, PA 10107 USA

Larry A. Donoso
Wills Eye Hospital Research Division
9th & Walnut Streets
Philadelphia, PA 10107 USA

ABSTRACT

Experimental autoimmune uveoretinitis (EAU) is a $CD4^+$ T-cell mediated autoimmune disease induced by S-antigen, a retinal photoreceptor cell protein. In order to identify T cell recognition sites responsible for pathogenicity, cyanogen bromide fragments and synthetic peptides were used to test uveitogenic T cell lines prepared against native S-antigen. Two non-overlapping synthetic peptides known to actively induce EAU did not induce proliferative responses in these T cell lines. In contrast, an adjacent synthetic peptide which was unable to actively induce EAU elicited strong proliferative responses from the T cell lines and gave rise to a uveitogenic line. Our results indicate that spatially distinct T cell epitopes are present in S-antigen which are responsible for the active induction of EAU, lymphocyte proliferation, and the ability to adoptively transfer EAU.

INTRODUCTION

Retinal S-antigen (S-Ag) elicits experimental autoimmune uveoretinitis (EAU) following immunization with antigen in complete Freund's adjuvant. S-Ag-specific T cell lines prepared from sensitized Lewis rats show that EAU can be adoptively transferred to syngeneic recipients by activated, $CD4^+$ T cells (Gregerson et al, 1986b, 1987). Identification of the T cell recognition sites in S-Ag, particularly uveitogenic sites, has been investigated by analysis of the specificity and uveitogenicity of T cell lines raised to bovine and human S-Ag using cyanogen bromide (CB) fragments of S-Ag

[1]This work was supported by NIH grants EY-05417 (D.S.G.), EY-05095 (L.A.D.), Research to Prevent Blindness, the Crippled Children's Vitreo-Retinal Research Foundation (L.A.D.), and the Pennsylvania Lions Sight Conservation and Eye Research Foundation (L.A.D.). D.S.G. is a Research to Prevent Blindness Senior Scientific Investigator.

NATO ASI Series, Vol. H 38
The Molecular Biology of Autoimmune Disease
Edited by A. G. Demaine et al.

(Gregerson et al, 1986a,b, 1987; Knospe et al, 1988), and by testing overlapping synthetic peptides corresponding to S-Ag for the ability to actively induce EAU (Donoso et al, 1986, 1988). By immunization with synthetic peptides, two non-overlapping uveitogenic sites, 12 residues in length, have been identified (Donoso et al, 1987, 1988). Both of these pathogenic sites are contained within a 123 residue peptide produced by CNBr cleavage of bovine S-Ag (CB123). CB123 is uveitogenic and a T cell line raised to CB123 adoptively transfers EAU (Gregerson et al, 1987). None of the other CB-peptides of S-Ag were uveitogenic.

In this study we have used synthetic peptides to further define the T cell sites in S-Ag. The results show that S-Ag contains multiple pathogenic and proliferative sites and that although the pathogenic and proliferative sites could be clearly dissociated into non-overlapping sites, T cells to one of the proliferative sites retained the ability to adoptively transfer EAU.

MATERIALS AND METHODS

Animals and immunizations. Specific pathogen-free female Lewis rats were immunized in a single footpad with 25 to 50 μg of peptides or S-Ag in complete Freund's adjuvant containing 2.5 mg/ml *M. tuberculosis* H-37Ra.

S-Antigen preparation. S-Ag's were isolated as described (Gregerson et al, 1986b). Peptides resulting from CNBr cleavage of bovine S-Ag were prepared as described (Gregerson et al, 1986a). These peptides are shown in (Fig.1).

Synthetic peptides. Synthetic peptides were made by conventional solid phase techniques. Where relevant, the amino acid sequences of the peptides are shown in the Tables; other peptides are shown on Fig. 1. Peptides are denoted by the origin of their sequence, whether bovine S-Ag (BSA) or human S-Ag (HSA) followed by the positions of the first and last residues.

Lymphocyte culture and proliferation assays. These were done as previously described (Gregerson et al, 1986b). The R9 line was selected from a rat immunized with bovine S-Ag by repeated selection in culture with bovine S-Ag while the R17 line was raised from a human S-Ag immunized rat by *in vitro* selection with human S-Ag. Both lines express T helper cell phenotype ($W3/13^+$, $W3/25^+$, $OX8^-$) and are class II MHC restricted. The potent uveitogenic activity of these two lines and their responses to bovine CB

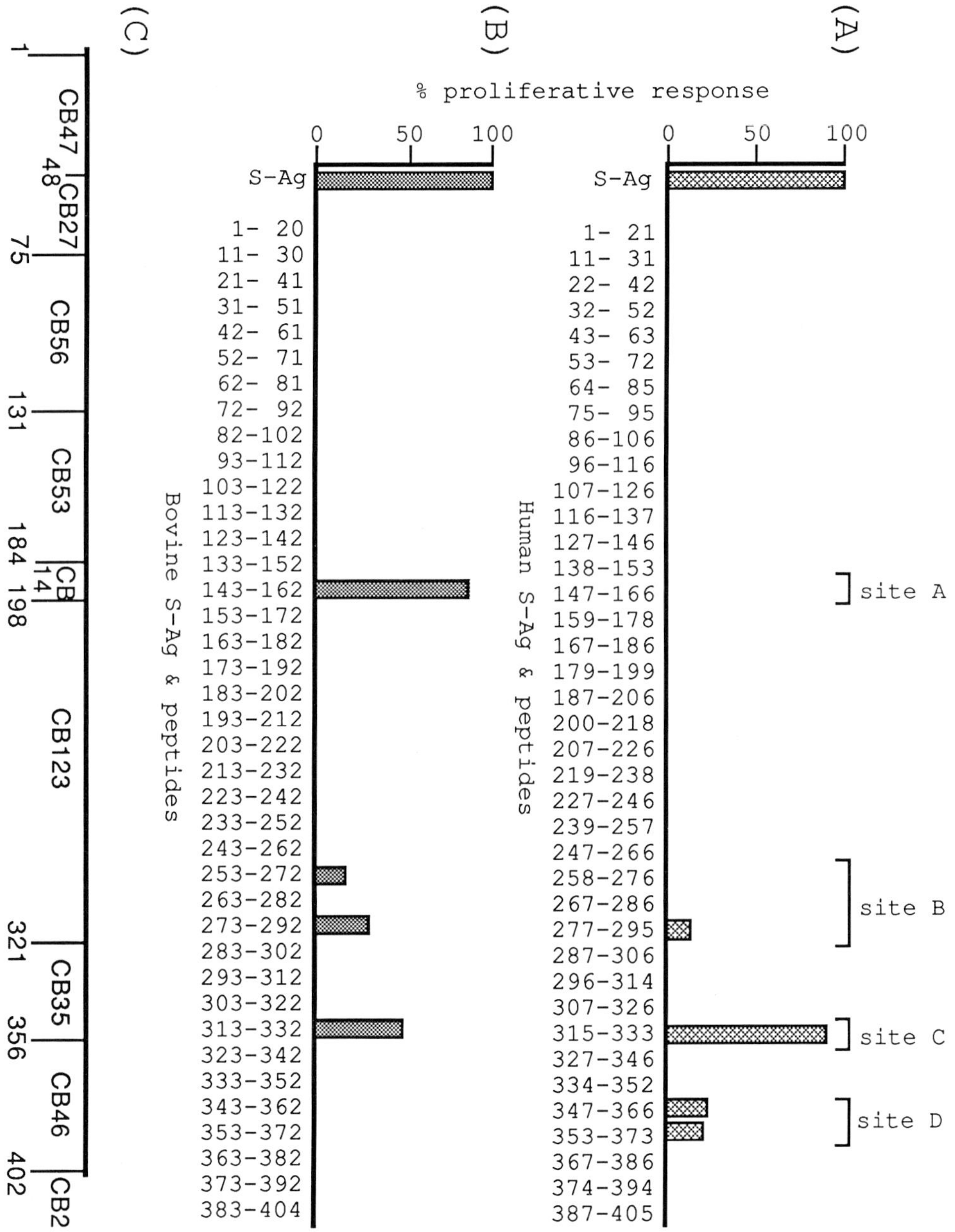

Figure 1. Identification of the major T cell proliferative sites in (A) human and (B) bovine S-Ag. T cell lines isolated from a bovine S-Ag immunized Le rat (R9 line) or a human S-Ag immunized rat (R17 line) were tested for proliferation to synthetic peptides corresponding to bovine and human S-Ag, respectively. Responses are shown as a per cent of the response to intact S-Ag. (C). Orientation of the cyanogen bromide (CB) peptides of bovine S-Ag. Peptides are designated by their lengths in residues.

peptides have been reported (Gregerson et al, 1986a,b). Routine screening was done at peptide concentrations of 0.25 and 1.25 µM. In experiments not shown here, concentrations between 0.01 and 10 µM were also used wherever any sign of response or evidence of pathogenicity was found.

RESULTS

Screening retinal S-Ag for T cell recognition sites. The ability of synthetic peptides to induce lymphocyte proliferative responses in the R9 and R17 T cell lines was tested. The results of multiple, separate screening experiments are summarized in Fig. 1. Four regions of S-Ag capable of eliciting significant proliferative responses from one or both of the T cell lines were identified. No peptide corresponding to the previously reported pathogenic sites, BSA 286-297 and BSA 303-314, tested over a wide concentration range, was able to stimulate a significant proliferative response in either T cell line. These four major proliferative sites were characterized more precisely, particularly those sites designated B and C, which are adjacent to known pathogenic sequences.

Characterization of site "B" in CB123. The results of proliferative assays of the R9 and R17 lines are shown in Table 1. Two adjacent, non-overlapping

TABLE 1. Proliferative Responses to Synthetic Peptides at Site B.

		Proliferation[a]			
		Lymph	R9 line		R17
Peptide	Sequence[b]	Node[c]	3X[d]	7X	7X
BSA 257-295	...KTVAAEEAQEKVPPNSSLTKTLTLVPLLANNRERRGIAL...	150	34	38	-[f]
HSA 261-299[e]	...*P**M**********T*******L***************...	-	-	-	78
BSA 253-272	...KTVAAEEAQEKVPPNS	12	13	-	2
HSA 258-276	..KPVAMEEAQEKVPPNS	-	-	-	2
BSA 261-280	AEEAQEKEPPNSSLTKTLTL	-	7	2	1
BSA 263-282	EAQEKVPPNSSLTKTLTLVP	38	5	1	1
HSA 267-286	EAQEKVPPNSTLTKTLTLLP	-	-	2	1
BSA 270-289	PNSSLTKTLTLVPLLANNRE	-	-	4	1
HSA 277-295	TLTKTLTLLPLLANNRERR	-	-	2	6
BSA 273-292	SLTKTLTLVPLLANNRERRG	43	20	12	2
BSA 281-302	VPLLANNRERRGIAL...	-	-	1	1
BSA 283-302	(pathogenic)[g] LLA<u>NNRERRGIAL..</u>.	8	6	3	1
control		5	4	2	1

[a]Cpm's x 10^{-3}. [b]Sequence and numbering of bovine S-Ag from Shinohara et al (1987). [c]Lymph node cells from bovine S-Ag sensitized animal. [d]Number of *in vitro* cycles of selection and propagation of the R9 and R17 lines on bovine and human S-Ag, respectively. [e]Sequence of human S-Ag (HSA) is from Yamaki et al (1988). [f](-), not determined. [g]The minimal pathogenic sequence is underlined.

peptides, BSA 253-272 and BSA 273-292, were found to stimulate the bovine specific R9 line, but not the human specific R17 line. The human sequence, HSA 277-295, corresponding to the bovine proliferation site BSA 273-292, induced a modest response in the R17 line. Peptides BSA 283-302 and HSA 287-306 actively induce EAU, but did not elicit proliferative responses from either line. The response to site B peptides was lost with repeated selections. BSA 273-292 partially overlaps the minimal uveitogenic sequence BSA 286-297, but was unable to actively induce EAU.

Analysis of proliferative site "C". Both T cell lines proliferated to the screening peptides from site C which overlap the uveitogenic site at BSA 303-314 by a single residue (Table 2). Further characterization showed that the full proliferative response could be elicited by BSA 317-328 which does not overlap the pathogenic site. The two residue differences between the human and bovine sequence had no effect on the responses. The pathogenic peptides BSA 303-322 and HSA 307-326 did not induce proliferative responses in either line. Neither BSA 313-332 nor HSA 315-333 actively induce EAU.

TABLE 2. Fine Specificity of the Proliferative Response at Site C.

		Proliferation[a]		
Peptide	Sequence[b]	Lymph Node[c]	R9 3X[d]	R17 8X
BSA 303-342	...DTNLASSTIIKEGIDKTVMGILVSYQIKVKLTVSGLLGEL...	-[f]	34	-
HSA 307-346[e]	...***************R**L****************F****...	-	-	117
BSA 303-322	DTNLASSTIIKEGIDKTVMG (pathogenic)[g]	12	5	1
HSA 315-333	IIKEGIDRTVLGILVSYQI	-	-	106
BSA 313-332	KEGIDKTVMGILVSYQIKVK	78	32	73
BSA 313-328	KEGIDKTVMGILVSYQ	88	-	94
BSA 313-326	KEGIDKTVMGILVS	25	-	22
BSA 313-324	KEGIDKTVMGIL	15	-	6
BSA 313-322	KEGIDKTVMG	8	-	2
BSA 315-332	GIDKTVMGILVSYQIKVK	84	-	94
BSA 317-332	DKTVMGILVSYQIKVK	65	-	99
BSA 319-332	TVMGILVSYQIKVK	27	-	96
BSA 321-332	MGILVSYQIKVK	5	-	48
BSA 323-332	ILVSYQIKVK	5	-	3
BSA 317-328	DKTVMGILVSYQ	23	-	98
BSA 323-342	ILVSYQIKVKLTVSGLLGEL	5	3	1
control		4	4	1

[a]Footnotes as in Table 1.

Long term selection of the R9 line on bovine S-Ag resulted in gradual loss of responsiveness to this epitope. Conversely, attempts to select a peptide-specific BSA 313-332 response from the lines using the synthetic peptides were successful, yielding sublines which were peptide specific.

R9 line cells selected with peptide BSA 313-332 *in vitro* were assessed for the ability to adoptively transfer EAU. Selected cells rapidly lost responsiveness to other peptides (Table 3) but were still able to transfer EAU to 4 of 6 recipients. These cells did not respond to peptides containing the BSA 303-314 pathogenic site which lacked the proliferative site (residues 317-328) and did not respond to CB123 which contains both the pathogenic sites and to which R9 cells are otherwise highly responsive.

Table 3. Selection of Peptide-Specific Lines.

In vitro Selection			Proliferative response									
					S-antigen		BSA Peptides				CBpeptides	
Line Cell	# of Cycles	Selective Antigen	Media	Con A	BSA	HSA	143-162	303-322	313-332	343-362	CB123	CB46
R9	7	BSA	7	285	217	46	68	7	46	6	143	44
R9[a]	4	313-332	18	135	119	-	27	20	103	-	-	-
R9	5	"	2	37	15	12	2	2	10	-	-	-
R9	6	"	1	50	12	-	-	-	16	-	1	1
R9	6	"	3	141	15	10	3	4	30	-	-	-

[a]The R9 cells had been through 7 cycles of selection and propagation on bovine S-Ag prior to this time.

Proliferative sites "A" and "D". The response to site D was unique to the R17 line (Table 4), although the bovine and human sequences are identical except for a two residue deletion in the human sequence which is apparently

TABLE 4. Specificity of the Response at Site D.

		Proliferation[a]		
Peptide	Sequence[b]	Lymph Node[c]	R9 4X[d]	R17 7X
BSA 339-380	...LGELTSSEVATEVPFRLMHPQEDPDTAKESFQDENFVFEEF...	140	34	-[f]
HSA 343-382[e]	...************************--****I**A*L*****...	-	-	140
BSA 339-355	LGELTSSEVATEVPFRL	-	-	3
BSA 343-362	TSSEVATEVPFRLMHPQPED	12	3	31
HSA 353-373	TEVPFRLMHPQPEDP--AKESYQ	-	-	44
BSA 352-372	FRLMHPQPEDPDTAKESFQD	3	3	26
BSA 363-382	PDTAKESFQDENFVFEEF	3	3	4
control		4	4	4

[a]Footnotes as in Table 1.

outside of the site. Stimulation by peptides HSA 353-373, HSA 347-366 and

BSA 353-373 indicates that the critical residues lie within the sequence FRLMHPQPEDP. None of these synthetic peptides actively induces EAU. Only the R9 line responded to BSA 143-162 in site A, and it did not cross-react with the human sequence which differs at 3 residues (data not shown). None of the synthetic peptides from this region are actively pathogenic.

DISCUSSION

The dissociation of proliferative and pathogenic sites emphasizes the complexity of the immune response to S-Ag, despite the ability of small peptides or peptide-specific T cell lines to mediate EAU. Synthetic peptides have also been used to map separate determinants for adoptive transfer, lymphocyte proliferation, and active induction of disease in EAE (Mannie et al, 1985; Offner et al, 1988; Sakai et al, 1988).

An explanation offered by Mannie et al (1985) and Fox et al (1987) regarding dissociation of pathogenic and proliferative responses is that the cell type which transfers disease is not a proliferative cell. While this point could be argued in their experiments which used unselected lymph node and spleen cells, our demonstration of pathogenesis in lines repeatedly selected *in vitro* would not be possible if the uveitogenic cells did not expand and remain in the population. Although it is a formal argument that a small population of cells could be carried along by lymphokines, our data regarding *in vitro* selection of lines with peptides show that such activities, even of cells with proliferative potential, are rapidly lost. It could be argued that the proliferative response helps the pathogenic response, although proliferative cells are fully able to transfer EAU.

In the results reported by Mannie et al (1985), the functional sites substantially overlapped; since unselected cells were used, the specificity and heterogeneity of the responding cells is not known. Also, activation for pathogenesis as opposed to proliferation could be a result of sub-threshold activation, as the epitopes were not shown to be significantly different in location. It is possible that the activation level required to confer pathogenicity on a cell need not drive it to proliferate *in vitro*. In S-Ag, the sites did not overlap, being separated by 3-4 amino acid residues.

An explanation for our finding of epitopes that are spatially separated and functionally distinct involves antigen processing. T cells must recognize the target antigen to mediate EAU. For a synthetic peptide to be pathogenic, it must represent, following its own potential processing (Fox et al, 1988), a peptide generated from the target autoantigen in its tissue site. Data from Offner et al (1988) are consistent with differences in processing affecting the generation of specificities to the encephalitogenic region of MBP. They found an encephalitogenic clone with specificity for a peptide that did not actively induce EAE.

REFERENCES

Donoso LA, Merryman CF, Sery TW, Shinohara T, Dietzschold B, Smith A, Kalsow CM (1987) S-antigen: characterization of a pathogenic epitope which mediates experimental autoimmune uveitis and pinealitis in Lewis rats. Curr Eye Res 6:1151-1159

Donoso LA, Merryman CF, Shinohara T, Dietzschold B, Wistow G, Craft C, Morley W, Henry RT (1986) S-antigen: identification of the MAbA9-C6 monoclonal antibody binding site and the uveitopathogenic sites. Curr Eye Res 5:995-1004

Donoso LA, Yamaki K, Merryman CF, Shinohara T, Yue S, Sery TW (1988) Human S-antigen: characterization of uveitopathogenic sites. Curr Eye Res 7:1077-1085

Fox BS, Carbone FR, Germain RN, Paterson Y, Schwartz RH (1988) Processing of a minimal antigenic peptide alters its interaction with MHC molecules. Nature 331:538-540

Fox GM, Redmond TM, Wiggert B, Kuwabara T, Chader GJ, Gery I (1987) Dissociation between lymphocyte activation for proliferation and for the capacity to adoptively transfer uveoretinitis. J Immunol 138:3242-3246

Gregerson DS, Fling SP, Wohlhueter RM (1986a) Characterization of immunologically active cyanogen bromide peptide fragments of bovine and human retinal S-antigen. Exp Eye Res 43:803-818

Gregerson DS, Obritsch WF, Fling SP (1987) Identification of a uveitogenic cyanogen bromide peptide of bovine retinal S-antigen and preparation of a uveitogenic, peptide-specific T cell line. Eur J Immunol 17:405-411

Gregerson DS, Obritsch WF, Fling SP, Cameron JD (1986b) S-antigen-specific rat T cell lines recognize peptide fragments of S-antigen and mediate experimental autoimmune uveoretinitis and pinealitis. J Immunol 136:2875-2882

Knospe V, Fling SP, Gregerson DS (1988) Assignment of several epitopes to cyanogen bromide peptides of bovine retinal S-antigen by immunoblotting with peptide-specific antibodies. Curr Eye Res 7:181-189

Mannie MD, Paterson PY, U'Prichard DC, Flouret G (1985) Induction of experimental allergic encephalomyelitis in Lewis rats with purified synthetic peptides: Delineation of antigenic determinants for encephalitogenicity, in vitro activation of cellular transfer, and proliferation of lymphocytes. Proc Natl Acad Sci USA 87:5515-5519

Offner H, Hashim GA, Chou YK, Celnik B, Jones R, Vandenbark AA (1988) Encephalitogenic T cell clones with variant receptor specificity. J Immunol 141:3828-3832

Sakai K, Sinha AA, Mitchel DJ, Zamvil SS, Rothbard JB, McDevitt HO, Steinman L (1988) Involvement of distinct murine T-cell receptors in the autoimmune encephalitogenic response to nested epitopes of myelin basic protein. Proc Natl Acad Sci USA 85:8608-8612

Shinohara T, Dietzschold B, Craft CM, Wistow G, Early JJ, Donoso LA, Horwitz J, Tao R (1987) Primary and secondary structure of bovine retinal S antigen (48-kDa protein). Proc Natl Acad Sci USA 84:6975-6979

Yamaki K, Tsuda M, Shinohara T (1988) The sequence of human retinal S-antigen reveals similarities with α-transducin. FEBS Lett 234:39-43

DISCUSSION

ALLEN: It is interesting that when you look at EAE, the 1-11 epitope of MBP recognized by the murine T cell clones is not predicted by the Berzofsky or the Rothbard algorithms. Are there any T cell epitopes on S-ag recgonized by your T cell lines that are not predicted by any of the algorithsms?

GREGERSON: The relationship between T cell sites and the predictions based on the Berzofsky or Rothbard algorithms can be summarized as follows. The proliferative site at residues 143-162 contains a Rothbard site (residues 150-154) but does not contain or overlap a Berzofsky site. The proliferative site at residues 253-272 contains a Rothbard site (residues 253-257) but no Berzofsky site. The proliferative site at 273-289 does not contain, or overlap, either type of predicted site. The pathogenic site at 285-297 contains a Rothbard site (residues 292-296). The pathogenic site at 303-314 slightly overlaps a Berzofsky site (residues 312-318) and the proliferative site at 317-328 partially overlaps the opposite end of the same Berzofsky site. Finally, the proliferative site at 352-364 contains a Rothbard site (residues 354-357) and a small Berzofsky site at 362-364.

At first glance, there seems to be a significant association of observed T cell sites with predicted sites; conversely, when one considers that 40% of S-Ag is predicted by the algorithms, there is not much room to accommodate sequences of 12-14 residues which do not overlap a predicted site. It may be more instructive to note that of the 28 predicted sites, only 6 are contained in or partially overlap known T cell sites. If one were to test the predictions by making 15 residue peptides corresponding to the predicted sites, approximately 90% of the entire sequence would be represented; this would not be a particularly strategic approach.

JANEWAY: You have mentioned that EAU in rats is much more severe when you immunize with S-ag in CFA whilst with activated T cell transfer, a milder lymphocytic infiltrate is apparent. Is there a role for antibody in the EAU model? Immunization with a soluble protein in CFA will induce large amounts of antibody whilst with the T cell transfer experiments, no antibody is detectable because, if transferred, T cell may actually switch off the antibody production?

GREGERSON: We did not intend to suggest that actively induced EAU is much more severe than that found following adoptive transfer of T cells. Certain T cell lines, including two presented at these meetings, do appear to be limited in their ability to transfer EAU, but this is not generally true of all the lines; some are highly pathogenic. No active role for antibody in the pathogenesis of EAU has been demonstrated to our knowledge and EAU cannot be transferred with antibody. There was one report several years ago suggesting that pre-treatment of animals with cobra venom C3 inactivator reduced the severity of EAU. Since the EAU elicited by T cell transfer as opposed to active induction has a different time course, it has been difficult to compare the histologic findings in any quantitative fashion. It has, however, been our subjective impression that PMN's are more prominent in the active disease than in EAU following adoptive transfer where a mononuclear infiltrate and hemorrhage seem more common. This would be consistent with some role for antibody in the pathogenesis.

AUTOREACTIVE CLONED T CELL LINES IN MURINE INSULIN-DEPENDENT DIABETES MELLITUS

Eva-Pia Reich, Satyajit Rath, Robert Sherwin, Hugh McDevitt, and Charles A. Janeway, Jr.
Section of Immunobiology
Howard Hughes Medical Institute, Yale University School of Medicine
New Haven, CT 06510

Cloned T cell lines expressing either CD4 or CD8 have been isolated from the islets of acutely diabetic NOD mice. These cloned T cell lines respond by proliferating specifically to islets from mice bearing MHC gene products of the NOD strain. Adoptive transfer of cloned T cell lines into irradiated recipients shows intense insulitis and occasional frank diabetes in recipients of both $CD4^+$ and $CD8^+$ cloned T cell lines, but only mild insulitis and no overt disease in recipients of either CD4 or CD8 cloned T cell lines alone. This experimental system will be used to probe three areas of insulin-dependent diabetes mellitus: first, what is the pathogenesis of ß cell destruction in IDDM. Second, what it the exact nature of the ligand recognized on ß cells by $CD4^+$ and $CD8^+$ cloned T cells. Third, what is the nature of the autoreactive T cell receptor, and are T cells mediating islet destruction in NOD mice homogeneous, oligoclonal, or highly variable in the expression of cell surface T cell receptors.

INTRODUCTION

Autoimmune diseases represent failures in normal mechanisms of self-tolerance, in which autoantigenic materials lead to a sustained immune response directed at the host. A great deal of effort has been expended in characterizing antibodies directed against host molecules,

NATO ASI Series, Vol. H 38
The Molecular Biology of Autoimmune Disease
Edited by A. G. Demaine et al.

and many autoantibodies have been defined in a variety of autoimmune diseases. However, only in certain cases can the autoantibody be proven to cause the pathology or symptomatology associated with the disease. Furthermore, certain autoimmune diseases can be transferred to genetically identical recipients using purified T cells. In such autoimmune diseases, it is clear that a complete understanding of the disease will require the isolation and analysis of such T cells, and the determination of the autoantigenic ligand the receptors on these cells recognize. In addition, as all sustained immune responses involve antigen-specific T cells, even those autoimmune diseases in which the pathology is mediated by autoantibody can only be fully understood when the helper T cells involved in autoantibody production are isolated and fully characterized.

The analysis of autoantigens using cloned T cells is significantly more difficult than is the analysis of autoantigens using autoantibodies. There are two major reasons for this difficulty. First, antibodies are soluble molecules that bind their ligand with high affinity, and can thus be used to isolate and characterize the autoantigenic ligand directly. Second, while antibodies recognize native protein conformations, T cells only recognize protein antigens as peptide fragments bound to the cleft of a major histocompatibility complex encoded (MHC) molecule. These technical problems have prevented the identification of autoantigens recognized by T cells in any spontaneous autoimmune disease to date.

To approach this problem, we have selected the sponataneous autoimmune disease insulin-dependent diabetes mellitus (IDDM) as a subject to study. The mouse strain non-obese diabetic (NOD) provides an excellent experimental model for the human disease, and has been well-characterized both physiologically and immunologically. In this report, we describe the production and characterization of cloned T cell lines specific for islets isolated from NOD mice, and capable of causing isulitis and ß cell destruction in mice adoptively transferred with these cloned T cell lines.

RATIONALE FOR APPROACH

Prior studies of both human and rodent IDDM have suggested a role for $CD4^+$ and $CD8^+$ T cells in ß cell destruction. A role for $CD4^+$ T cells is strongly supported by the finding that susceptibility to IDDM is extremely tightly linked to the presence of a particular DQ ß class II MHC gene (Todd et al., 1987, 1988). T cells responding to class II MHC presented antigens invariably express CD4 on the cell surface (Swain, 1983). Further evidence for an involvement of $CD4^+$ T cells in IDDM comes from studies showing that anti-CD4 antibody injections can prevent diabetes (Shizuru et al., 1988), and from the finding that $CD4^+$ T cells are required to adoptively transfer rapid onset of IDDM in young irradiated NOD mice (Miller et al., 1988). Evidence for an involvement of $CD8^+$ T cells comes from the exquisite specificity of ß cell destruction, a property most likely to be associated with class I MHC-specific cytolytic T cells expressing the $CD8^+$ co-receptor molecule. Additional support for an involvement of $CD8^+$ T cells in the immunopathogenesis of IDDM comes from identical twin pancreas grafts, in which ß cell destruction was accompanied by a T cell infiltrate dominated by $CD8^+$ T cells (Sutherland et al., 1989), from the finding that combined injection of anti-CD4 and anti-CD8 was most effective in inhibiting IDDM in experimental animals (Hayward et al., 1988), and from the finding that both $CD4^+$ and $CD8^+$ T cells are required for the adoptive transfer of IDDM to young irradiated NOD mice (Bendelac et al., 1987; Miller et al., 1988). Because of these findings, we set out to clone both $CD4^+$ and $CD8^+$ islet-specific T cell lines from recently diabetic NOD mice.

Effective growth of cloned T cell lines required repeated exposure to the autoantigenic ligand. This requirement raises significant problems, particularly in the case of $CD8^+$ cloned T cells which recognized autoantigens presented by self class I MHC molecules. While antigens presented in association with class II MHC molecules are generally believed to be derived from cell surface or extracellular proteins taken up and degraded via the endocytic pathway, peptides presented by class I MHC molecules are thought to be derived from proteins synthesized within the cell's own biosynthetic pathways. Thus, in order to present our cloned lines with the appropriate autoantigenic complex ligand, we elected to use syngeneic NOD islets as a source of autoantigen. Islets are purified by repetitive handpicking, treated with mitomycin C, and added to the cloned T cell lines followed by the addition of exogenous interleukin 2 two days later.

RESULTS

Cloned T cell lines expressing CD4 or CD8 respond to syngeneic islets.

The cloned T cell lines produced in this study express either CD4 or CD8 on the cell surface. When such cells are stimulated with freshly isolated, mitomycin C-treated islets and given interleukin 2 two days later, significant proliferation by both sets of cells in response to syngeneic NOD islets is observed. Allogeneic $H\text{-}2^d$ islets from BALB/c mice do not stimulate the $CD4^+$ cloned T cell lines, suggesting that the response of the $CD4^+$ cloned T cell line is MHC-restricted. However, it is also possible that the cloned T cells lines are responding in a non-MHC-restricted fashion to islet antigens presented by MHC molecules expressed only in the inflamed NOD islet and not in the normal BALB/c islet. To examine this question, BALB/c and NOD were crossed, and F1 hybrid iselts isolated and used to stimulate the cloned T cell lines. Such islets are not in any way inflamed, and yet they stimulate the $CD4^+$ cloned T cell line nearly as well as the inflammed NOD islet. Thus, the failure of our cloned T cell lines to respond to BALB/c and $H-2^d$ B10.BR islets, almost certainly reflects MHC restricted recognition of an islet autoantigen. Spleen cells from all strains fail to stimulate our cloned T cell lines, demonstrating the islet specificity of this response.

The $CD8^+$ cloned T cell lines respond to both NOD and BALB/c islets, but not to islets derived from B10.BR mice. NOD mice express the BALB/c class I antigen $H-2K^d$, so this crossreactivity may reflect recognition of an autoantigen presented by this class I MHC molecule. Thus, both cloned T cell lines recognize islet-specific autoantigens and appear to show MHC restriction.

<u>In vivo activity of cloned T cell lines.</u>

In order to determine whether the islet-specific cloned T cell lines isolated in this study may be relevant to the immunopathogenesis of IDDM, we attempted to induce disease in irradiated syngeneic recipient mice by adoptive transfer of the cell lines. These studies sought to answer four questions: First, can the long-term cultured T cell lines home to iseles? Second, is homing to islets specific? Third, what are the cellular requirements to produce lymphocytic infiltrates in islets? And fourth, do the cloned T cell lines cause ß cell destruction in vivo? These experiments were carried out using an experimental protocol developed by Wicker and colleagues, in which populations of $CD4^+$ and $CD8^+$ T cells were shown to be required to adoptively transfer diabetes to irradiated young NOD recipient mice.

These studies may be summarized as follows. The most critical finding is that intense lymphocytic infiltration is observed in islets, but not in exocrine pancreas, liver, thyroid, or other tissues, when a mixture of $CD4^+$ and $CD8^+$ cloned T cells is adoptively transferred to irradiated syngeneic recipients. Control mice receiving no cells show no inflammation, and mice receiving either $CD4^+$ or $CD8^+$ T cells alone show minimal inflammation and no ß cell destruction. These in vivo results strongly support the argument that the cloned T cell lines isolated in this study are representative of T cells participating in the immunopathogenesis of IDDM in NOD mice. They are thus excellent candidates for studying the detailed immunobiology of this autoimmune disease. Future studies will focus on in vitro effector functions of the various cloned T cell lines, on the exact nature of the infiltrating cells in adoptive recipients of cloned T cells lines, and on the ratio of CD4 to CD8 T cells needed to optimally transfer disease, the route of delivery, and the timing of these separate cellular events. Our working hypothesis is that $CD4^+$ T cells are required for the effective activation and optimal effector function of $CD8^+$ T cells, the latter being directly involved in ß cell destruction.

Identification of a ß cell tumor line able to stimulate proliferation by cloned islet-specific T cells lines.

A principle goal of these studies is to identify and fully characterize the autoantigens recognized by autoreactive T cells in IDDM. In addition, we seek to identify a tumor line expressing autoantigens for use as a substitute for freshly isolated islet cells in the growth and analysis of islet-specific T cells. To this end, we have screened a number of murine islet cell tumors derived from mice, transgenic for the SV40 T antigen under the control of the rat insulin 1 promoter (RIP-TAg). RIP-TAg transgenic mice have been shown by Hannahan (1985) to develop insulin-secreting ß cell tumors at high frequency. McDevitt and co-workers have retrogressively backcrossed the RIP-TAg transgene onto NOD mice. Such NOD mice develop insulinomas at high frequency, and we have explanted and tested dissociated cultures of these insulinomas for their ability to stimulate our cloned T cell lines. Two tumor lines stimulate proliferation by both $CD4^+$ and $CD8^+$ cloned islet-specific T cell lines. Specific cell lines are now being established in culture, and will have four uses: First, they may be useful for antigen-specific stimulation of these and other freshly isolated T cells from NOD mice; thus, they may replace the tedious procedure of handpicked islets for the growth of such cells. Second, such cells may be useful as targets in chromium^{51} release assays used to characterize the effector function of the cloned T cell lines. Third, cDNA libraries constructed from such cells should carry sequences encoding the specific autoantigens recognized by $CD4^+$ and $CD8^+$ T cells. Finally, antigen loss variants of such cells perhaps selectable by co-culture with the cloned T cell lines may help in direct characterization of autoantigenic ligands, and could also serve as recipient cells for cDNA transfection in searching for genes encoding the autoantigenic ligand.

DISCUSSION

The studies presented here represent our approach to the characterization of autoantigens and autoreactive T lymphocytes in a spontaneous autoimmune disease, murine IDDM. While the major goals of this study remain to be achieved, the procedures and reagents we have assembled to date should lead directly to the accomplishment of these goals.

In addition to studies of immunopathogenic mechanisms and the identification of ß cell autoantigens, the analysis of the T cell receptors on such cloned T cell lines may also prove to be valuable in approaching a variety of outstanding issues in the area of spontaneous autoimmunity. For instance, do T cell receptor genetics play a critical role in the susceptibility to spontaneous autoimmune disease? By analyzing the germ line encoded elements in receptors of our autoreactive cloned T cell line, we can ask whether the NOD mouse has unique V, D or J gene elements utilized in generating autoreactive T cell receptors. If this were the case, one would expect to find that all T cells involved in IDDM in the NOD mouse bear the unique polymorphic form of the receptor. Second, in both spontaneous IDDM and in recipients of adoptively transferred cloned T cell lines, how many of the invading T cells are specific for ß cells, thus bearing the same receptor as the cloned T cell lines that can transfer the disease? This will determine the extent of T cell recruitment to such lesions, and also the homogeneity of the infiltrate.

Our studies appear to have already shed light on one issue, namely, the protective effect of I-E expression in IDDM in the NOD mouse (Nishimoto et al., 1987). BALB/c by NOD F1 hybrids do not develop IDDM or insulitis. Nevertheless, their ß cells appear to express the islet-specific autoantigens recognized by our cloned T cells lines. Thus, I-E is not grossly altering expression of ß autoantigens in these mice. Thus, it seems more likely that I-E is altering the T cell receptor repertoire. Once we know the nature of the autoreactive T cell receptor, we can directly ask whether T cells bearing this receptor type are deleted during T cell development in mice expressing I-E molecules. T cells bearing TCR encoded by certain Vß gene segments are preferentially deleted in mice expressing I-E molecules, due to proteins of a class we refer to as co-ligands (Janeway et al., 1989). By examining Vß expression on our cloned T cell lines, in NOD mice, and in NOD x BALB/c mice, it should be possible to determine whether the expression of I-E deletes all T cells bearing the Vß gene segment encoded TCR required to mediate autoimmune IDDM. Such studies should shed light on many issues having to do with IDDM.

Ideally, such studies should be carried out directly in human IDDM patients. However, a source of human islets sufficient to conduct such studies is not available. Two approaches are being taken to this problem. First, mice transgenic for the appropriate HLA-DQ antigens have been produced, and islets from such mice may allow the cloning and long-term growth of islet-specific T cells from human IDDM patients. Second, the identification of the gene encoding the islet specific autoantigen should allow isolation and characterization of the homologous gene in man. If such a gene can then be expressed in a cell carrying the appropriate MHC gene products, this cell line could be used for the growth and analysis of T cells from human IDDM patients, leading to the eventual identification of cells involved in this disease as well.

In summay, the approach we have adopted to IDDM could be adapted to virtually any spontaneous autoimmune disease in mouse or man. Technical considerations will govern the feasibility of such approaches, and studies in model animal systems may allow us to devise efficient strategies for the analysis of autoimmunity in human patients. Ultimately, it is to be hoped that the complete molecular characterization of T cells and T cell autoantigens will lead to strategies for the prevention of such autoimmune diseases without affecting other aspects of the adaptive immune response. The development of a comprehensive understanding of the immunobiology of normal T cell responses to antigens has been of fundamental importance in developing strategies to approach the role of T cells in spontaneous autoimmune disease. By applying these same approaches to the analysis of spontaneous autoimmune disease, the detailed understanding of these complex and medically important processes should soon be available.

ACKNOWLEDGEMENTS

The authors wish to thank Denise Scaringe and Janet Williams for invaluable technical assistance, Liza Cluggish for preparation of the manuscript, and many colleagues for invaluable discussions and reagents. NOD mice were initially donated by Masakazu Hatori. This work is supported by a grant from the Juvenile Diabetes Foundation, No. 187512 to

CAJ, and a grant from the American Diabetes Association, No. 187764, to RS, by the Howard Hughes Medical Institute, and by NIH Training Grant AI-07019 to P-ER.

REFERENCES

Bendelac AC, Carnaud C, Boitard C, Bach JF (1987) Syngeneic transfer of autoimmune diabetes from diabetic NOD mice to healthy neonates. Requirement for both L3T4$^+$ Lyt-2$^+$ T cells. J exp Med 166:823-832

Hanahan D (1985) Heritable formation of pancreatic ß cell tumors in transgeic mice expressing recombinant insulin/simian virus 40 oncogenes. Nature 315:115-122

Hayward AR, Cobbald SP, Waldmann H, Cooke A, Simpson E (1988) Delay in onset of insulitis in NOD mice following a single injection of CD4 and CD8 antibodies. J Autoimmunity 1:191-96

Janeway CA Jr, Yagi J, Conrad PJ, Katz, ME, Jones B, Vroegop S, Buxser S (1989) T cell responses to Mls and to bacterial proteins that mimic its behavior. Immunol Rev 107:61-88, 1989.

Miller BJ, Appel MC, O'Neil JJ, Wicker LS (1988) Both the Lyt-2$^+$ and L3T4$^+$ T cell subsets are required for the transfer of diabetes in nonobese diabatic mice. J Immunol 140:52-58

Nishimoto H, Kikutani H, Yamamura K, Kishimoto T (1987) Prevention of autoimmune insulitis by expression of I-E molecules in NOD mice. Nature 328:432-434

Shizuru JA, Taylor-Edwards C, Banks BA, Gregory AK, Fathman CG (1988) Immunotherapy of the nonobese diabetic mouse: treatment with an antibody to T-helper lymphocytes. Science 240:659-62

Sutherland DER, Silbey R, Xu XZ, Michael A, Srikanta S, Taub F, Najarian J, Goetz FC (1984) Twin-to-twin pancreas transplantation: reversal and reenactment of the pathogenesis of type I diabetes. Trans Assoc Am Physicians 97:80-87

Swain SL (1983) T cell subsets and the recognition of MHC class. Immunol Rev 74:129-142

Todd JA, Acha-Orbea H, Bell JI, Chao N, Fronek Z, Jacob CO, McDermott M, Sinha AA, Timmerman L, Steinman L, McDevitt, HO (1988) A molecular basis for MHC class II-associated autoimmunity. Science 240:1003-1009

Todd JA, Bell JI, McDevitt HO (1987) HLA-DQ$_{\beta}$ gene contributes to susceptibility and resistance to insulin-dependent diabetes mellitus. Nature 329:559-604

DISCUSSION

ALLEN: Aren't you surprised by the high percentage - 13% of your IA molecules are bound with a single ligand? You would think that they don't have that much room for other foreign antigens

JANEWAY: Yes, I think that's the most surprising thing about it but on the other hand, as far as I'm aware, IA and IE are brought into the same endosome of B cells. Now some people who don't believe that IA recycles would expect perhaps that the substance most present in those endosomes is going to be IE. As you know, you can get very good presentation in F1 beta cells of the IE of one haplotype by the IA of the other, but the percentage is stunning. Yes, absolutely, but it is tethered and I think that may be the explanation. There may be some specific binding, one thing we have observed is that there is competition because we have taken a positive strain 5R and crossed it with certain negative strains and there is tremendous variation in expression of this determinant independent of the expression of IA and IE genes.

ALLEN: That was the second question, have you taken peptides from IE in corresponding sequences?

JANEWAY: So far we haven't found the right one, but since we don't have any positive control, this is a bit like working with the autoantigens - you don't have a positive control.

PAPADOPOLOUS: Two quick questions, first did I understand you correctly, you transferred the disease through these two lines to NOD mice or NON?

JANEWAY: We haven't done NON, as we don't have any NON mice. We have done it to irradiated NOD and irradiated Balb/C by NOD, although I have to say in the latter case the inflammation is less severe.

PAPADOPOLOUS: And second, do you have any explanation now that you have lines that can transfer the disease as to the female preponderance for NOD mouse diabetes?

JANEWAY: No, we haven't really paid much attention to that we have only recently got this anti V beta 5 antibody that allowed us to identify the clones. We've looked at it in a limited number of clones because you have to prove that they're pathogenic, and we haven't looked for instance at V beta 5 representation in the two lines so I will say in our colony the incidence of diabetes in males is 40 to 50% and females 80% so its not such a big effect.

EISENBARTH: These clones look like they're a great deal of fun to work with, I guess one question related to the IE namely, if one breeds IE into the NOD you hardly prevent insulitis at all? Very different from Ishimoto's transgene so the expression of IE's still gives tremendous insulitis and probably quite a bit of beta cell destruction that would be one general comment; the other question is are you transferring diabetes?

JANEWAY: As I say we do get diabetes but its nowhere near as high as the pathology I showed you where we see intense insulitis and beta cell destruction but we tend to kill the mice after awhile to look at their pancreases because we have used that as our end point. We do get diabetes but we haven't done enough mice yet to give a statistical value on it.

EISENBARTH: And the trick that you used to keep them going longer?

JANEWAY: We just gave fewer cells. I think actually we are seeing some kind of bone marrow death that is my suspicion. At first, we got really excited and thought we were seeing hypoglycaemia with acute rupture of the beta cells and release of so much insulin that the mice died but it didn't look like that and we simply reduced the cell dose and now they get much more profound inflammation and you can keep them longer.

NEPOM: On this interesting V beta 5 antibody, have you been able to do any kind of competition even though you don't know the source of the peptide sequence?

JANEWAY: We've done those experiments and so far interestingly enough they've been negative but on the other hand, you know our system is a positive B cell that is turning IA and IE around like crazy and people tell me that when you add peptides they mainly will go into new sites and so on and so forth. I think physically its not a likely one we thought of it and tried it. In fact every peptide we make is screened both for generating and for inhibiting reactivity and so far the answer is no.

RATANACHAIYAVONG: The adoptive transfer was performed in the same inbred strain of NOD mice?

JANEWAY: As well as into F1s.

RATANACHAIYAVONG: Yes but why do you need to irradiate the mice first?

JANEWAY: Yes, well that's an interesting question; we do it for a very simple reason if we don't irradiate the mice we're going to find a certain number of lymphocytes in the islets because these are NOD mice, that's not a problem with Balb by NOD but the other thing is and this has never been adequately explained that all adoptive transfers seem to require irradiation for the full flourishing of the effect - that's not actually true of all of them there are some rat diseases I know that you can transfer without irradiation but antibody responses and so on seem to require irradiation but we haven't studied that as an isolated issue. We have followed the published procedures of Miller & Wicker because their system works.

RATANACHAIYAVONG: Could differences in infection susceptibility account for the protective effects you have demonstrated?

JANEWAY: Well I don't know of any evidence for that. That V beta deletion is associated with an increased infection. I think Ann Pullen should comment on that but I think her point today was actually that deleting V betas protects you from some of these pathogenic effects of the enterotoxins rather than causing it.

C A JANEWAY - SESSION CHAIRMAN'S SUMMING UP AND GENERAL DISCUSSION

Are there questions people want to bring up relating to the general theme of how the T cell and B cell get together, we could talk about CD4, if not I had lunch with Alan McGregor and he sort of said where are you going to go in the future and so I made a quick trip to Delphi and saw the Delphi Oracle. The Delphi Oracle told me three things; the first was to finish with this business which I think is a bit of a disease now which we call liganditis, its being preoccupied with receptors and ligands as the be all and end all of immunology. There is a very real issue which is, what was years ago called second signals, and I briefly outlined thinking on that in my comment on Steve Fling's talk that understanding the activation of T cells once you have finished liganditis is largely a matter of second signals and I would like to just recount if you will one of the interesting diabetes studies that's been published in the last year and that's in transgenic mouse experiments. Many people have put alien MHC genes into the pancreatic islets and as far as I am aware to date, no-one has produced an immunological diabetes by that means, in other words the ligand is not sufficient to generate the disease. Its necessary but its not sufficient, what I thought was particularly intriguing was that in transgenic mouse into which were introduced the gamma interferon gene with a rat insulin promoter you get a most dramatic inflammatory disease that leads to immunological beta cell destruction and because the animals had destroyed their own beta cells they lost the expression of interferon gamma

NATO ASI Series, Vol. H 38
The Molecular Biology of Autoimmune Disease
Edited by A. G. Demaine et al.

some months before and were diabetic. When you now transplant in normal syngeneic islets they were immediately attacked by lymphocytes and destroyed so that islets which would normally be tolerated were what I would call antigenic going back to the old terms of antigenic and immunogenic so liganditis has to do with antigenicity but it does not explain immunogenicity and immunogenicity is going to require that we understand these so-called second signals. Now I put this in quote because its my personal belief that second signals come first and first signals come second but anyway they are traditionally called second signals and then the third thing the Oracle told me was that we ought to understand suppression if we want to deal with autoimmune disease. I am now interpreting what you do when you go the Delphi Oracle I think they throw some entrails on the ground and blow a few smoke rings and then tell you these cryptic phrases which always initiated Greek tradegies and may be this will help us to understand suppression and my interpretion of that is that there are many systems in which dominant antigen specific suppression of immune responses can be demonstrated and if one wants to turn off an active immune response its too late to work on the second signal. The ligand is there you can't get away from it and so we have got to have some way to shut off the response and the only thing I know that does that is activated suppressor T cells now I say that in the broadest possible terms. I don't mean that these are IJ or anything specific simply the phenomenon of down regulating active immune responses which I think are going to be an important thing in the future and obviously the Delphi Oracle agrees with me. Ann do you want to make a comment, it doesn't have to be about this - nobody argues with the Oracle?

PULLEN: I just wanted to make a couple of comments on your model for MLS and the entertoxins that you showed in the beginning. These aren't just my problems with the model. A lot of people have asked me questions about your model so I thought maybe I would ask you some of them. Really, if this MLS is sitting on the outside how come so many people have been trying to make monoclonals for so long and not a single antibody has been made against it? The only way MLS can be detected is by T cell responses.

JANEWAY: I think that is a good question and it is an obvious problem with the model. The only answer I can give you, to go back to the Oracle, is that if you look at the literature on the injection of MLS into dispersed cells it results in complete inhibition of all immune reactivity. So for some reason these cells and substances including Staphylococcus entertoxins are profoundly immunosuppressive. So my defence is that perhaps we have done the wrong immunisation, we've done a suppressive immunisation rather than an immunising immunisation. I think we need to learn how to make these immunisations. Until that is done, and we can make antibodies against it since it is a physical structure, whether its a peptide in the groove or an outside binding molecule it doesn't matter, you ought to be able to make an antibody to it. The failure to raise antibody must have some other explanation.

PULLEN: Why do you think MLS is attached?

JANEWAY: Well, either its attached or not, but I'm not sure if its attached or if its actually peripheral.

PULLEN: We don't want to propose a particular model, we don't think we are ready to do that yet. We were wondering why you can't turn it through 90°, then you could have MLS or the toxins coming into the groove at one end and the V betas would still be coming into contact?

JANEWAY: Your laboratory is well known for its championship of MLS's peptide. Its been published in many places. In fact its previously well known for saying that the T cell receptor wasn't involved in the MLS response which fortunately you have thoroughly refuted. We can't say what the precise orientation is. I will however say the following; its known that SEs binds very stably to class II and they bind in a fixed orientation as intact proteins. If you cleave SE's with any reagent they lose the ability to stimulate so its known that if you fix APC's both in the mouse and in the human there is no diminution in response although you ablate antibody antigen recognition it is now known that if you mutate any residue in the cleft certain of those mutations will disrupt peptide recognition but none of them disrupt SE recognition so I think all of that points very strongly at least for class II binding taking place outside the cleft. CD4 seems to be a critical element and we think it has to be bound in the proper orientation. We think SEs bind to V beta because the only thing that we can inhibit it with is anti V beta antibodies. The reason for postulating that MLS works the same way is that if I handed you a tube of spleen cells and said tell me if this tube is from an MlsA animal or does it have staphylococcus enterotoxin B in it you would have a hard time until you actually went and sequenced the individual V betas that were responding because they are absolutely identical in their behaviour so it seems likely to us that the SE's and MLS are basically doing the same thing. I would add since we're on the SE's just one little bit of experimental detail because it fits nicely with what you were saying earlier today. One of the beautiful things you can do with SE's is you now have total control over the dose of these molecules (we'll call them molecules OK) and unlike MLS where you don't really know what it is or how much is there and so if you look at V beta deletion and by SE's and thymocyte culturing and compare it to what is required for T cell activation there is at least a one log difference that is V beta deletion is at least a log more sensitive than activation in our hands for the SEs we have studied. So I think the thymus seems to be set up to play it safe.

NEPOM: I wanted to pose a question related to both you, Ann and Paul. Instead of refining and simplifing the model what about expanding it. You have got a handle on a mechanism for deletion of T cell specificities, but what are the arguments against this also operating as a primary mechanism in the negative selection events in the thymus. Could the self antigen component not be represented as molecules like Mls/SE which bind outside the groove and be a mechanism of negative selection?

<u>JANEWAY</u>: You're raising the possibility that specific clonal deletion operates not by presenting the same ligand in the thymus as you would find in the periphery but by presenting some analogue of it, is that right?

<u>NEPOM</u>: Right, of course that has been suggested by many people but the problem with this particular model would be that the presentation of that peptide need not occupy the usual peptide groove.

<u>JANEWAY</u>: I don't like that idea at all because it seems to me that in as much as tolerance is deletional, it always looks identical to recognition. It also says that a T cell receptor can recognize one thing in one place and recognize the same thing in a completely different configuration in another place. That sort of undermines my understanding of stereo specificity in protein-protein interactions which is a very precise.

<u>EISENBARTH</u>: I'm just wondering whether perhaps, some of these super antigens might be involved in autoimmunity. We have been concentrating on the complementarity determining region of the T cell receptor and we really have no clear data on what is involved in the derivation of type I diabetes, even in the NOD mouse. To throw a monkey wrench, we've discussed our data of V beta T cell receptor transgene animals - basically one gets allelic exclusion in these animals. One gets allelic exclusion of utilisation of almost all V beta T cell receptors within a lesion, yet one gets insulitis just as dramatic as in NOD mouse and I am wondering whether it might either be the alpha chain which is determining the specificity or there

might be some other explanation for the experimental result or perhaps the possibility that we're not going to have classical presentation for the generation of autoimmunity?

JANEWAY: I think you need to make T cell clones from those mice and describe the pathogenic receptor, then we can talk about it and we'll try and do the same with ours and then we can compare notes. We are a long way from being there but I would argue if we can isolate the peptide that is presented by class I and the peptide that is presented by class II and find that they stimulate pathogenic clones then you would have a hard time.

EISENBARTH: I'm not quite so sure there. I guess part of it is what determines the natural disease. For instance, we have clearly a whole series of antigens that can be used to immunise mice and transfer disease yet we are not at all sure for instance, that the EAE peptide is the basis for any clear disease so the ability to generate a clone in culture is extremely useful but it doesn't prove that it is that antigen which creates the disease.

JANEWAY: The reason we studied spontaneous autoimmune disease is that we don't want to bias the outcome, but of course the clones that we have do cause disease. If it is a polyclonal disease someone might come up with a different receptor. I really don't think one can say, just as if you find one autoantigen that it is 'the' autoantigen.

HLA CLASS II SEQUENCE POLYMORPHISM AND AUTOIMMUNITY

Henry A. Erlich, Teodorica L. Bugawan, and Stephen J. Scharf
Department of Human Genetics
Cetus Corporation
Emeryville, CA 946081 USA

INTRODUCTION

Specific alleles at the HLA-DR and -DQ loci have been associated with a variety of autoimmune diseases. The role of HLA-DP polymorphism in susceptibility has not been as fully explored as that of the other class II antigens due to the complexity of the primed lymphocyte typing (PLT) method for determining DPw specificities. These class II loci encode a heterodimer consisting of an alpha (ca 32 kDa) and a beta (ca 29 kDa) glycoprotein chain. These α-β heterodimers are highly polymorphic transmembrane proteins which bind peptides derived from the processing of foreign antigens (Babbitt et al., 1985; Guillet et al., 1987; Sette et al., 1987; Unanue et al., 1987; Watts et al., 1986). The activation of $CD4^+$ T lymphocytes results from the recognition of this class II-peptide complex by the alpha-beta T cell receptor. In addition to their role in peptide binding on antigen-presenting cells, the polymorphic class II molecules present on thymic stromal cells influence the specificity of the mature T cell repertoire (Kappler et al., 1987; Kappler et al., 1988; MacDonald et al., 1988; Teh et al., 1988).

Our approach to examining the relationship between HLA class II polymorphism and autoimmune diseases has been to use the polymerase chain reaction (PCR) (Mullis and Faloona, 1987; Saiki et al., 1985; Saiki et al., 1988) method of specific DNA amplification to define the allelic diversity at these loci. The DNA-defined polymorphisms subdivide the serologically defined haplotypes (e.g., DRw6, DQw1) and thus allow one to ask whether a particular DNA-defined subtype is more strongly associated with the disease than is the serological specificity. If so, the locus (e.g., DQβ) that provides this

NATO ASI Series, Vol. H 38
The Molecular Biology of Autoimmune Disease
Edited by A. G. Demaine et al.

informative "subdivision" may account for the observed disease association with the serotype. However, given the strong linkage disequilibrium that characterizes the HLA class II region, it is sometimes difficult to identify specific alleles on a haplotype which are candidates for directly conferring susceptibility.

In this paper, we discuss the role of allelic variation at the HLA class II and genetic susceptibility, using the disorders Celiac disease (CD) and *Pemphigus vulgaris (PV)* as illustrative examples. Both these diseases are associated with two DR serotypes (CD with DR3 and DR7 and PV with DR4 and DRw6). This pattern could mean that either that an allele or epitope *shared* on the two associated haplotypes confers predisposition or, alternatively, that *different* sequences on the two haplotypes are responsible for the observed disease associations.

PEMPHIGUS VULGARIS

In PV, we have previously shown that the DR4 association appears to be conferred by the Dw10 allele at the DRβI locus (Scharf et al., 1988). This DRβI allele differs from the other non-associated DR4 subtypes (Dw4, Dw14, Dw13, and Dw15) primarily in the polymorphic residues encoded in the third "hypervariable" region, in particular at residues 67, 70, and 71. The DRβI allele on most DRw6 haplotype shares this epitope, however, it is not this allele that is responsible for the observed DRw6 association since it is less frequent in $DRw6^{+}$ patients than in $DRw6^{+}$ controls. Rather, it is a specific DQβ allele, DQB1.3, on the DRw6 haplotype which shows the highest association (RR of ~100 vs. RR of 2.5 for the DRw6 serotype) (Scharf et al., 1988). This allele differs from another non-susceptible DQβ allele found on DRw6 haplotypes (DQB1.1) only by a Val to Asp substitution at position 57, suggesting that the charge of this polymorphic residue, like those of the DRβI third hypervariable region, is a critical element in susceptibility. However, other DQβ alleles found on DRw6 haplotypes with Asp-57 *do not* confer susceptibility so that it is the entire *allele* not an isolated residue that is involved in genetic predisposition. As a result of linkage disequilibrium, it is often difficult to determine whether a disease-associated allele (e.g., DQB1.3) is simply a marker for a "disease haplotype" or whether it confers susceptibility directly. In the case of PV and the DQB1.3 β chain, we have found four different DRw6, DQw1 haplotypes in PV patients, all of which encode the same β chain (Scharf et al., 1989). This observation suggests that it is this DQB1.3 allele that accounts for the DRw6 susceptibility to PV.

In PV, we found no evidence for a DP association. In celiac disease, however, we have observed an association with specific polymorphic variants at the DPβ locus, in addition to the well-known DR3 and DR7 associations.

CELIAC DISEASE

Celiac disease is an autoimmune disease of the intestinal mucosa, elicited by ingestion of wheat gluten in genetically susceptible individuals (Booth, 1974). Susceptibility to celiac disease has been associated with the serologically defined variants DR3 and DR7 encoded by the HLA-DRβI locus. Recently, we have described a new method for typing polymorphism at the DPβ locus (Bugawan et al., 1988) using the polymerase chain reaction (PCR). The analysis of the distribution of DPβ alleles in a group of celiac disease patients and healthy controls revealed that two specific DPβ alleles (DPB4.2 and DPB3) are increased in the patient population. Comparison of the DPβ sequences suggests that the polymorphic residues at position 69 and at 56 and 57 may be critical in conferring susceptibility. Further, the contribution of the susceptible DPβ alleles appears to be independent of linkage to the previously reported DR3 and DR7 markers for celiac disease. The distribution of DQα and β alleles in patients suggests that a specific DQ heterodimer may be responsible for the observed DR associations. Individuals with this DQ antigen *and* a specific DPβ allele are at increased risk for celiac disease.

In general, the 21 sequence defined DPβ alleles represent new combinations of the previously described DPβ sequences. The second exon of the DPβ locus contains 6 variable regions with a limited number of polymorphic residues (n = 2 or 3) at each position. This patchwork pattern of polymorphism suggests that recombination may have played an important role in generating DPβ allelic diversity. These alleles can all be identified using a panel of 15 sequence specific oligonucleotide (SSO) probes. The distribution of DPβ alleles was determined by SSO probe analysis in 23 CD patients from Italy and in 19 ethnically matched controls, as well as in 150 other control individuals (Bugawan et al., 1989).

The frequency of the DPβ 4.2 allele is significantly increased in the CD patients relative to the ethnically restricted Italian controls (52% vs. 10.5%; p = .005) as well as the other controls. The calculated relative risk (RR = 9.3) for the DPB4.2 allele is higher than for the classic DR3 and DR7 markers (RR = 2.8 and 3.0, respectively) for this group of patients. Similar risk estimates for DR3 and DR7 were reported by Tosi et al (1983). Six of the 11 (55%) non-DPB4.2 patients carry the DPB3 allele. Most (78%) of the CD patients carry either DPB4.2 or DPB3 compared to only 21% of the Italian controls. The relative risk for the presence of either of these markers is 13.5. The observation of a specific DPβ allele associated with CD could simply reflect linkage disequilibrium, with the DPB4.2 (or DPB3) allele being a marker for a particular "disease" haplotype. Alternatively, the association could reflect the contribution of the DPβ allele to susceptibility independent of the well-known DR3 and DR7 CD associated haplotypes. The finding that the same proportion of DR3+ patients and DR7+ patients carry the DPB4.2 and DPB3 alleles as do all CD patients suggests that the association of these DPβ alleles is independent of linkage to the DR3 and DR7 associated susceptibility haplotypes. In control haplotypes, there is no evidence for linkage disequilibrium between DPB4.2 (or DPB3) and DR3 or DR7. In one pedigree tested, the DPB4.2 allele in the patient was on a paternal DR5 haplotype and the DPB3 allele on a maternal DR7 haplotype. A similarly independent relationship between the disease-associated class II alleles DPB2.1 and DR5 and DRw8 was observed in our recent study of pauciarticular Juvenile Rheumatoid Arthritis (Begovich et al., submitted).

Because most DPw4 typed cells have the DPB4.1 allele, not DPB4.2, and because many cells with the DPB4.2 allele have been PLT typed as DP-blank (Bugawan et al., 1988), it is not surprising that no DPw specificity has been previously associated with CD. In addition to its capability of subdividing immunologically or RFLP defined variants, PCR/SSO typing has the virtue of revealing *how* alleles differ not simply *that* they are different. The DPB4.2 allele differs from the DPB2.1 allele only by a Lys to Glu change at position 69 (Bugawan et al., 1988), suggesting that this residue may play a critical role in susceptibility to CD. As discussed previously (Bugawan et al., 1988), the charge of this residue must be important in T cell recognition because cells with the DPB4.2 allele have the PLT-defined specificity DPw4 (or blank) while cells with DPB2.1 type as DPw2. The nature of the polymorphic residues in this region of the DRβ-I chain has also been implicated in susceptibility to IDDM and PV (Erlich et al., 1989; Horn et al., 1988; Scharf et al., 1988). However, not all DPβ alleles with Lys-69 confer susceptibility; thus it is the allelic structure of the beta chain, not simply an isolated residue that appears most highly associated with disease. The DPB3 allele which is also associated with CD is present on over half (6/11) of the non-DPB4.2 patients. This allele shares not only the Lys-69 with DPB4.2 but is the only other common DPβ allele with both Asp-Glu at position 56-57 *and* Lys-69. The nature of the polymorphic residue at position 57 of the DQβ chain appears to be an important element in susceptibility to IDDM and PV (Erlich et al., 1989; Horn et al., 1988; Scharf et al., 1988; Sinha et al., 1988; Todd et al., 1987). In the structural model for class II antigens proposed by Brown et al. (Brown et al., 1988), the polymorphic residues at these locations point in toward the putative peptide binding cleft and may, therefore, serve as peptide contact sites.

Another study of DP polymorphism and a group of U.S. CD patients revealed a somewhat different pattern of DPβ association (Kagnoff et al., 1989). In these patients, who were predominantly B8, DR3 with no significant increase in DR7, an increase in the DPB1 allele frequency as well as that of the DPB3 and the DPB4.2 alleles was observed. Thus, in different ethnic groups, different DPβ alleles may be associated with susceptibility to CD.

In both studies, however, virtually all the patients have the DQw2 serotype. While 78% (18/23) of the CD patients in this study are DPB4.2 or 3, 91% (20/22) are DQw2 (DR3 or DR7). DR3 and DR7 haplotypes each have the DQB2 allele at the DQβ locus (Horn et al., 1988) which encodes the DQw2 specificity. This observation suggests that the DQ antigen is a major determinant of susceptibility and that specific combinations of DQβ alleles (DQB2) and DPβ alleles (DPB4.2 or 3) may confer increased risk for CD. A specific DQα allele (DQA4) common to DR3, DR5, and DRw8 haplotypes (Horn et al., 1988) has also been implicated in CD susceptibility by serologic (Tosi et al., 1983), RFLP (Roep et al., 1988), and more recently, by oligonucleotide (Sollid et al., 1989) studies. Thus, the same DQ heterodimer (DQB2 and DQA4) is encoded in *cis* by the DR3 haplotype and in *trans* by the DR5/DR7 or the DRw8/DR7 genotypes.[1] Of the 11 DR7$^+$ CD patients, 6 were DR5/DR7

---

[1]The sequence of the DQα allele (DQA4.1) on DR3 and DR5 haplotypes is identical and differs from the sequence of the DQα allele on DRw8 haplotypes (DQA4.2 or DQA4.3) by only one or two amino acids.

heterozygotes compared to an expected number of 2, based on the DR5 allele frequency in patients ($p<.05$). Of the other 5 $DR7^+$ patients, 3 had DR3, and 1 had DRw8 on the other haplotype. Of the 9 $DR5^+$ patients, 6 had DR7 and 3 had DR3 on the other haplotype. This distribution is consistent with the notion that it is this particular DQ heterodimer (DQB2 and DQA4), in combination with the DPβ4.2 (or 3) allele, which confers high risk for CD. Similarly, it appears that specific combinations of DQβ alleles (DQB3.2) and DRβI alleles (Dw4 or Dw10) account for most of the observed DR4 association with insulin dependent diabetes (Erlich et al., 1989; Sheehy et al., 1989). This putative joint contribution of different class II molecules could be mediated at the level of peptide binding and presentation, at the level of T cell repertoire, or at both. Whatever the mechanism, polymorphic residues of the DPβ chain, as well as those of the better characterized DR and DQ antigens, appear to confer susceptibility to autoimmune diseases.

ACKNOWLEDGMENTS

We thank Corey Levenson, Chu-An Chang, Dragan Spasic, and Lauri Goda for the synthesis of oligonucleotides, and Ann Begovich for helpful discussions, and Kathy Levenson for careful preparation of this manuscript.

REFERENCES

Babbitt BP, Allen PM, Matsueda G, Huber E, Unanue E (1985) Nature 317:359.
Begovich A, et al. Manuscript submitted.
Booth CC (1974) in Proceedings of the 2nd International Celiac Symposium (Stenfert Kroese) p 17.
Brown JH, et al (1988) Nature 332, 845-850.
Bugawan, TL, Horn GT, Long CM, Mickelson E, Hansen JA, Ferrara GB, Angelini G, Erlich H (1988) J Immunol 141:4024-4030.
Bugawan T, Angelini G, Larrick J, Auricchio S, Ferrara GB, Erlich HA (1989) Nature 339:470-472.
Erlich HA, Horn G, Scharf SJ, Bugawan T (1989) in Molecular Biology of HLA Class II Antigens, J. Silver (ed.), CRC Press.
Guillet J-G, et al (1987) Science 235:865.

Horn G, Bugawan T, Long C, Erlich H (1988) Proc Natl Acad Sci USA 85:6012-6016.
Kagnoff M, et al. (1989) Proc Natl Acad Sci USA, in press.
Kappler JW, Roehm N, Marrack P (1987) Cell 49:273.
Kappler JW, Staerz U, White J, Marrack PC (1988) Nature 332:35.
MacDonald HR, et al (1988) Nature 332:40.
Mullis K, Faloona F (1987) Meth Enzymol 155:335-350.
Roep BO, Bontrop EE, Pena AS, van Eggermond MCJA, van Rood JJ, Giphart MJ (1988) Human Immunology 23:271-279.
Saiki RK, Scharf S, Faloona F, Mullis KB, Horn GT, Erlich HA, Arnheim NA (1985) Science 230:1350-1354.
Saiki R, Gelfand DH, Stoffel S, Scharf SJ, Higuchi R, Horn GT, Mullis, Erlich HA (1988) Science 239:487.
Scharf S, Friedmann A, Brautbar C, Szafer F, Steinman L, Horn G, Gyllensten U, Erlich H (1988) Proc Natl Acad Sci USA 85:3504-3508.
Scharf S, Friedmann A, Steinman L, Brautbar C, Erlich HA (1989) Proc Natl Acad Sci USA, in press.
Sette A, et al (1987) Nature 328:395.
Sheehy MJ, Scharf SJ, Rowe JR, Neme de Gimenez NH, Meske LM, Erlich HA, Nepom BS (1989) J Clin Invest 83:830-835.
Sinha AA, et al (1988) Science 239:1026.
Sollid LM, Markussen G, Ek J, Gjerde H, Vartdal F, Thorsby E (1989) J Exp Med 169:345-350.
Teh HS, et al (1988) Nature 335:229.
Todd JA, Bell JI, McDevitt HO (1987) Nature 329:599.
Tosi, et al (1983) Clin Immunol Immunopathol 28:395-404.
Unanue ER, Allen PM (1987) Science 236:551.
Watts TM, McConnell HM (1986) Proc Natl Acad Sci USA 83:9660.

HLA-DQ AND DIABETES MELLITUS: A GENETIC AND STRUCTURAL PARADIGM FOR MODELS OF DISEASE SUSCEPTIBILITY

Gerald T. Nepom
Immunology Research Program
Virginia Mason Research Center
1000 Seneca
Seattle, WA 98101 USA

David M. Robinson
Section of Clinical Immunology
Virginia Mason Clinic C2-N
1100 Ninth Avenue
Seattle, WA 98101 USA

Approximately 70% of patients with Type I diabetes (IDDM) carry a specific HLA gene, called HLA-DQ3.2, representing one specific allele at the DQß (DQB1) locus within the HLA-D region of chromosome 6. HLA-DQ3.2 is linked to nearby HLA-DR locus genes which encode the HLA-DR4 specificity, accounting for the fact that the "DR4 type" is the most common HLA specificity associated with IDDM (Nepom, 1986). HLA-DQ3.2 is therefore an excellent candidate for a "disease susceptibility gene", contributing to important pathogenic events in the induction or progression of autoimmunity in IDDM.

One of the DR4-associated genes linked to HLA-DQ3.2, called HLA-Dw4, is also found on closely related haplotypes which carry a different DQ gene, called HLA-DQ3.1 (Kim, 1985). The importance of this linkage for understanding the HLA contribution to IDDM stems from the observation that DR4-positive haplotypes which carry a DQ3.1 gene are extremely rare in diabetics, and are negatively correlated with disease. We summarize below some of the key structural and genetic distinctions between the DQ3.1 and DQ3.2-positive haplotypes, which lead to explicit models for understanding the contribution of specific HLA genes, such as DQ3.2, to disease susceptibility.

The DQß polymorphism which distinguishes between the two haplotypes DR4(Dw4),<u>DQ3.2</u>, and DR4(Dw4),<u>DQ3.1</u> can be easily

NATO ASI Series, Vol. H 38
The Molecular Biology of Autoimmune Disease
Edited by A. G. Demaine et al.

detected using serologic markers (Kim, 1985; Maeda, 1986), restriction fragment length polymorphisms (Kim, 1985; Nepom, 1986; Michelsen, 1987; Schreuder, 1986; Monos 1988) and oligonucleotide probes (Holbeck, 1986; Robinson, 1989; Todd, 1987; Horn, 1988; Morel, 1988). There are several nucleotide sequence differences between the DQ3.1 and DQ3.2 genes (Holbeck, 1988; Michelsen, 1987); however, within the second exon of the gene, corresponding to the functionally polymorphic first domain of the DQß molecule, there are only four codons which encode amino acid polymorphisms. These four residues, at codons 13, 26, 45, and 57 of the DQß polypeptide, are excellent candidates for functionally important sites of interaction between the class II molecule and antigen and/or T cell receptor in the immunogenetic events associated with IDDM. Site-directed mutagenesis has been employed to substitute DQ3.1-like residues at each of these four positions in the DQ3.2 molecule (Kwok, 1989). Such studies demonstrate a complex set of intramolecular interactions, in which some immunologic specificities associated with DQ3.2 are attributed to a single amino acid substitution (i.e., codon 45 is critical for the DQw7(3.1) and DQw8(3.2) allospecificities) but others may involve additional residues on both the alpha and beta chains of the molecule.

Precisely how these limited structural changes correspond to the genetic susceptibility phenotype is not known. In general, there are two theoretical paradigms which relate DQß structure to genetic models of autoimmunity: *[1] The HLA-DQ3.2 molecule may be critical for antigen presentation.* In structural terms, polymorphic sites on the DQ3.2 molecule would be responsible for determinant selection associated with antigens or peptides important in the triggering of disease. This model predicts a genetic mechanism in which the DQ3.2 molecule would be permissive for disease, but not sufficient (Nepom, 1986). This susceptibility phenotype would be inherited as a dominant trait. *[2] The observation that DQ3.1 is not associated with IDDM has been interpreted as indicating a "protective" role of this allele*

(Todd, 1987). Mechanisms associated with such "protection" could potentially involve an innate tolerance toward DQ3.1-associated epitopes, or a role for the DQ3.1 molecule in T cell repertoire selection during the development of the immune system. A prediction of this model is that genetic susceptibility to IDDM would be recessive, since the "protective allele" would be dominant.

To begin to address the questions posed by these two models, we analyzed the segregation of different DQ3.1 and DQ3.2-positive HLA haplotypes among diabetic and non-diabetic siblings. The data base for this study was derived from the Fifth Genetics Analysis Workshop (Spielman, 1989), in which 87 multiplex IDDM families were analyzed for a combination of immunologic and genetic markers, including RFLP analysis for HLA-DQß polymorphisms. As previously reported (Robinson, 1989), 75 of 87 families (86%) studied carried at least one DR4-positive haplotype. Of the 75 DR4-positive multiplex families, the DQ3.2 gene was present in 70 (93%) and the DQ3.1 gene was present in nine (13%). Since each family had multiple affected individuals, the data was analyzed to determine DQß markers on haplotypes which segregated with disease; that is, which were present in all affected individuals. The DR4,DQ3.2 haplotype segregated with disease in 58 of the 70 families in which a DQ3.2 gene was present, accounting for 133/163 (82%) of the total DR4-positive IDDM-affected individuals among the 87 families studied. Some DR4,DQ3.1 haplotypes were identified in the analysis; however, in no case was this the sole haplotype segregating with the disease in a family. To directly test the "dominant resistance" model, we identified all 14 siblings in nine families which carried a DR4,DQ3.1-positive haplotype. Of these 14 siblings, 7 were affected with IDDM, and 7 were clinically non-diabetic. This analysis thus fails to support the hypothesis that the DQ3.1 gene confers a protective effect.

A similar analysis among the families in this study highlighted two other haplotypes which, like the DR4,DQ3.1 haplotype, are negatively correlated with IDDM, but which, unlike the DR4,DQ3.1 haplotype, do appear to confer some element of relative resistance to disease. Fifteen families in this study carried DR2-positive haplotypes; among 24 siblings inheriting a shared DR2 haplotype, only five had IDDM. Similarly, among 11 families in which a DR5,DQ3.1 haplotype was found, only five of 21 siblings with this haplotype had IDDM. Notably, nine out of ten of these affected individuals carried a DQ3.2 gene on the other haplotype. Thus, while these data do not support the idea that HLA genes confer "resistance" in a dominant fashion, these studies do suggest significant variation in genetic susceptibility to IDDM associated with specific HLA haplotypes carrying DR2 and/or DR5. In the affected individuals, the presence of a DQ3.2 gene was apparently sufficient, in spite of the second DR2 or DR5 haplotype, to contribute to disease, consistent with the model in which the DQ3.2 gene is a dominant, permissive genetic element.

The distribution of DR3-positive haplotypes in this study of multiplex families confirmed previous observations suggesting that the presence in a heterozygous individual of both DR3 and of DR4,DQ3.2 confers an extremely high degree of associated risk (Bertrams, 1984). In 23 of the 87 families, all IDDM patients were heterozygous for DR3 and DQ3.2 (26%). A DR3-positive haplotype co-segregated with DQ3.2 in almost half of the families in which DQ3.2 segregated with disease, indicating that, in DQ3.2-heterozygous individuals, a DR3-positive haplotype may contribute some additional permissive susceptibility element(s) which augment the HLA-associated risk.

The most straightforward way to interpret these genetic data is to view the HLA-DQ3.2 gene as a dominant susceptibility gene, which functions as a permissive element contributing to disease susceptibility. In this model, other HLA genes, often found on a second inherited haplotype in heterozygous patients, contribute significant secondary genetic factors which either increase or decrease relative risk of IDDM in an individual carrying one susceptibility gene. It should be noted, however, that the specific genes on such "secondary" haplotypes which modify disease susceptibility are entirely unknown. That is, whereas DR3 haplotypes provide synergistic elements of risk for IDDM and DR2 and DR5 haplotypes provide relatively protective contributions, it is not known what genes on these haplotypes are responsible for these phenomena and, indeed, whether such genes are themselves HLA class II genes or other linked elements.

ACKNOWLEDGMENTS

We thank our collaborators and colleagues involved in the laboratory studies and the Genetics Analysis Workshop summarized above, especially Drs. Barbara Nepom, Jerry Palmer, David McCulloch and Richard Spielman, and thank Nan Knitter-Jack for technical assistance. This work was supported by grants from the Juvenile Diabetes Foundation and the National Institutes of Health. DMR is the Rowland Pearsall Fellow in Immunology at Virginia Mason Medical Center and the Senior Fellow in Allergy and Immunology at the University of Washington (Seattle).

REFERENCES

Bertrams J, Baur M. (1984) Insulin dependent diabetes mellitus. In: Albert E, Baur M, Mayer W, eds. Histocompatibility Testing. Berlin: Springer-Verlag, p. 348-358

Holbeck SL, Nepom GT. (1988) Molecular analysis of DQβ3.1 genes. Human Immunol 21:183-192

Holbeck SL, Nepom GT. (1986) Exon-specific oligonucleotide probes localize HLA DQ beta allelic polymorphisms. Immunogenetics 24:251

Horn G, Bugawan T, Long C, and Erlich H. (1988) Allelic sequence variation of the HLA DQ loci: Relationship to serology and to IDDM susceptibility. Proc Natl Acad Sci USA 85, 6012-6016

Kim SJ, Holbeck SL, Nisperos B, Hansen JA, Maeda H, Nepom GT. (1985) Identification of a polymorphic variant associated with HLA-DQw3 and characterized by specific restriction sites within the DQ beta-chain gene. Proc Natl Acad Sci USA 82:8139

Kwok, WW, Lotshaw C, Milner ECB, Knitter-Jack N, and Nepom GT. (1989) Mutational analysis of the HLA-DQ3.2 IDDM susceptibility gene. Proc Natl Acad Sci USA, 86:1027-1030

Maeda H, Hirata R, Kambayashi H, Koning F, Schreuder G. (1986) Multiple epitopes on a single DQ molecule from the DQw3-carrying haplotypes. Tissue Antigens 29:136-145.

Michelsen B, and Lernmark A. (1987) Molecular cloning of a polymorphic DNA endonuclease fragment associates insulin-dependent diabetes mellitus with HLA-DQ. J Clin Invest 79:1144-1152

Monos DS, Spielman RS, Gogolin KJ, Radka SF, Baker L, Zmuewski CM, Kamoun M. (1987) HLA-DQw3.2 allele of the DR4 haplotype is associated with insulin-dependent diabetes; correlation between DQß restriction fragments and DQß chain variation. Immunogenetics 26:299-303

Morel P, Dorman JS, Todd JA, McDevitt HO, and Trucco M. (1988) Aspartic acid at position 57 of the HLA-DQß chain protects against type I diabetes: A family study. Proc Natl Acad Sci USA 85:8111-8115

Nepom GT, Palmer J, Nepom B. (1986) Specific HLA class II variants associated with IDDM. In: Immunology of Diabetes Mellitus, M. Jaworski, G. Molnar, R. Rajotte, B. Singh, eds. Excerpta Medica, Amsterdam, pp. 9-20

Robinson DM, Holbeck S, Palmer J, Nepom GT. (1989) HLA DQß3.2 identifies subtypes of DR4+ haplotypes permissive for insulin-dependent diabetes mellitus. Genetic Epidemiol, 6:149-154

Schreuder GM, Tilanus MG, Bontrop RE, Bruining GJ, Giphart MJ, van Rood JJ, de Vries RR. (1986) HLA-DQ polymorphism associated with resistance to type I diabetes detected with monoclonal antibodies, isoelectric point differences, and restriction fragment length polymorphism. J Exp Med 164:938-43

Spielman RS, Baur MP, and Clerget-Darpoux F. (1989) Genetic Analysis of IDDM: Summary of GAW5-IDDM Results. Genetic Epidemiol 6:43-58

Todd JA, Bell JI, McDevitt HO. (1987) HLA-DQß gene contributes to susceptibility and resistance to insulin-dependent diabetes mellitus. Nature 329:599-604

DISCUSSION

THORSBY: This is very nice data Gerry. I would just like to elaborate on your point that the DQ alpha chain has to be taken into account concerning recognition of T cell epitopes on DQ beta. There are some T cell clones which have been generated in my own lab by Dr Lundine and his associates which recognize an epitope with determinants around residue 57 of a DQ beta chain as it recognizes DQW8 but not DQW9 and as you said the only difference between these two molecules is an amino acid substitution at position 57. These T cell clones are completely dependent upon a given alpha chain because if you exchange an alpha chain from the DQW8 type for one from DQW2 or any other, the reactivity is lost. Therefore, this is a T cell clone which is recognizing something around residue 57 the one we all, or somebody thinks is involved in diabetes. But these T cell clones are independent of a particular DQ alpha chain. We cannot just focus on the beta chain and residues of the beta chains, these have to be considered together with the alpha chain residues or the alpha chain itself.

NEPOM: Absolutely, that's very nice data.

JANEWAY: Position 45 looked to be out on one of the elbows of the beta plated sheet. My question is, is that substitution likely to alter the interaction between the beta pleated sheet and the alpha helix?

NEPOM: That's a very important point, the residue at 45 in the A2 model just precedes the short alpha helical loop on the long free standing loop which precedes the proline at 55-56 which precedes the long alpha helical loop. In the class II A2 structure the side chain at the equivalent of position 45 points in towards the helix and is a small residue like the glycine. In fact it is a glycine just like the glycine on the DQ 3.2 molecule. It is the only residue outside the binding pocket which has a side chain pointing sufficiently into the groove to actually interact with things that are opposing. One of the important points with respect to position 45 is that if that orientation is correct, based on the class I structure, with the side chain pointing in, and you substitute the glycine for the glutamic acid that characterises the DQ 3.1 gene, there is no way that glutamic acid could fit so that if it substitutes a glutamic acid you can predict and we have modelled this so that the entire loop would actually move away from the molecule and would actually change dramatically the confirmation of this entire portion of the molecule including the orientation of the side chain at position 57 emphasizing the close interaction between different aspects of the structure and the fact that you cannot just put your finger on a single residue.

EISENBARTH: Gerry, are there haplotypes with DQ 3.2, for instance with DW13, that are not diabetes associated?

NEPOM: The question relates to the fact that there is a preference in diabetics for a specific haplotype which occurs with a DQ 3.2 gene compared to other haplotypes which also carry a DQ 3.2 gene. Now when we look at recent published data we realise that all the controls are DR4 positive as are all the diabetics. The control frequency of DR4 is about 27%

and the frequency in diabetics is around 70%, therefore if you want to get absolute population frequencies you have to multiply these numbers by about 0.27 and 0.7 respectively. When you do that the relative risk, or the increased risk associated with this haplotype is quite large for diabetes. This haplotype, the DQ 3.2 DW14 haplotype is also increased in diabetes relative to controls. There are several things we don't know one of which is whether there are other genes on DQ 3.2 positive haplotypes which contribute to diabetes. Another thing is that haplotypes other than DR4-DQ 3.2, are associated with diabetes, predominantly DR3 haplotypes and to a lesser extent, some DR1 haplotypes. We have no idea what gene or genes on those haplotypes accounts for the association with diabetes. There is good reason to think its not in fact DQ. It could be anything, even a non class II gene. Further, in the heterozygote recombination there is yet a third category of things we don't know - modifying the DQ 3.2 beta gene depending on what's in trans on the heterozygote.

RATANACHAIYAVONG: Does the amino acid substitution residue at the 45 glycine correspond with the TA10 seriology positive or IIB3?

NEPOM: Glutamic acid at 45 accounts for TA10 activity.

RATANACHAIYAVONG: Are the TA10 and the IIB3 mutually exclusive?

NEPOM: IIB3 is equivalent to DQ, within the DQ3 family and is equivalent to the DQ8 antibody which I showed you.

JANEWAY: There is a suggestion and evidence for a role for CD8 positive cells in diabetes implicating that there might be class I polymorphisms of interest. Have you picked up anything in your linkage analysis that point to class I polymorphisms playing a role?

NEPOM: We haven't at all. My suspicion is that its going to be difficult to pick up anything of the linkage problem in humans. That is, the DQ 3.2 DW4 haplotype that is most prevalent in diabetes also has a common HLA B specificity and if that is playing some role it will be masked by the fact that it is linked to DQ 3.2.

ERHLICH: One point I would like to make, is that the simplest interpretation of the DR4 haplotype effect that is the 3.2 with DW4 or 3.2 with DW10 having a much higher risk than 3.2 with DW14, is that there need not be one HLA class II gene that confer susceptibility. You get a combination of alleles on class II loci that confers to susceptibility so one can have DQ and DP as in coeliac disease contributing or for the DR4 haplotype in IDDM DR and DQ contributing. Finally, with respect to the relevant gene on other haplotypes I fully agree that there is no way at the moment of knowing what's going on with respect to DR3, but I think on DR6 it is fairly clear that it is the DQ beta allele as there are different DR6 haplotypes some of which are associated with IDDM and some which aren't. They have the same DR beta 1 but they have a different DQ beta and in fact one of the reasons that some people feel that position 57 may be an important element is that the susceptible DQ beta and the non-susceptible DQ beta allele on DR6 haplotypes differ only at 57 and at 70.

<u>NEPOM</u>: The potential to have two genes contributing to these HLA and disease associations is really dramatic. Henry's data on coeliac disease and diabetes, and our own data on diabetes clearly demonstrates this particularly for DR3 or 4 heterozygotes in diabetes and potentially this cis effect where certain DQ 3.2 haplotypes are more prevalent than others all might point towards a 2 gene effect. If those are structural HLA genes we could speculate and say that one gene might be related to selection and antigen presentation, whilst the other might have more to do with repertoire selection, skewing or something like that. There truly might be a mechanistic synergy as well as genetic synergy. Its a very attractive way to think about these things.

<u>TROWSDALE</u>: Could you comment on your allotypic clones - they presumably all see transfectants of B cells. Do you see the same fidelity for these clones if you use other types of class II transfected cells. Is it possible that the clones are seeing a peptide in the groove associated with particular residues?

<u>NEPOM</u>: One of these clones is probably seeing a peptide as an allele determinant, the others we can't really tell. Its potentially an important point in our justification for using alloreactivity as a model system but as I say with the one exception it doesn't tell us anything else. We have transfected these genes into human B cells and into monocyte lines. We haven't done anything in mouse lines. Only in the one case does it look like there is an endogenous peptide in the binding pocket.

<u>DEMAINE</u>: Have you looked in other racial groups for any interaction between DQW 3.2 and the DQ alpha chain?

<u>NEPOM</u>: The contribution of the DQ 3.2 to diabetes is not by any stretch of the imagination the whole story. In Caucasians it is the dominant HLA susceptibility allele and accounts for two thirds of the HLA susceptibility of diabetes. That is not true when you look at other ethnic groups. For instance, in the oriental populations which we have studied diabetes is associated with the DQ 3.2 gene which carries an aspartic acid at position 57 and therefore contradicts the popular model. It is the dominant major susceptibility allele in these populations. There are other ethnic groups where DQ 3.2 is very rare and in those cases other alleles are associated with diabetes. I think the bottom line is that there are going to be multiple immunogenetic types of the disease leading to a common phenotypic type I diabetes. The context that I regard these data in is that we need to create a model system for how type I diabetes occurs in humans and the best candidate gene for a pathway that will get us to that and its by no means the only pathway to that end.

A SINGLE RECESSIVE NON-MHC DIABETOGENIC GENE DETERMINES THE DEVELOPMENT OF INSULITIS IN NOD MICE

Masakazu Hattori, Masahiro Fukuda and Fumihiko Horio

Joslin Diabetes Center
One Joslin Place
Boston Massachusetts 02215
U. S. A.

NATO ASI Series, Vol. H 38
The Molecular Biology of Autoimmune Disease
Edited by A. G. Demaine et al.

Introduction

Insulin-dependent diabetes of man, the BB rat and the NOD mouse appears to result from autoimmune β cell destruction in a setting of genetic predisposition. The NOD mouse develops insulin-dependent diabetes secondary to islet β cell destruction by infiltrating lymphoid cells (insulitis), resulting in lack of intrinsic insulin secretion, hyperglycemia, loss of body weight and ketosis as seen in human insulin-dependent diabetes (Makino S, et al. 1980). Insulitis appears as early as 5 weeks of age. The lymphoid cells invade islets and are often seen adjacent to the ducts and blood vessels (Figure 1). The inceidence of insulitis is 90% in NOD females and 70% in NOD males at 9 weeks of age. The incidence and degree of insulitis increase with age. The NOD mouse develops diabetes usually by 6 months of age. The cumulative incidence of diabetes in our NOD/ShiJos colony is 80% in NOD females and less than 20% in NOD males at 7 months of age. In some other colonies, the incidence of diabetes in males is higher (approximately 50%) than that in our NOD/ShiJos colony (Prochazka M, et al. 1987). This could be due to differences in diets, environments and NOD-lines.

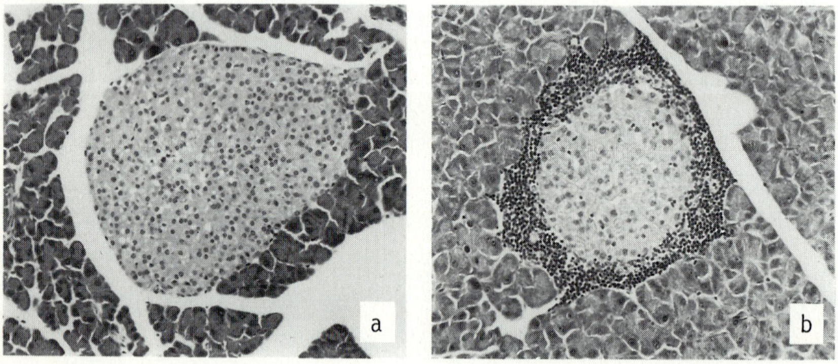

Figure 1. Histology of pancreatic islets. a) islet of a nondiabetic ICR mouse with H.E. staining, and b) islet of a diabetic NOD mouse with H.E. staining (Note infiltrating lymphoid cells).

Genealogy of the NOD Mouse and its Sister Strain

The nonobese diabetic (NOD), nonobese nondiabetic (NON), cataract Shionogi (CTS) and ICR-L-Ishibe (ILI) mice were originally derived from outbred Institute of Cancer Research (ICR) mice (Makino S, et al. 1980; Katoh H. 1988) (Figure 2). Briefly, one mouse with cataracts and small eyes was fortuitously found in outbred ICR mice. An inbred CTS strain was established and characterized by cataracts and microphthalmia. Cataracts are often observed in diabetic patients. During the process of establishing the CTS starin, two substrains were separated at the 6th generation according to fasting blood glucose levels; one with euglycemia (100 mg/dl) and the other with slight hyperglycemia (150 mg/dl). One female mouse in the former euglycemic line spontaneously developed diabetes at the 20th generation and the inbred NOD was established by selective breeding for diabetes. From the latter line the inbred NON strain was established. The ILI mouse is inbred and directly derived from outbred ICR mice.

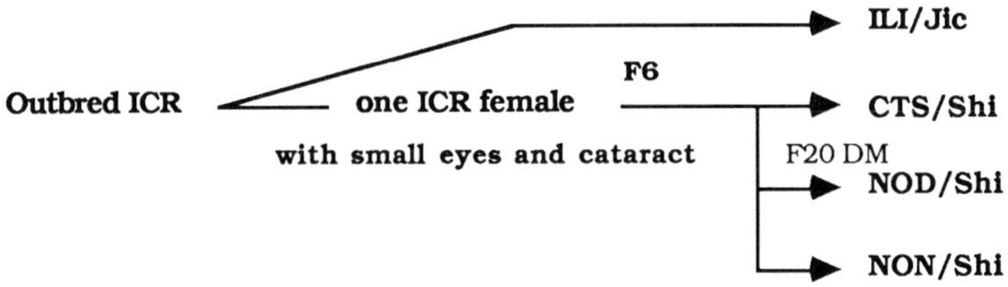

Figure 2. Genealogy of the NOD mouse and its sister strains.

Major Histocompatibility Complex (MHC) of the NOD and ILI Mouse

With the use of a panel of monoclonal antibodies and restriction fragment length polymorphism (RFLP) analysis, it has been shown that the NOD mouse possesses a recombinant class I (K^d, D^b) and unique MHC class II molecules with no expression of surface I-E molecules and different I-A molecules from any known I-A (Hattori M, et al. 1986; Ikegami H, et al. 1988). Lack of surface I-E molecules is due to absence of messenger RNA for I-Eα. Sequence studies (Acha-Orbea H and McDevitt HO. 1987) indicate that the I-Aβ chain is unique in NOD mice. The amino acid residue at position 57 of the I-Aβ chain is serine in NOD mice and asparatic acid in nondiabetic inbred laboratory mouse strains.

The ILI mouse in our colony is inbred (F43) and directly derived from outbred ICR mice. We characterized the MHC class I and class II of the ILI mouse using monoclonal antibodies (mAb) and a flow cytometer. MAb 31-3-4S (specificity: K^d) reacted with ILI, NOD, CTS and BALB/c mice. MAb 28-14-8S (D^b, L^d) reacted with ILI, NOD, NON, BALB/c and C57BL/6, but not with CTS and C3H. Regarding the MHC class II, mAb 10-2-16 (I-$A^{k,f,r,s}$) reacted with

ILI, NOD, CTS and NON. MAb 39B and 40A (I-$A^{k,f,r,u}$) reacted with ILI, NOD and CTS mice, sharing the same I-A. MAb 14-4-4S, which recognize any I-E molecules expressed on the cell surface, did not react with ILI, NOD, CTS and C57BL/6, indicating a lack of I-E molecules. In the mixed lymphocyte reactions (two ways) between ILI, NOD, NON and C57BL/6 mice, ILI and NOD mice showed the same stimulation indices against each other and high stimulation indices against NON and C57BL/6. Thus, the ILI and NOD mice share the same MHC class I and class II (K^d, unique I-A, absence of I-E molecules and D^b).

MHC-Linked Diabetogenic Gene

The development of diabetes in NOD mice is controlled by at least 2 or more recessive genes (Hattori M, et al. 1986; Prochazka M, et al. 1987; Wicker L, et al. 1987). Environmental factors such as viruses, diets and hormones can also influence the development of diabetes (Makino S, et al. 1981; Scott FW, et al. 1985; Yoon JW, et al. 1979). One of the recessive diabetogenic genes is tightly linked to the major histocompatibility complex on chromosome 17 (MHC-linked diabetogenic gene, Figure 3) (Hattori M, et al. 1986). It is suggested that the unique sequence of I-Aβ alle in NOD mice make the animals susceptible to diabetes (Acha-Orbea H and McDevitt HO. 1987). Recent breeding studies in crosses of NOD with I-E expressing C57BL/6 [B6(I-Eα of d)] transgenic mice suggest that I-Eα gene expression prevents the development of insulitis (Nishimoto H, et al. 1987). It is still unkown whether the unique I-Aβ or a lack of I-E molecules is diabetogenic in NOD mice.

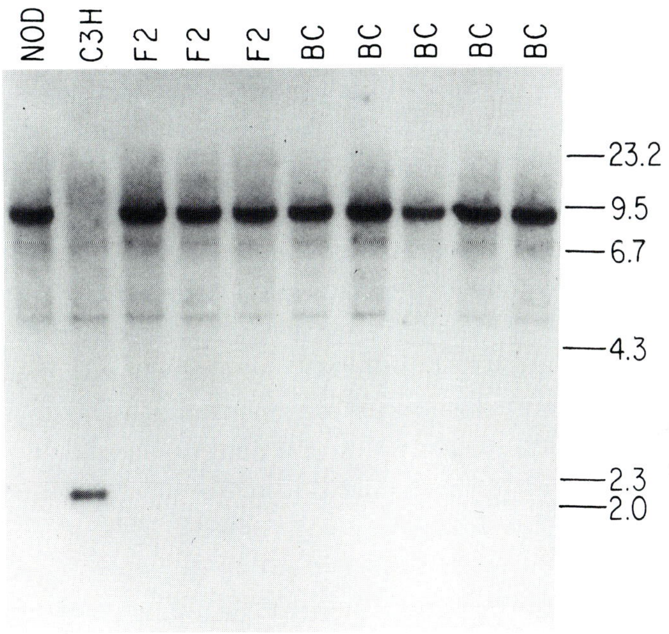

Figure 3. Restriction fragment length polymorphism analysis of NOD and C3H (parental strains) and diabetic F2 and backcross (BC) animals with BamHI and an Aβ probe. All diabetic animals were homozygous for the NOD 9.5-kb fragment and lacked the C3H 2.1-kb fragment. Size of DNA marker fragments are shown in kilobases.

NON-MHC-Linked Diabetogenic Gene

Backcrosses of NOD with NON and C3H/He developed insulitis at 39-50% incidence over 1-year-period. The F1 animals did not develop insulitis. It is suggested that a single recessive gene determines the development of insulitis regardless of MHC haplotypes. Backcrosses of NOD with C57BL/6 developed insulitis at an incidence of 24%. This was a half of the incidence of insulitis in the other backcross groups, suggesting a suppressed development of insulitis.

The ILI and NOD mice serologically shared the same MHC class I and class II molecules. The ILI mice, however, did not develop insulitis or diabetes. ILI females were mated with NOD males to produce F1 animals. The F1 females were mated with NOD males to produce backcross animals. The backcross animals were sacrificed at 9 weeks of age, typed for MHC class I and class II, and the pancreata were subjected to histological examination. The incidence of insulitis was 0% in F1 females (0/7) and 40% in backcrosses (8/20). Crosses of NON with NOD, and C3H/He with NOD were also typed for MHC class I and class II and subjected to histological examination at 1 year of age. Insulitis was not found in F1(NONxNOD) and F1(C3HxNOD). Insulitis was found in BC[(NONxNOD)F1xNOD] females at the incidence of 50% (12/24) regardless of NOD's MHC homozygosity or heterozygosity. In BC[(C3H/HexNOD)F1xNOD] females, insulitis was found at the incidence of 48% (14/25) regardless of NOD's MHC homozygosity or heterozygosity. The results suggest that a single recessive non-MHC gene determines the development of insulitis in NOD mice.

Thy-1-Linked Diabetogenic Gene

Breeding studies in crosses of NOD with NON mice demonstrated a second diabetogenic gene, Thy-1(T-cell surface marker)-linked gene on chromosome 9 in addition to the MHC-linked diabetogenic gene on chromosome 17 (Ikegami H, et al. 1986, Prochazka M, et al 1987). In our breeding studies [99 female and 58 male backcrosses] of NON (Thy-1.1) with NOD (Thy-1.2), 14 backcrosses developed diabetes and were homozygous for NOD's MHC. Among the 14 diabetic animals typed for Thy-1 phenotype on chromosome 9, 12 diabetic backcrosses were homozygous for NOD's Thy-1.2. This suggests a contribution of another diabetogenic gene linked to Thy-1 on chromosome 9 to diabetes susceptibility in NOD mice. Two out of the 14 diabetic backcrosses were heterozygous (Thy-1.1/1.2) and had a recombinant event between Thy-1 and the malic enzyme-1 (Mod-1) locus. This observation indicates that the map distance containing the Thy-1-linked diabetogenic gene is 14 cM (2/14=14%, approximately 14 million base pairs). This map distance is too large to further localize the diabetogenic gene on chromosome 9.

To further define the localization of the Thy-1-linked diabetogenic gene on chromosome 9, we performed linkage analyses of P-450, T3 delta, T3 epsilon, dilute and Mod-1 locus with the inheritance of diabetes in BC[(NONxNOD)F1 xNOD] using RFLP and enzymatic (biochemical markers) analyses. In the RFLP analysis, polymorphisms were found between NOD and NON with Thy-1 probe (restriction enzymes: Kpn I, Bgl II) and P-450 probe (Pvu II). There was, however, no linkage of the loci with the inheritance of the development of diabetes. We tested dilute, T3 delta, T3 epsilon and NCAM probes with 20 restriction enzymes, but have been unsuccesful in finding polymorphisms between NOD and NON. In the analysis of biochemical marker genes, Mod-1 was polymorphic between NOD and NON, but unlinked to the inheritance of the development of diabetes. Regarding the possibility of loci on other chromosomes, Idh-1 on chromosome 1, β-2 microglobulin on chromosome 2, Car-2 and Amy-2 on chromosome 3, and T-cell receptor gamma on chromosome 13 were polymorphic between NOD and NON, but not linked to the inheritance of the development of diabetes. To date, we have been unsuccessful in finding any other loci linked to the inheritance of the development of diabetes. This could be due to a lack of polymorphism between NOD and NON, or a lack of linkage even if there was a polymorphism.

Genetic distortion of Thy-1 phenotype and MHC haplotype in diabetic and nondiabetic backcrosses [(NONxNOD)F1xNOD)]

The ILI mouse possesses Thy-1.1 phenotype as well as the NON mouse. We, therefore, have typed nondiabetic backcrosses [(ILIxNOD)F1xNOD] for Thy-1 phenotype and compared with nondiabetic backcrosses [(NONx NOD)F1 xNOD] typed for Thy-1 phenotype and MHC haplotype. The NOD and ILI mice share the same MHC class I and class II. Among 20 nondiabetic backcrosses [(ILIxNOD)F1xNOD], 9 animals were homozygous for Thy-1.2 (45%) and 11 heterozygous for Thy-1.1/1.2 (55%). Among 53 nondiabetic backcrosses [(NONxNOD)F1xNOD] homozygous for NOD MHC, 37 animals were homozygous for Thy-1.2 (70%) and 16 heterozygous for Thy-1.1/1.2 (30%). This indicate a genetic distortion of Thy-1 phenotype in backcrosses [(NONx NOD)F1xNOD]. The Thy-1 linkage of the inheritance of diabetes in NOD mice showed a recombination frequency of 14%. This means that the Thy-1-linked gene is located at 14 cM from Thy-1 locus. When we consider the genetic distortion of Thy-1 phenotype (homozygosity:heterozygosity= 70:30%) in backcrosses [(NONxNOD)F1xNOD], the Thy-1-linkage becomes looser than we thought initially. The Thy-1-linked gene may be located at approximately 30 cM (14cMx70/30%) from Thy-1 locus. Further analysis is required to confirm the Thy-1-linkage of the development of diabetes in NOD mice.

Conclusion

Breeding studies of NOD mice with C3H/He, NON and ILI mice suggest that a single recessive non-MHC gene is required for the development of insulitis regardless of MHC homozygosity or heterozygosity. The genetic distortion of Thy-1 phenotype could exaggerate the linkage of NOD's Thy-1.2 phenotype with the development of diabetes in backcrosses of NOD with NON mice.

Acknowledgements

This work was supported by grants of NIH DK-33641, NIH 1P30 AM368378 (Diabetes and Endocrinology Research Center, Animal Core Facility and Tissue Culture Core) and Juvenile Diabetes Foundation International (187400). M.F. is a recipient of a JDF fellowship.

Literature Cited

Acha-Orbea H, McDevitt HO (1987) The first external domain of the non-obese diabetic mouse class II I-Aβ chain is unique. Proc Natl Acad Sci USA 84: 2435-2439

Hattori M, Buse JB, Jackson RA, Glimcher L, Dorf ME, Minami M, Makino S, Moriwaki K, Kuzuya H, Imura H, Strauss WM, Seidman JG, Eisenbarth GS (1986) The NOD mouse: recessive diabetogenic gene in the major histocompatibility complex. Science 231:733-735

Ikegami H, Jackson RA, Makino S, Watts DE, Eisenbarth GS, Hattori M (1986) Homozygosity for two genes (H-2:chromosome 17 and Thy-1: chromosome 9) linked to the development of Type I diabetes of the NOD mouse. Clin Res 34: 683A

Ikegami H, Makino S, Harada M, Eisenbarth GS, Hattori M (1988) The cataract Shionogi mouse, a sister strain of the non-obese diabetic mouse: similar class II but different class I gene products. Diabetologia 31:254-258

Katoh H (1988) MHC genes of inbred strains derived from outbred ICR mice. In:Yoshida T (ed) Annual Report 1987 by the Research Committee of Experimental Models for Intractable Diseases. The Ministry of Health and Welfare of Japan, Tokyo, p139

Makino S, Kunimoto K, Muraoka Y, Mizushima Y, Katagiri K, Tochino Y (1980) Breeding of a non-obese, diabetic strain of mice. Exp Anim 29:1-13

Makino S, Kunimoto K, Muraoka Y, Katagiri K (1981) Effect of castration on the appearance of diabetes in NOD mice. Exp Anim 30:137-140

Nishimoto H, Kikutani K, Yamamura K, Kishimoto T (1987) Prevention of autoimmune insulitis by expression of I-E molecules in NOD mice. Nature 328:432-434

Prochazka M, Leiter ED, Serreze DV, Coleman DG (1987) Three recessive loci required for insulin-dependent diabetes in nonobese diabetic mice. Science 237:286-289

Scott FW, Mongeau R, Kardish M, Hatina G, Trick KD, Wojcinski Z (1985) Diet can prevent diabetes in the BB rat. Diabetes 34:1059-1062

Wicker LS, Miller BJ, Cocker LZ, McNally SE, Scott S, Mullen Y, Appel MC (1987) Genetic control of diabetes and insulitis in the nonobese diabetic (NOD) mouse. J Exp Med 165:1639-1654

Yoon JW, Austin M, Onodera T, Notkins AL (1979) Virus induced diabetes. Isolation of a virus from the pancreas of a child with diabetic ketoacidosis. N Engl J Med 300:1173-1179

DISCUSSION

NEPOM: Why do you think it is that the MHC homozygous animals have a high incidence of IDDM?

HATTORI: One possibility is that the MHC-linked gene is amplified and therefore amplifies the immune process once the insulitis gene has got to work.

NEPOM: Do you think that the non MHC gene encodes for the islet autoantigen?

HATTORI: This seems very unlikely to us from the bone marrow transplant data.

COOKE: Is the gene for insulitis also the gene which controls the induction of infiltration in all the other organs in your mice?

HATTORI: The only thing we do know is that the salivary gland infiltration is not linked to the insulitis gene.

AUTOIMMUNITY - MORE THAN THE MHC?

A.G. Demaine, B.A. Millward, N.Willcox[1], A. Thompson, J. Newsom-Davis[1].

Department of Medicine,
King's College School of Medicine,
Denmark Hill,
London SE5 8RX.

and

Department of Neurological Sciences[1],
Institute of Molecular Medicine,
John Radcliffe Hospital,
Oxford.

NATO ASI Series, Vol. H 38
The Molecular Biology of Autoimmune Disease
Edited by A. G. Demaine et al.

Analysis of human genetic polymorphisms, has succeeded in uncovering variability at many gene loci, which determine cell surface antigen structures, enyzme proteins, and serum proteins with many different, and in some cases unknown function. These polymorphisms have been used as markers to investigate the genetic susceptibility to many diseases. At least one-third of the known structural genes which determine blood enzymes exsist as polymorphisms. Estimates on the number of structural proteins in man range from 50-150,000. Therefore, thousands of polymorphisms presumably exsist in the population, however, to date fewer than 150 have been described. Therefore, the search for diseases associated with exsisting polymorphisms will usually be fruitless unless a pathophysiological relationship can be established.

There have been many reports of associations between blood groups and autoimmune disease. For instance, insulin dependent diabetes mellitus (IDDM) has been shown to be associated with the Kidd blood group, whilst rheumatoid arthritis has been reported to be associated with certain allotypes of alpha-1-antitrypsin. A lot of attention has been focused on finding associations with the Major Histocompatibility Complex (MHC) by comparing the frequency of HLA class I and II antigens between disease and control populations. The search for other immunogenetic markers which might be important in determining susceptibility to autoimmunity has until recently, been restricted to the allotypes of immunoglobulin (Ig). These had previously been used to investigate the genetic restriction of antibody responses

(Whittingham et. al., 1980), and soon lead to their application to disease susceptibility studies. One of the earliest reports of either Gm (IgG) or Km (Ig kappa chain) allotypes being associated with autoimmune diseases was by Farid et. al. (1977), who showed that the Gm haplotype Gm(3,5) or Gm(3,5,23) was present in all 40 patients with Graves' disease studies and only 20/31 patients with Hashimoto's thyroiditis. This soon led to many other studies investigating Gm and Km allotypes frequencies in disease.

The cloning of the genes coding for the Ig genes has now allowed diseases associations to be investigated in more detail. In particular, it is now possible to analyse the role of the variable (V) region genes and the immune response. The first studies used restriction fragment length polymorphism (RFLP) analysis and Ig-C gamma probes to investigate the extent of linkage disequilibrium within the human Ig-CH loci. Extensive linkage disequilibrium was found between Gm allotypes and RFLPs of the Ig-C gamma loci (Bech-Hansen et. al., 1983; Hoover et. al. 1986). Since then, a number of RFLPs have been described which span the whole of the Ig-CH loci from $C\mu$ to $C\alpha 2$. These have been used to extend the studies using Gm allotypes. The results are summarised in Table 1.

The association of Ig switch region RFLPs with myasthenia gravis (MG) is particularly intriguing. MG is a classic autoimmune diseases characterised by autoantibodies directed towards the acetylcholine receptor (AChR). There are 4 main subgroups of MG based on clinical presentation and thymic histology:

Young onset - age at onset <40 years, tend to be female and HLA-B8,DR3

Old onset - age at onset >40 years, tend to be male and HLA-B7, DR2.

Thymoma - associated with thymic hyperplasia, no HLA association.

Ocular - no HLA association, symptoms confined to the ocular muscle, may progress to more generalised MG.

Gm allotypes have previously been shown to be asociated with MG in Japanese populations, although the reports in Caucasian patients have been difficult to confirm. Therefore, probes to the Ig-Sμ, Sα1 and D14S1 loci have been used to investigate the role of the IgH region in MG. No association was found with the Sα1 or the downstream D14S1 loci and any of the subgroups of MG. However, a highly significant association was found between the Sμ locus and old onset MG; 53.3% of these patients had the Sμ 2.6;2.6 kilobase (kb) genotype compared to 19.9% in normal controls ($p < 0.0005$, corrected). There was also a significant increase of the Sμ 2.6 kb allele in these patients. Further, there is a clear increase in the frequency of the Sμ 2.6;2.6 kb genotype with age at onset of all patients with generalised MG (young and old onset MG).

TABLE 1: RESTRICTION FRAGMENT LENGTH POLYMORPHISM ASSOCIATIONS OF THE Ig HEAVY CHAIN GENES

LOCUS	DISEASE	ASSOCIATION
Sμ	Membranous nephropathy	2.6;2.6 and 2.1;2.1 kb Sst-I genotype
	Psoriatic arthropathy	2.6;2.6 kb Sst-I genotype
Sα1	IgA nephropathy	7.4 kb Sst-I allele
Cγ3	Multiple sclerosis	5.9 kb Bst-EII allele

There is no correlation of the Sμ, Sα1 or D14S1 genotype with the titre of the anti-AChR antibody. Preliminary analysis of the Ig-VH loci using probes to VH2 subgroup has shown no association with any of the subgroups. This may be because the VH2 RFLPs are located at the distal end of the VH loci. The human IgVH loci may contain a number of recombinatorial hot-spots resulting in little linkage disequilibrium between Ig-VH2 and the downstream Ig-CH loci.

The recent cloning of the T-cell antigen receptor (TCR) now allows the tri-molecular complex of TCR-antigen-MHC to be analysed in detail. There is already a wealth of information on the role of the MHC in autoimmune disease. However, the penetrance of associations with alleles of MHC molecules in disease populations is low because these alleles also occur at a high high frequency in the normal population. For instance, HLA-DR3 is found in approximately 30% of the normal caucasian population and yet is associated with many autoimmune diseases.

This would suggest that either the association with MHC is poorly defined and with better analysis, e.g. sequence comparisions an absolute marker with disease will be found, or, that other genes such as those coding for the TCR also contribute to the immunogenetic background. As the immune (or autoimmune) response depends upon the recognition of antigen+MHC molecular complex by a T-cell expressing a particular TCR it is likely that the TCR will contribute to the genetic susceptibility to autoimmune disease.

The classical TCR consists of two chains - alpha and beta, both chains have a variable (V) and constant (C) region which are coded for by separate genes (Acuto et. al., 1985; Kronenberg et. al. 1986). At the present time, studies have been carried out investigating the association of RFLPs of the TCR-C_β and -C_α genes with autoimmune disease. Table 2 summarises the results.

TABLE 2: RESTRICTION FRAGMENT LENGTH POLYMORPHISM ASSOCIATIONS OF THE T-CELL RECEPTOR (TCR) BETA AND ALPHA CHAIN GENES

LOCUS	DISEASE	ASSOCIATION
TCR-C_β	Graves' disease (Newfoundland)	10;9.2 kb Bgl-II genotype
	Membranous nephropathy	10;9.2 kb Bgl-II genotype
TCR-C_α	Multiple sclerosis	
	Myasthenia gravis	
TCR-V_α	Hypothyroidism/Graves' disease	1.4 kb Taq-I fragment

The association of RFLPs of TCR-C_β with insulin dependent diabetes mellitus (IDDM) has been investigated and associations have been found in both Caucasian and Japanese patients (Hoover et. al., 1986; Ito et. al., 1988). In our own study, we have investigated singletons as well as identical twins concordant or discordant for IDDM. The results are summarised in Table 3.

Perhaps the most interesting finding is that identical twins who are concordant for IDDM have the most striking RFLP association with the TCR-C_β, whilst those identical twins who have remained discordant for IDDM for at least 11 years have no significant association with the TCR-C_β.

TABLE 3: T-CELL RECEPTOR C_β GENOTYPE FREQUENCIES (%) IN INSULIN DEPENDENT DIABETES MELLITUS

	TCR-C_β GENOTYPE (Kb)		
	10.0;9.2	10.0	9.2
Singletons (n = 116)	56.0	21.6	22.4
Identical twins concordant for IDDM (n = 24)	79.2*	8.3	12.5
Identical twins discordant for IDDM >11 years (n = 20)	60.0	5.0	35.0
Controls (n = 126)	42.1	24.6	33.3

* versus frequency in controls $p = < 0.005$

The association between TCR-C_β and IDDM has been pursued further using probes to the TCR-V_β genes. A problem of investigating the TCR-V_β loci has been the lack of probes and suitable RFLPs. Using the restriction endonuclease Msp-I and the V_βS97 probe a number of RFLPs have been detected. RFLPs of 1.5, 1.6, 3.8, 4.1, 4.4 and 4.8 kb have been shown to segregate in families and at least 8 different genotypes can be detected, although 2 of these account for more than 50% of all genotypes.

The frequency of the $V_\beta S97$ genotypes of IDDs and controls differ significantly, the results are shown in Table 4. Therefore, the TCR-V_β genes may themselves confer susceptibility to IDDM - suggesting that the germ line polymorphism may have a significant role in determining the immune response. Recent sequence data on the $V_\beta S97$ clone shows that it belongs to the $V_\beta 1$ subgroup.

TABLE 4: FREQUENCY OF $V_\beta S97$ GENOTYPES IN INSULIN DEPENDENT DIABETES MELLITUS

	$V_\beta S97$	GENOTYPE(kb)	
	3.8;4.4;4.8	4.4;4.8	OTHER
Patients (n = 61)	43.3	22.4	34.3
Controls (n = 58)	27.6	48.3	24.1

p = <0.01, 3 X 2 contingency table.

In the non-obese diabetic (NOD) mouse there are thought to be at least three genes which confer susceptibility to IDDM (Hattori et. al., 1986; Wicker et. al., 1987). Backcross experiments suggests that one of these genes may be linked to the Thy-I locus on chromosome 9 of the mouse. In man, the Thy-I locus resides on chromosome 11. The organisation of these regions of chromosome 9 and 11 is syngeneic between mouse and man - Thy-I, Apo-I, P450-3, TCR-CD3 gamma-delta-episilon. The search for the analagous NOD mouse Thy-I associated gene in man has so far proved inconclusive. However, using a probe to the CD3 episilon gene and the restriction endonuclease Taq-I, RFLPs have been detected which have an interesting distribution within the diabetic population. Two allelic fragments are detected of 9.0 or 8.0 kb - the frequency of the 8.0 kb fragment is significantly increased in female diabetics compared to male diabetics (Table 5), and this increase is reflected in the genotype frequencies. Further confirmation of this result is required.

TABLE 5: FREQUENCY OF CD3 EPSILON ALLELES OF FEMALE AND MALE INSULIN DEPENDENT DIABETICS

	Allele (kb)	
	8.0	9.0
Male (n = 46)	0.239	0.761
Female (n = 46)	0.500	0.500

$p < 0.01$.

In conclusion, whilst genes residing in the MHC are known to confer susceptibility to a number of diseases, it is unlikely that a disease specific allele will be found. Further, it is likely that other genes outside of the MHC such as TCR and Ig will be important, particularly when considered in relation to the MHC. Also, we are just beginning to elucidate at the molecular level the mechanism of tolerance induction and selection in the thymus, and the mechanism of MHC restriction. It may then become clear how tolerance breaks down, the relationship to the immunogenetic background, and the process leading to autoimmunity.

REFERENCES

Acuto, O and Reinherz, E.L. (1985) The human T-cell receptor. Structure and function. N Engl J Med 17; 1100-1111.

Bech-Hansen, N.T., Linsley, P.S., Cox. D.W. (1983) Restriction fragment length polymorphisms associated with immunoglobulin C gamma genes reveal linkage disequilibrium and genomic organisation. Proc Natl Acad Sci 80; 6952-6956.

Farid, N.R., Newton, R.M., Noel, E.P., Marshall, W.H. (1977) Gm phenotypes in autoimmune thyroid disease. J Immunogenet 4; 429-432.

Hattori, M., Buse, J.B., Jackson, R.A., Glimcher, L., Dorf, M.E., Minami, M., Makino, S., Moriwaki, K., Kuzuya, H., Imura, H., Strauss, W.M., Seidman, J.G., Eisenbarth, G.S. (1986) The NOD mouse: recessive diabetogenic gene in the Major Histocompatibility Complex. Science 231; 733-735.

Hoover, M., Angelini, G., Ball, E., Stastny, P., Marks, J., Rosenstock, J., Raskin, P., Ferrara, G.B., Tosi, R., Capra, J.D. (1986) T-cell receptor genes in insulin dependent diabetes mellitus. Cold Spring Harbor Symp Quant Biol Ll; 803-809.

Ito, M., Tanimoto, M., Kamura, H., Yoneda, M., Morishima, Y., Takatsuki, K., Itatsu, T., Saito, H. (1988) Association of HLA-DR phenotypes and T-lymphocyte-receptor beta-chain-region RFLP with IDDM in Japanese. Diabetes 37; 1633-1636.

Johnson, M.J., de lange, G., Cavill-Sforza, L.L. (1986) Ig gamma restriction fragment length polymorphisms indicate an ancient separation of Caucasian haplotypes. Am J Human Genet 38; 617-640.

Kronenberg, M., Siu, G., Hood, L., Shastri, N. (1986) The molecular genetics of the T-cell antigen receptor and T-cell antigen recognition. Ann Rev Immunol 4; 529-591.

Whittingham, S., Mathews, J.D., Schanfield, M.S., Mathews, J.V., Tait, B.D., Morris, P.J., Mackay, I.R. (1980) Interactive effect of Gm allotypes and HLA-B locus antigens on the human antibody response to a bacterial antigen. Clin Exp Immunol 40; 8-15.

Wicker, L.S., Miller, B.J., Coker, L.Z., McNally, S.E., Scott, S., Mullen, Y., Appel, M.C. (1987) Genetic control of diabetes and insulitis in the nonobese diabetic (NOD) mouse. J Exp Med 165; 1639-1654.

DISCUSSION

EISENBARTH: Have you performed sib-pair analysis particularly for the CD3 or any of the other associations?

DEMAINE: No we haven't done this, and the chromosome 11 work is still preliminary. Obviously, the next stage will be to show segregation in multiplex families. We don't know whether sib-pair analysis is the right approach, since only about 10% of diabetics come from multiplex families and the other problem is the availability of family material. There are problems in obtaining multiplex families in London.

THORSBY: Can I ask you a question about your genomic studies on the T cell receptor. I always find these studies very interesting, but I am a little bit puzzled about what sort of interpretation one can make of them. I take it that your RFLPs have been done at the germ line level and one wonders what one can detect by RFLPs in the germ line level in the first place? Are these polymorphisms in the intron or are they in the exon parts of the variable genes?

DEMAINE: The RFLPs are at the 5' end of CB2 in the intron. We have no information on the position of the RFLP of the VBS97 gene.

THORSBY: So my general question is actually what do we know about polymorphisms or variations between variable alpha and variable beta genes in the exon parts?

DEMAINE: Well all the mouse and human V beta genes and many of the human V alpha genes have been sequenced but I don't think anyone has published any studies on structural polymorphisms. One of the areas which we are pursuing is to try and look at this at the level of expression of these genes. I haven't shown that data today because its preliminary but we know that VbS97 is expressed in around 5% of peripheral T cell receptors in normal individuals.

QUESTION: I would like to raise a similar question about immunoglobulin genes - an important feature of this human locus is its lack of polymorphism this comes from the work of many groups. However, we get the impression from your work that its highly polymorphic? Do you want to comment on that?

DEMAINE: I don't think I said it was highly polymorphic. I don't think you can actually say that it's not polymorphic at this early stage. You can't dismiss polymorphism at VH genes as no-one has worked on it significantly.

QUESTION: When human VH genes are sequenced we see little polymorphism I think everybody agrees on that?

DEMAINE: The other point looking at this region is simply you don't know how many of those genes are perhaps inherited and maintained in the germ line and how many are not. It may be that certain VH genes are inherited and maintained in the population which would alter the polymorphism because you might have certain VH genes which are conserved the ones that are not might increase polymorphism.

QUESTION: Another possibility with the kinds of studies you are performing is that they may show us a major alteration of these loci.

DEMAINE: Yes, I'm sure that's a possibility.

G S EISENBARTH - SESSION CHAIRMAN'S SUMMING UP

I think for our understanding of autoimmunity we are going to have to know what the genes are that are involved in susceptibility to the development of these diseases. In relation to type I diabetes, 3 species develop the disease, the BB rat, the NOD mouse and man. Its clear that there are at least two genes conferring susceptibility; one is a gene that destroys or leads to the absence of all RT6 positive T lymphocytes and the other is an MHC gene which has been very well localized to the class II region where there are recombinants on both sides of the class II region and the disease is carried within the class II region. It is not known whether its an IA or IE like gene. In addition, in the BB rat there is a severe T cell lymphopenia gene that is inherited as a simple autosome recessive gene creating an immunodeficient rat which has in the order of a 100 to a 1000 times greater incidence of diabetes compared to a rat which only has the MHC susceptibility gene. Also I might just mention that BB rats have no CD8 T lymphocytes. They are apparently killing their beta cells without any of the classic CD8+ T cells. Hence, it has been virtually impossible to breed a strain that consistently develops type I diabetes in the absence of the T cell lymphopenia gene. One can have animals which sporadically develop type I diabetes without the T lymphopenia gene or one can inject the antibody to RT6 into a non-lymphopenic diabetes resistent strain that has the MHC for type I diabetes and create a diabetic animal. In relation to the NOD mouse, I would take caution in assigning the gene

NATO ASI Series, Vol. H 38
The Molecular Biology of Autoimmune Disease
Edited by A. G. Demaine et al.

within the MHC creating diabetes suceptibility. I think the sequence data is extremely interesting, its very clear that IA alpha has the same sequence as Balb/c which is not diabetogenic, the lack of IE by itself is not diabetogenic. Breeding studies, with C57 mice suggest that IA beta with its unique sequence will be involved but its only a suggestion. The proof of that suggestion would be breeding studies with natural recombinants for instance, workers have identified the CTS mouse as a natural recombinant within the IA region of NOD but differing in K and E. I think we need direct tests in the mice to determine the actual susceptibility gene. An antibody has been discovered which stains the pole region of the RIN islet beta tumour cells. The presence of this antibody in NOD mouse is inherited as a simple autosome recessive trait. The antibody appears by 7 days of age in mice and essentially all NOD mouse have this antibody. No F1 mice have this antibody, and no mouse of any normal strain which has been looked at have the antibody. But if one does backcross experiments, for instance, with B6PL, 50% of these have this antibody. If one looks at the animals who go on to develop diabetes either from a cross of B6PL or a cross of NON with NOD, one gets up to 97% of the mice expressing this antibody. If one then looks at a second backcross generation one winds up with more mice having the antibody but you can segregate the animals. If a parent mouse of the backcross has the anti polar antibodies then essentially 100% of their offspring will have this antibody. The presence of this antibody is independent of the MHC which suggests that it is a very simple Mendelian inheritance of an antibody that for some reason is correlating with the development of type I diabetes. With a disease model as simple as the BB rat and NOD mouse we clearly need to know what the genes are which confer susceptibility. In man, I would say that no extra MHC gene has been identified which segregates the way these and other genes segregate in the BB rat or the NOD mouse. Either its because no such gene has been found for instance, or that its just going to take more studies to blanket the rest of the human genome to find it or that the human disease is a complex mixture of different diseases. I suspect though that another gene will be found which will be just as important as the insulitis gene in the NOD mouse and the lymphopenia gene in the BB rat. Finally, I would just like to speculate and go from the question of genetic susceptibility to genetic activation. I think we have very little information for type I diabetes in particular of what activates the autoimmunity or what takes a genetically susceptible individual and leads to development of active autoimmunity and the best example of that we've heard a little about are identical twins. About 50% of identical twins will remain discordant for type I diabetes for life and in essence the question that is being asked is what determines penetrance for an identical twin for the activation of disease and I would just like to try out a suggestion that it might be something like the retinablastoma gene story, that there might be genetic activation of the autoimmune process. Basically one inherits a dominant gene determining disease susceptibility but the gene is only activated in a cell that mutates the alternative allele so the hypothesis that we are pursuing, but very slowly as we don't know the genetic localization of the cell is that in type I diabetes and autoimmunity it might be similar. In all the autoimmune diseases we have heard about there are none that have a 100% concordance in identical twins, at least, none that I'm aware of. Now the one other interesting point that I would like to make about activation is that in man one could have such a genetic mechanism that occurs in retinoblastoma because humans who develop these disease are diallelic, obviously of multiple alleles but in our animal models we can't have that mechanism and as best I can tell in the twins that we studied the twin who doesn't activate the disease process stays non-activated over many years and we now finally have some pathologic data from twins from their pancreas who did not activate the disease and the pancreases are normal. If you take Sutherland and co-workers they have now begun doing, as we heard a little about, living related donor pancreas transplants and one of things they do when they take the pancreas from the twin that didn't develop diabetes is look at the pancreas and it is normal. In NOD mice if we had a mouse that didn't develop diabetes the pancreas wouldn't be normal it would have insulitis essentially all the mice. In the BB rat there are a few rats who don't activate the autoimmune process. Our antibody data in twins go along very much with no activation in the autoimmunity though there is some controversy between our twin studies and the twin studies in Great Britain. I think Sutherland's twin data looking at the pancreas is very important. As I say, contrary to man, the animal strains we work with are identical at certain loci by their breeding process and they should all activate the disease.

THE IDIOTYPIC NETWORK IN EXPERIMENTAL AUTOIMMUNE THYROIDITIS (EAT): TOWARDS A NEW CONCEPTION OF AUTOIMMUNE REACTIVITY.

C. Bédin, B. Texier, C. Roubaty, J. Charreire
INSERM U. 283
Hôpital Cochin
27, rue du Fg St-Jacques
75674 Paris Cedex 14
France

Thyroiditis is an autoimmune disorder resulting in hypofunction of the thyroid gland because of its damage. This disease occurs either spontaneously in various species of animals including the OS chicken or the Buffalo rat, or experimentally after immunization of susceptible animals with thyroglobulin (Tg) or defined Tg tryptic fragments. Transfer of experimental autoimmune thyroiditis (EAT) can also be achieved by Tg specific helper T cell lines or clones (for review, see J. Charreire, 1989).

In the last years, the ability of anti-idiotype antibodies (anti-id Abs), of antigen-specific T cell lines or of their specific anti-id Abs to prevent experimentally induced autoimmune disease has been proven in EAT (Maron et al., 1983), encephalomyelitis (Lider et al., 1988; Ellerman et al., 1988), collagen arthritis (Kakimoto et al., 1988), uveoretinitis (De Kozak et al., 1987) and myasthenia gravis (Agius and Richman, 1986).

In a recent work, we described the protective immunity against EAT induced by injection into syngeneic CBA ($H-2^k$) mice of a mitomycin-inactivated Tg-specific cytotoxic T cell clone: HTC2 (Remy et al., 1989). We demonstrated that this

NATO ASI Series, Vol. H 38
The Molecular Biology of Autoimmune Disease
Edited by A. G. Demaine et al.

protection occurred through an idiotypic network, bridging T and B lymphocytes, both exhibiting a specificity for the same EAT inducer determinant of the Tg molecule (Salamero et al., 1987). More precisely, in the protected animals, anti-id auto-Abs (A-Abs) Ab2 beta (Roubaty et al., submitted), which recognize the paratope of a monoclonal anti-Tg (m anti-Tg) Ab1 specific for the pathogenic epitope of the Tg molecule, were detectable three weeks after HTC2 cell inoculation and before Tg immunization. Therefore, we hypothesized that prevention resulted from the appearance of anti-T cell receptor (TCR) A-Abs which behave like anti-id A-Abs to Ab1 specific for the EAT inducer epitope of the Tg molecule. To test this hypothesis, we produced and selected two sets of m anti-id A-Ab, specific for HTC2 TCR and anti-Tg paratope, both recognizing the same EAT inducer Tg epitope. Then, these anti-id A-Abs were injected into syngeneic naive recipients seven days prior to immunization with Tg. Histological examination of the thyroids was performed on day 28 post-immunization.

Materials and methods.

Production of mA-Abs: Spleen cells from immunized CBA ($H-2^k$) mice were fused with the BALB/c myeloma cells X63 Ag 8.653 at a ratio of spleen to myeloma cells 5:1 by using polyethylene glycol 1500 according to Kohler and Milstein (1976). Characteristics of the different mAbs used in this study are shown on Table 1. They were used after purification on Protein A-(Ig2a) or Protein G-(IgG1) coupled-Sepharose.

Designation	Characteristics	Binding to	Specificity
E1 (unrelated)	IgG1	Cryptococcus neoformans	Cryptococcal polysaccharide
18A8H2	IgG2a, Kappa	B cell producing IgG specific for EAT inducer epitope	Ab1 paratope
18A8A1	IgG1, Kappa		Ab1 idiotope
AG7	IgG1, Kappa	HTC2-cell specific for EAT inducer epitope	Ti
AC8	IgG2a, Kappa		Ti

Table 1: Characteristics of mAb used for protection of CBA mice against EAT.

Experimental protocol for EAT prevention: Forty µg of mAb were injected i.p. into naive CBA mice. Each experimental group included 5 to 8 mice. Seven days later, mice were immunized in both hind foot pads with 50 µg of porcine Tg (PTg) emulsified in complete Freund's adjuvant and boosted two weeks later with 50 µg of PTg in incomplete Freund's adjuvant. Twenty-eight days after Tg priming, the animals were bled before killing and their thyroids and kidneys were fixed in Bouin's solution.

Histopathological studies: Five µm thick sections were stained with Masson-Goldner's trichrome solution. The histological incidence of EAT was graded as function of the mononuclear cell thyroid infiltration indexes (Salamero et al., 1987): 1: interstitial accumulation of inflammatory cells distributed between two or more follicles; 2: one to two loci of inflammatory cells of at least the size of one follicle; 3: 10 to 40% of the thyroid replaced by inflammatory cells; 4: > 40% of the thyroid replaced by inflammatory cells. Mean grades of EAT were assigned as follows: 0 to 1: negative; 1 to 2: mild; 2 to 3: severe; 3 to 4: acute.

Results and Discussion.

In a first set of experiments, we induced EAT prevention by injection of 1×10^6 cloned cytotoxic T cell hybridoma, HTC2, specific for a Tg determinant inducing EAT, and MHC class I restricted. The mitomycin-inactivated HTC2 cells were injected 21 days before Tg immunization (Table 2A).

The fact that we detected anti-Tg and anti-id (Ab2 beta) A-Abs on day 0 (three weeks after HTC2 injection and before Tg immunization), and on day 28 post-immunization led us to hypothesize that HTC2 cells bearing specific receptors for the autoantigen prevented the induction of EAT through two possible mechanisms. The first one supposed the generation of anti-TCR A-Abs, structurally similar to the anti-id (Ab2 beta) Abs which would represent the internal image of pathogenic Tg epitope and would result in the production of specific Ab3 A-Abs. These Ab1-like A-Abs would in turn block the specific pathogenic epitope at the time of immunization and therefore the specific helper T cell response that induces EAT. Consequently, they would protect against EAT. An other explanation would envision that injected cytotoxic HTC2 cells specifically migrated to the thyroid gland,

Inoculation Nature	Day	Tg challenge	No. of mice		Infiltration index ± SEM	
A. Tg specific cytotoxic T cells						
None	None	None	5		0.40 ± 0.04	
None	None	+	8	**	4.20 ± 0.40	
BW 5147	- 21	+	8		3.10 ± 0.30	
HTC2	- 21	+	8		1.00 ± 0.23	
B. m anti-idiotype autoantibody						
Unrelated IgG	- 7	+	5		2.60 ± 0.2	
Ab2 alpha	- 7	+	5	*	2.40 ± 0.12	
Ab2 beta	- 7	+	5		1.20 ± 0.30	*
AC8	- 7	+	5		1.25 ± 0.12	

Table 2: Prevention of CBA mice EAT by Tg specific cytotoxic T cell hybridoma or anti-idiotype A-Abs. ** $p < 0.0001$; * $p < 0.001$ (Student's t test).

destroyed it, thus liberating syngeneic Tg. In this latter alternative, the anti-Tg A-Abs that we called Ab3 would become conventional anti-Tg A-Abs which would further stimulate "in vivo" anti-id A-Abs production.

We further investigated the potential role of specific anti-id A-Abs in EAT prevention by injecting mice, seven days prior to immunization with Tg, with m anti-id A-Abs, Ab2 beta, or with one m anti-id A-Ab to HTC2 TCR (Table 2B, Figure 1). Anti-id Ab2 alpha and an unrelated IgG were used as controls. Therefore we supposed, when protection occurred, that it would be obtained by the presence at the time of immunization of anti-Tg A-Abs blocking the pathogenic Tg epitopes. As anticipated from our previous data, only mice receiving Ab2 beta or anti-HTC2 TCR mAb were significantly protected against EAT, while those injected with control mAb or Ab2 alpha were not.

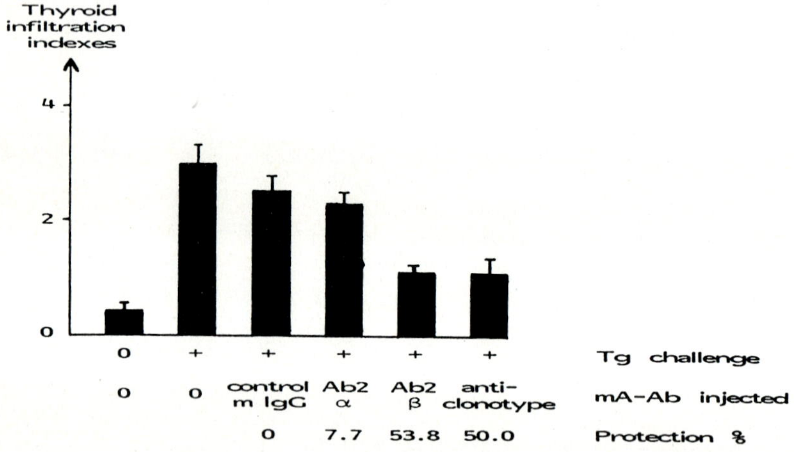

Figure 1: EAT protection by anti-clonotypic Abs directed against Tg specific cytotoxic T cells.

This last series of experiments even further established that a physiological idiotypic network bridging T and B lymphocytes could represent a regulatory mechanism for EAT. In these experiments, Ab2 beta directed against m anti-Tg A-Ab would play a pivotal role because they bind to the B cell producing the Ab1 specific to the EAT inducer epitope as well as to the T cells specific to this epitope; furthermore, they would represent the internal image of the nominal antigen.

Attention must be drawn to the fact that it requires

the simultaneous recognition of a crucial epitope by both T and B cells. More precisely, the basic question raised by the existence of this specific id network and its potential in regulating EAT concerns the relationship between the TCR carried by Tg-specific T cells and the Igs borne by specific B cells. In this network, a given epitope of the Tg molecule must be recognized by both the specific B and specific T cells. Up to now, such a "natural" coincidence has proven to be exceptional and only a few reports have been published (Eichmann et al., 1978; Ertl et al;, 1982; Singhai and Levy, 1987). However, in the past few years, the homology of sequences and residues corresponding to important structures has been demonstrated between alpha- and beta-chains of the TCR and L and H chains of the Igs (Novotny et al., 1986; Claverie et al., 1989), revealing that these products belong to the same superfamily and thus could present similar secondary conformations. Homology between T and B cell surface products would favor similar antigenic recognition by these cells particularly for autoantigens.

In conclusion, it can be envisioned that thyroiditis and, to a broader extend, autoimmune reactivity, would only occur when a pathogenic autoantigen can be recognized by T and B cells which share a same specificity. This simultaneous recognition would strongly dysregulate the homeostatic id network present in any normal individual or animal.

Acknowledgments.

We wish to thank Ms. E. Lallemand for her excellent technical assistance and Mrs. J. Decaix for designing the figure and typing the manuscript.

Agius MA, Richman DP (1986) Suppression of development of experimental autoimmune myasthenia gravis with isogeneic monoclonal antiidiotopic antibody. J Immunol 137:2195-2198.

Charreire J (1989) Immune mechanisms in autoimmune thyroiditis. Adv Immunol 46 (in press).

Claverie JM, Prochnicka-Chalufour A, Bougueleret L (1989) Implications of a Fab-like structure for the T-cell receptor. Immunol Today 10:10-14.

Eichmann K, Falk I, Rajewsky K (1978) Recognition of idiotypes in lymphocyte interactions. II. Antigen-independent cooperation between T and B lymphocytes that possess similar and complementary idiotypes. Eur J Immunol 8:853-857.

Ellerman KE, Powers JM, Brostoff SW (1988) A suppressor T-lymphocyte cell line for autoimmune encephalomyelitis. Nature 331:265-267.

Ertl HCJ, Greene MI, Noseworthy JH, Fields BN, Nepom JT, Spriggs DR, Finberg RW (1982) Identification of idiotypic receptors on reovirus-specific cytolytic T cells. Proc Natl Acad Sci USA 79:7479-7483.

Kakimoto K, Katsuki M, Hirofuji T, Iwata H, Koga T (1988) Isolation of T cell line capable of protecting mice against collagen-induced arthritis. J Immunol 140:78-83.

Kozak Y de, Mirshahi M, Boucheix C, Faure JP (1987) Prevention of experimental autoimmune uveoretinitis by active immunization with autoantigen-specific monoclonal antibodies. Eur J Immunol 17:541-547.

Köhler G, Milstein C (1976) Derivation of specific antibody-producing tissue culture and tumor lines by cell fusion. Eur J Immunol 6:511-519.

Lider O, Reshef T, Beraud E, Ben-Nun A, Cohen IR (1988) Anti-idiotypic network induced by T cell vaccination against experimental autoimmune encephalomyelitis. Science 239:181-183.

Maron R, Zerubavel R, Friedman A, Cohen IR (1983) T lymphocyte line specific for thyroglobulin produces or vaccinates against autoimmune thyroiditis in mice. J Immunol 131:2316-2322.

Novotny J, Tonegawa S, Saito H, Kranz DM, Eisen HN (1986) Secondary, tertiary and quaternary structure of T-cell-specific immunoglobulin-like polypeptide chains. Proc Natl Acad Sci USA 83:742-746.

Remy JJ, Texier B, Chiocchia G, Charreire J (1989) Characteristics of cytotoxic thyroglobulin-specific T cell hybridomas. J Immunol 142:1129-1133.

Salamero J, Remy JJ, Michel-Béchet M, Charreire J (1987) Experimental autoimmune thyroiditis induced by a 5-10-kDa tryptic fragment from porcine thyroglobulin. Eur J Immunol 17:843-848.

Singhai R, Levy JG (1987) Isolation of a T-cell clone that reacts with both antigen and anti-idiotype: Evidence for anti-idiotype as internal image for antigen at the T-cell level. Proc Natl Acad Sci USA 84: 3836-3840.

DISCUSSION

WEKERLE: Is it possible to use this anti T cell receptor antibody to stain T cells and so to isolate the positive cells by FACS in order, for example, to establish T cell lines which you could use to transfer disease?

CHARREIRE: We have not done this experiment but intend to do so.

DEMAINE: Have you had time to look at the rearrangement of your T cell receptor genes?

CHARREIRE: Not yet.

FRICKE: I really like your result which you got when you took your antibody 2 beta in order to protect the mice from getting thyroiditis. We did similar experiments in our SLE model. We also got anti-idotypic antibodies which also gave us an internal image of our first antigen but could use these antibodies to induce SLE in mice so they did not protect but rather induced the disease.

CHARREIRE: Our protocol is under investigation since we thought if we used exclusively antibody 2 beta we would induce wonderful murine experimental thyroiditis

FRICKE: Have you also been able to establish a monoclonal antibody properly which is the antibody 3?

CHARREIRE: Yes, we have but we don't yet have this fully characterised

WEKERLE: Did I understand correctly that the pathogenic epitope on the thyroglobulin is the epitope recognized by this particular T cell hybridoma in conjunction with class I?

CHARREIRE: Yes.

<u>WEKERLE</u>: Does the monoclonal antibody against this epitope block the T cell receptor?

<u>CHARREIRE</u>: We have not done the experiment.

FACTORS AFFECTING DIABETES IN RODENT MODELS OF INSULIN DEPENDENT DIABETES MELLITUS

L. O'Reilly, P.R. Hutchings, N. Parish, *E. Simpson, *T. Tomonari, T. Lund, **P. Crocker and A. Cooke

Department of Immunology,
University College & Middlesex School of Medicine,
Arthur Stanley House,
40-50, Tottenham Street,
London, W1P 9PG,
U.K.

*Clinical Research Centre,
Northwick Park ,
Harrow,
Middx., U.K.

**Sir William Dunn School of Pathology,
Parks Road,
Oxford, U.K.

NATO ASI Series, Vol. H 38
The Molecular Biology of Autoimmune Disease
Edited by A. G. Demaine et al.

Introduction

Insulin dependent diabetes mellitus (IDDM) is a disease with an autoimmune aetiology . The mechanism by which selective beta cell destruction occurs is not understood. Although T cells are clearly involved in the disease process it is not known whether they are effector cells directly mediating destruction via a class I or class II cytotoxic mechanism or via the production of cytokines or whether they are indirectly involved either by producing lymphokines which synergise with macrophage products in the destruction of the beta cell or by providing help for B cells to make antibody which affects beta cells by ADCC. The non obese diabetic (NOD) mouse strain and the BB rat spontaneously develop IDDM and provide excellent animal models of the human autoimmune disease (Makino et al. 1980, Nakhooda et al. 1977). These two animal models complement one another , it being easier to carry out some manipulations in the NOD e.g. genetics, while other manipulations e.g. pancreatic biopsies are easier in the BB rat.

In the NOD mouse it has been shown that the development of the disease is under the control of three recessive genes, one of which Idd-1 is linked to the MHC. Another gene has been located on chromosome 9 while the chromosomal location of the third gene remains unknown (Wicker et al. 1987, Hattori et al. 1986, Prochazka et al.1987). Selective beta cell destruction occurs in this animal following progressive pancreatic infiltration from 5-6 weeks of age by mononuclear cells, predominantly $CD4^+$, $IL\text{-}2R^+$ T cells and macrophages (Signore et al. 1987) and IDDM develops in 70% animals by 28 weeks of age. Infiltration itself is under the control of one incomplete dominant gene which is not linked to MHC (Wicker et al.1987). In the BB rat the genetic linkages for disease onset are not so well defined but the phenotypic characterisation of the mononuclear cell infiltration is perhaps more complete. The combination of longitudinal studies and pancreatic biopsy has made it possible to identify the sequence of cellular events in the pancreas which culminates in beta cell destruction. Macrophages and Th cells are the first cells to infiltrate the pancreas (Dean et al. 1985) with class II MHC antigen expression being observed on vascular endothelium perhaps suggesting local production of gamma interferon (γ-IFN). Tc/s cells, NK cells and B cells were present in the infiltrates at a later stage. The infiltrating macrophages can be phenotypically distinguished from resident tissue macrophages , the former being ED1+ and the latter ED2+ (Dijkstra et al. 1985, Walker et al.1988). The disease in both the BB rat and the NOD mouse is prevented by T cell depletion (Like et al.1986, Harada and Makino,1986) or agents e.g. Cyclosporine (Bone et al.1986,Mori et al. 1986) which are known to affect T cell function. The disease furthermore can be transferred by a combination of $CD4^+$ and $CD8^+$ splenic T cells in both rats and mice (Koevary et al. 1983,Wicker et al.1986). In the NOD mouse IDDM can be transferred into irradiated syngeneic young recipients by a combination of $CD4^+$ and $CD8^+$ splenic T cells from diabetic donors. By carrying out time course studies using this transfer system it has been possible to demonstrate that CD4+ and CD8+ T cells enter the recipient pancreas between 1 and 2 weeks after transfer. This T cell infiltration is accompanied by an influx of macrophages bearing the type 3 complement receptor (CR3). Disease transfer has usually been accomplished within 4-5 weeks following T cell transfer at which point no beta cells can be found in the pancreas whereas the glucagon and somatostatin containing cells remain intact.

We have further used this transfer system to show that treatment of irradiated recipients up to two weeks after diabetic spleen transfer with anti-CD8 antibodies prevents the onset of diabetes and interestingly also halts the massive pancreatic infiltration by T cells and inflammatory macrophages (Hutchings et. al. J.Autoimmunity,in press).

In the NOD mouse there is a sex bias in disease incidence, females developing the disease at a much higher frequency than males although both sexes develop infiltration from 6 weeks of age. We have used a panel of antibodies to a variety of T cell and macrophage antigens to further analyse the infiltrates in the two sexes. Additionally using an antibody which depletes Vβ8-positive T cells, we have analysed the role of T cells which use this common Vβ family in their receptor.

Materials and Methods

Mice.

A breeding nucleus of NOD mice was established at the CRC, Northwick Park from mice provided by Dr.E.Leiter, Jackson Laboratory, Bar Harbor,USA. Diabetic female mice were standardly used as donors of spleen cells and the recipients were young male NOD mice, 2-4 months of age and always negative for glucose in the urine at onset of the experiment.

Monitoring for diabetes. The clinical onset of diabetes was ascertained by the presence of glucose in the urine and in the blood. Urine was tested by "Diastix" reagent strips (Miles Laboratories Ltd.) and blood glucose assessed weekly using a Glucometer

(Ames). A consistent reading of >10mMols/litre coupled with a positive test by Diastix was taken to be an indication of overt diabetes. All positive animals eventually displayed weight loss which progressed to death unless sacrificed earlier.

Cell transfer. Spleen cells from overtly diabetic NOD mice were prepared as a single cell suspensions in Hanks balanced salt solution (HBSS) and 20×10^6 injected intravenously into disease free male recipients which were given 650 rads earlier the same day using a Cobalt source. After transfer, recipients were monitored closely for the development of overt diabetes.

In vivo Vβ8 depletion. Mouse monoclonal F23.1 which recognises Vβ8.1+8.2+8.3 (Staerz et al. 1985) was used to deplete the Vβ8+ cells in the donor spleen cell preparation and also in the recipient following transfer. Donor animals were injected with 500ug F23.1 i.p. 3 days before transfer to deplete Vβ8+ cells. 24 hours after transfer of diabetogenic spleen cells into 650 rad irradiated recipients these animals were also injected with 500ug F23.1 i.p. to ensure depletion. Control mice (donors and recipients) were injected with a comparable volume of phosphate buffered saline (PBS).

Tissue preparation. Pancreata were excised from mice at the appropriate time and snap frozen in isopentane. 5um cryostat sections were cut, air dried and fixed in 100% acetone at room temperature for 10 minutes. These were then air dried and stored at -70°C.

Immunohistology. Cryostat sections of pancreatic tissue were stained for T cell subsets by a two layer peroxidase technique using the rat anti-mouse monoclonal antibodies anti-L3T4 (YTS191.4),anti-Ly2 (YTS169.4) and anti-Thy-1 (YTS154.7) and a goat anti-rat IgG biotin conjugate followed by avidin biotin horse radish peroxidase. These antibodies were a generous gift from Dr. H. Waldmann, Dept. Pathology, University of Cambridge, Cambridge, UK.

Dual fluorescent staining of beta cells and T cells/macrophages:Beta cells were detected by a guinea pig anti-porcine insulin monoclonal antibody followed by a rhodaminated anti-guinea pig antibody. Infiltrating T cells/macrophages were detected by an indirect fluorescence technique utilising the following rat anti-mouse antibodies: M1/70 (Mac-1detects the c3biR present on neutrophils, macrophages and NK cells). The rat hybridoma cell line making this antibody was obtained from Dr.T.Springer (Dept. of Pathology, Harvard Medical School, Boston,MA. USA), F4/80 (specific for mature macrophages, Hume et al. 1984), anti-vβ8.1.+8.2 (KJ16;Haskins et.al. 1984), F23.1 anti-vβ8.1+8.2+8.3, (F23.1; Staerz et al.1985)44.22.1 anti-vß6 (44.22.1; MacDonald et al.1988), anti-vβ11 (KT11, Tomonari and Lovering, 1988), followed by a fluorescein conjugated goat anti-rat antibody.

Results

1. Phenotypic analysis of pancreatic infiltrates of normal male and diabetic NOD mice

The infiltrates of non diabetic and diabetic pancreas can clearly be distinguished by the presence of peripheral infiltrates only in the former and destructive intra-islet infiltration in the latter. Using antibodies which identify different T cell subsets both CD4+ and CD8+ T cells can be demonstrated in the infiltrated pancreas of both non diabetic and diabetic NOD mice. Analysis of Vβ usage by these T cells using available antibodies clearly showed that T cells were present which expressed Vβ8, or Vβ6 or Vβ11also in both diabetic and non diabetic animals. However examination of the infiltrating T cells for IL2 receptor expression showed very few positive cells in the non diabetic infiltrates compared to very large numbers of IL2R+T cells in the intra-islet infiltration of the diabetic pancreas. Thus although the infiltrating T cells in normal and diabetic NOD mice cannot be distinguished on the basis of Vβ usage they are clearly different with regard to state of activation.

2. Effect of depletion of Vb8 bearing T cells on the transfer of diabetes.

The monoclonal antibody F23.1 is a complement fixing antibody which is specific for murine Vβ8 TCR chains (Staerz et al. 1985). Donor diabetic mice were pretreated with 500ug of monoclonal antibody three days prior to spleen transfer to deplete Vβ8+ cells in the donor inoculum. Following transfer of the depleted diabetic spleen cells to 650 Rads irradiated mice the recipients were treated with 500ug F23.1. The treated and control animals were monitored weekly for changes in blood glucose levels and on sacrifice the numbers of F23.1+ cells present in the periphery was established and the pancreas subjected to histological analysis. From Table 1 it can be seen that depletion of

TABLE 1

Incidence of IDDM in recipients of Vβ8 deleted diabetic spleen cells

	% Incidence of diabetes			
	Expt1*		Expt 2*	
Donor	F23.1 depleted	Control	F23.1 depleted	Control
Time				
wk 1	0	0	0	0
wk 2	20	20	0	0
wk 3	30	20	20	100
wk 4	30	30	80**	100**
wk 5	60**	80**		

* 5 recipients in each group
** animals sacrificed for histological analysis

Vβ8 bearing T cells did not significantly diminish the incidence of diabetes. Analysis of blood and pancreas showed that depletion of Vβ8 bearing cells had been accomplished and that the intra-islet infiltrate of the diabetic pancreas of the depleted recipient was free of Vβ8+ cells but contained large numbers of Vβ6 bearing cells. Vβ11 bearing cells were also present intra-islet. Thus Vβ8 bearing cells are not necessary for beta cell destruction.

Discussion

The underlying basis for the development of rodent and human IDDM and the mechanism by which beta cells are destroyed by the immune system remains unknown. Several authors have suggested that there might be a viral trigger for the autoimmune destruction of the NOD beta cell (Fujita et al.1984, Suenaga and Yoon, 1988) and the demonstrable involvement of CD8+ T cells in the autoimmune disease is suggestive of a class I restricted killing mechanism. Indeed the ability of NOD bone marrow to destroy NON or C57Bl/10 pancreas is consistent with this hypothesis (Wicker et al.1988, Serreze et al. 1988). Our own studies suggest that CD8+ T cells may play an additional role controlling the influx of mononuclear cells into the pancreas since treatment of animals with anti-CD8 antibodies prevents diabetes and also affects infiltration of pancreas by T cells and macrophages (Hutchings et al. J. Autoimmunity in press)
Comparison of the infiltrates of non diabetic and diabetic male mice revealed that the only phenotypically significant differences were the wholly peripheral infiltration in the non diabetic animal and the virtual absence of IL-2R bearing T cells. Otherwise it appeared that all the relevant cell types were present. Diabetes can only be transferred into young non diabetic male mice by diabetic spleen cells if the recipients are subjected to at least 650 rads irradiation (Wicker et al. 1986, Hutchings, unpublished observations) or given a high dose (300 mg/Kgm) of cyclophosphamide (Hutchings, unpublished observations). In non diabetic animals it has also been shown that T cell mediated destruction of the beta cell can be precipitated by pretreating the animals with this high dose of cyclophosphamide (Harada and Makino,1982). The necessary dose of irradiation required to facilitate disease transfer and the necessary doses of cyclophosphamide employed are far greater than those required to abrogate any conventional immunological suppressor mechanism. Since irradiation at this level can affect vascular permeability and 300mg/Kgm cyclophosphamide can cause retroviral

expression in beta cells (Suanaga and Yoon,1988) it seems more likely that these agents are perturbing some system other than the immune network.

In vivo treatment of animals with antibodies to Vβ 8 has been shown to prevent the induction of experimental autoimmune disease (Acha-Orbea et al. 1988). As we found large numbers if Vβ8+ T cells intra-islet in diabetic animals we decided that it would be worthwhile attempting to modulate disease in NOD mice by deleting T cells bearing this Vβ. Our results suggest that Vβ8+ T cells are not necessary for the effector phase of beta cell destruction in the NOD mouse. We propose to extend our T cell receptor studies by examining the effects of other antibodies in vivo which recognise different Vβ. In addition we have now started to analyse the Vβ usage in transgenic NOD mice which we have generated expressing I-E due to the introduction of the $E\alpha^{d}$ transgene.

Acknowledgements

We would like to thank Drs.H. Waldmann and P.Crocker for their helpful discussions and the generous provision of reagents. We are also indebted to Drs. Marrack and Hengartner for the provision of cell lines producing antibodies to murine Vβ. We are grateful to Phil Chandler and Susan Fairchild for their assistance. Anne Cooke is a Wellcome Trust Senior Lecturer. This work has been made possible by support provided by the Wellcome Trust, the BDA and the MRC.

References

Acha-Orbea H, Mitchell DJ, Timmermann L, Wraith DC, Tausch GS, Waldor MK, Zamvil SS, McDevitt HO, Steinman L (1988) Cell 54:263-273

Dean BM, Walker R, Bone AJ Cooke A , Baird JD (1985) Diabetologia 28:464-466

Dijkstra CD, Dopp EA, Joling P, Kraal G (1985) Immunology 54:589-599

Fujita H, Fujino H, Nonaka K, Tarui S, Tochino Y (1984) Biomed Res 5:67-70

Harada M, Makino S (1986) Jikken-Dobutsu 35:501-504

Haskins K, Hannum C, White J, Roehm N, Kubo R, Kappler J, Marrack P (1984) J Exp Med 160:452-471

Hattori M, Buse JB, Jacobsen RA, Glimcher L, Dorf ME, Minami M, Makino S, Moriwake K,

Kuzuya H, Imura H, Strauss WM, SeidmanJ.D. Eisenbarth GS.(1986) Science 231,733-735

Koevary SB, Rossini A, Stoller W, Chick W, Williams RM (1983) Science 220, 727-728

Like AA, Biron CA, Weringer EJ, Byman K, Sroczynski E, Guberski DL (1986) J Exp Med 164:1145-1159

MacDonald HR, Schneider R, Lees RK, Howe RC, Acha-Orbea H, Festenstein H, Zinkernagel RM, Hengartner H (1988) Nature 332:40-44

Makino S, Kunimoto K, Muaoka Y, Mizushima Y, Katagiri K, Tochino Y (1980) Exp.Anim.29:1-13.

Mori Y, Suko M, Okudaïra H, Matsuba I, Tsuruoka A, Sasaki A, Yokoyama H, Tanase T, Shida T, Nishimura M (1986) Diabetologia 29:244-247

Prochazka M, Leiter EH, Serreze DV, Coleman DL (1987)Science 237:286-289

Serreze DV, Leiter EH, Worthen SM, Schultz LD (1988) Diabetes 37:252-255

Signore A, Cooke A, Pozzili P,Butcher G,Simpson,E, Beverley PCL (1987) Diabetologia 30:902-905

Staerz JD, Rammansee H, Benedetto J, Bevan M (1985) J Immunol 134:3994-4000

Suenaga K, Yoon JW (1988) Diabetes 37:1722-1726

Tomanari K, Lovering E (1988) Immunogenetics 28:445-451

Walker R, Bone AJ, Cooke A, Baird JD (1988) Diabetes 37:1301-1304

Wicker,L.S, Miller,B.J & Mullen,Y.(1986) Diabetes 35, 855-860

Wicker LS, Miller BJ, Coker LZ, McNally SE, Scott S, Mullen Y, Appel MC (1987) J.Exp.Med. 165: 1639-1654

Wicker LS, Miller BJ, Chai A, Terada M, Mullen Y (1988) J Exp Med 167:1801-1810

DISCUSSION

WEKERLE: May I ask what do the peri-islets immune cells see when they aggregate around the islets and on what antigen presenting cells do they see it?

COOKE: What do you mean what do they see? That was one of the things that I was trying to ask earlier today about the infiltration because the infiltrations are not restricted just to the pancreas. You get infiltrations in the salivary gland and also in the adrenal gland and also the thyroid gland. One thing I didn't mention actually is this transfer system is really good because what we now do using the system is to infect T cells with a retrovirus with Beta galactosidase on it and you can pick it up in salivary gland and in the pancreas but I don't why they are in there and I don't know what causes them to come in.

PAPEDOPOULOS: In your passive transfer experiments do you see class II expression in the appropriate epithelial cells before, during or after the infiltration of the cells into the islets?

COOKE: It's a good point. The problem is you don't know what that 650 rad irradiation is doing just as you don't know what the cyclophosphamide is doing. I don't happen to feel that its necessary getting rid of suppressor cells I think it could be doing something else may be making the system much more permeable.

KOLB: Ann, have you looked to see whether the transfer is MHC restricted. Could you transfer to semi allogeneic or totally allogeneic recipients?

COOKE: It would be very difficult to do. In the Wicker NOD mouse experiments its certainly clear the killing is not class II restricted at that level.

WILCOX: I'm interested in the difference between the sexes, is that a hormonal thing?

COOKE: It seems very clear, probably Dr Hattori knows much more about these experiments than I, but certainly if you castrate the males and give them female hormones they get the disease and likewise if you oophorectomise with females and give them testosterone they don't get the disease.

WEKERLE: Would it be possible to modulate disease in NOD mouse by neonatal or adult treatment with staphylococcal enterotoxin?

COOKE: It doesn't look like it.

CELLS AND IMMUNE PROCESSES CONTRIBUTING TO PANCREATIC ISLET INFLAMMATION

H. Kolb, V. Kolb-Bachofen
Diabetes Research Institute and
Institute for Biophysics and Electron Microscopy
University of Düsseldorf
D-4000 Düsseldorf 1
Fed. Rep. Germany

ABSTRACT

Macrophages precede lymphocytic infiltration of pancreatic islets during the development of insulin dependent diabetes in BB rats. Concomitant with macrophage invasion, local hyperexpression of class I MHC antigens and vascular defects are seen in afflicted islets. A macrophage produce, TNF, was shown to enhance transcription and cell surface expression of class I MHC antigens on rat insulinoma cells. Another monokine, interleukin 1 beta, was found to be a potent inducer of vascular permeability increase. Thus macrophages may be responsible for early lesions seen in inflamed islets.

The clinical onset of type 1 (insulin-dependent) diabetes is preceded by mononuclear infiltration of pancreatic islets with progressive destruction of insulin-producing beta cells. Studies on the natural history of islet inflammation in the prediabetic phase as yet have not been

NATO ASI Series, Vol. H 38
The Molecular Biology of Autoimmune Disease
Edited by A. G. Demaine et al.

performed in humans due to the risks of pancreatic biopsies. We therefore undertook a semiquantitative analysis of pancreata from diabetes prone BB rats.

BB rats spontaneously develop insulin-dependent diabetes around puberty or later. As in humans a genetic predisposition is found inside and outside the major histocompatibility gene complex, and mononuclear infiltration of islets precedes beta cell loss and diabetes onset (Mordes, Desemone, Rossini; 1987). The disease is immune-mediated because T-lymphocyte directed immune intervention prevents insulitis and manifestation of disease (Laupacis et al., 1983; Like et al., 1986). Furthermore, adoptive transfer of the disease by concanavalin A-activated spleen cells to normal recipients has been demonstrated (Koevary et al., 1985; Like et al., 1985).

Natural history of islet inflammation

Our study on islet inflammation in diabetes prone BB rats, 70 - 90 days of age, comprised a total of 201 islets from 21 rats (Hanenberg et al., 1989). Serial cryostat sections were stained by the indirect peroxidase technique with antibodies to class I or class II major histocompatibility (MHC) antigens (Ox18, 0x3, Ox6, Ox17), to macrophages (ED1, ED2), to T-cells (Ox19),to CD4 positive cells (W3/25), to CD8 positive cells (Ox8), to kappa chain positive cells (Ox12). More than 98 % of islets could be classified to one of four different grades of islet infiltration, indicating that islet inflammation follows a specific, non-random sequence of events:

<u>Stage 1a:</u> Focal macrophage (ED1$^+$, W3/25$^+$, Ox3$^+$, Ox6$^+$, Ox17$^+$, ED2$^-$) infiltration at the periphery of islets.
At the same site: focal hyperexpression of class I MHC antigens on all cell types.
At the same site: vascular damage, or dilated or shrunken endothelia.
Absence of lymphocyte infiltration and class II MHC antigen expression on islet cells.

<u>Stage 1b:</u> Macrophage infiltration throughout the islet.
Hyperexpression of class I MHC antigen throughout the islet.
Vascular damage, enhanced vascular permeability.
One T-lymphocyte (Ox19$^+$) detectable per mean islet section.

<u>Stage 2:</u> Macrophage infiltration throughout the islet.
T-lymphocyte (Ox19$^+$, W3/25$^+$) and T-/NK-cell (Ox8$^+$) infiltration throughout the islet.

<u>Stage 3:</u> Macrophage infiltration throughout the islet.
T-, NK-cell infiltration throughout the islet.
Focal B-lymphocyte (Ox12$^+$, Ox19$^-$) infiltration.

These results imply that macrophages precede lymphocyte infiltration in islet inflammation. T-lymphocytes precede B-lymphocytes. Macrophages seen in inflamed islets differ from resident islet macrophages in that they lack the ED2 marker.

Macrophages may induce class I MHC antigen hyperexpression

Since hyperexpression of class I MHC antigens was seen concomitantly with macrophage infiltration of islets and prior to the occurrence of T-lymphocytes we determined whether macrophage products may induce MHC antigen expression in islet cells.

Table 1
TNF alpha induces class I MHC hyperexpression in rat insulinoma cells[a]

	Time	-TNF	+TNF
Transcription of class I MHC genes[b]	24 hours	(+)	++
Expression of class I MHC antigens[c]	7 days	+	++

a, modified after G. Kantwerk-Funke, K. Kawai, H. Rothe, K. Reske, H. Kolb, K. Fehsel (submitted for publication)
b, RIN cell RNA, isolated by acid guanidium thiocyanate - phenol-chloroform extraction, was hybridized against a 2.5 Kb Bam H1 fragment of the 3'-region of the mouse D^b gene including exons 4 to 8.
c, cells were fixed in acetone and stained with Ox18 (anti RT-1A) by indirect immunocytochemistry (peroxidase method).

Recombinant human tumor necrosis factor alpha (100 units) was added to a rat insulinoma cell line (RIN m5f) followed by incubation at 37°C. As shown in Table 1 enhanced transcription of class I MHC genes was observed at 24 hours and enhanced staining of cells with Ox18 antibody was seen at day 7. Similar results were recently also reported by Cambell et al. (1988).

Further evidence for macrophage products as inducers of class I MHC hyperexpression during early islet inflammation comes from the observation that class I MHC hyperexpression is absent in islets from BB rats treated with silica particles to prevent macrophage infiltration of islets (Hanenberg et al., 1989; Lee et al., 1988).

Macrophages may induce enhanced vascular permeability

A second pathological change associated with macrophage infiltration of islets is the occurrence of vascular defects such as endothelial damage (Hanenberg et al., 1989) and enhanced vascular permeability within islets (Shinzato, Burkart, Kolb; 1989).

We determined whether cytokines produced by macrophages may cause leakage of vessel walls by injection of test substances into rat skin and quantitative analysis of serum protein-dye conjugates accumulating over the injection site (Martin et al., 1988).

Table 2
Interleukin 1 increases vascular permeability[a]

Cytokine injected	Permeability increase[b]
Buffer	0
Interleukin 1 alpha (10 U)	0.8 ($p < 0.05$)
Interleukin 1 beta (10 U)	1.4 ($p < 0.001$)
TNF alpha (10 U)	0.6 (n.s.)

a, modified after Martin et al. (1988)
b, Evans blue was injected 5 min prior to cytokines and dye extracted from the site at 30 min and determined by photometry at 620 nm of wavelength.
Permeability increase is given as $E_{sample} - E_{buffer}$ by E_{serum}.

As shown in Table 2 injection of interleukin 1 beta caused strong dye accumulation in the skin, reflecting enhanced vascular permeability.

Conclusions

An analysis of the natural history of islet inflammation in diabetes prone BB rats showed that early lesions are devoid of lymphocytes but are characterized by the infiltration of macrophages with concomitant hyperexpression of class I MHC antigens and vascular defects. Data reported here demonstrate that macrophage products may be responsible for pathological changes in islets: Tumor necrosis factor alpha was found to enhance transcription of class I MHC gene products and their expression on the cell surface. Another macrophage product, interleukin 1 beta, was shown to be a potent inducer of enhanced vascular permeability.

The contribution of macrophage activity to diabetes development is underscored by reports that the inhibition of macrophage invasion of islets by i.p. silica administration to BB rats also prevents later lymphocytic insulitis and insulin deficiency (Hanenberg et al., 1984; Lee et al., 1988). Further support comes from our recent finding that macrophages from diabetes prone but not from diabetes resistant BB rats show a regulatory defect in TNF production. In response to macrophage activating stimuli, secretion of TNF is enhanced by at least one order of magnitude and is not rapidly down regulated (Rothe, Fehsel, Kolb; 1989).

As speculated earlier (Kolb-Bachofen, Kolb; 1989) a macrophage defect may be decisive for islet inflammation, T-cell autoimmunity and diabetes development in BB rats.

ACKNOWLEDGEMENTS

This work was supported by the Deutsche Forschungsgemeinschaft (SFB 113, B 5 and Ko 806/2-2), by the Bundesministerin für Jugend, Familie, Frauen und Gesundheit and by the Ministerin für Wissenschaft und Forschung des Landes Nordrhein-Westfalen and by Nordisk-price grant to Dr. V. Kolb-Bachofen.

REFERENCES

Campbell IL, Oxbrow L, West J, Harrison LC (1988) Regulation of MHC protein expression in pancreatic ß-cells by interferon- and tumor necrosis factor- . Mol Endocrinol 2: 101-107

Hanenberg H, Kolb-Bachofen V, Kantwerk-Funke G, Kolb H (1989) Macrophage infiltration precedes and is a prerequisite for lymphocytic insulitis in pancreatic islets of pre-diabetes BB rats. Diabetologia 32: 126-134

Koevary SB, Williams DE, Williams RM, Chick WL (1985) Passive transfer of diabetes from BB/W to Wistar-Furth rats. J Clin Invest 75: 1904-1907

Kolb-Bachofen V, Kolb H (1989) A role for macrophages in the pathogenesis of Type 1 diabetes. Autoimmunity, in press

Laupacis A, Gardell C, Dupre J, Stiller CR, Keown P, Wallace AC, Thibert P (1983) Cyclosporin prevents diabetes in BB Wistar rats. Lancet 1: 10-12

Lee KU, Pak CY, Amano K, Yoon JW (1988) Prevention of lymphocytic thyroiditis and insulitis in diabetes-prone BB rats by the depletion of macrophages. Diabetologia 31: 400-402

Like AA, Weringer EJ, Hosdash A, McGill P, Atkinson D, Rossini AA (1985) Adoptive transfer of autoimmune diabetes mellitus in BioBreeding/Worcester (BB/W) inbred and hybrid rats. J Immunol 134: 1583-1587

Like AA, Biron CA, Weringer EJ, Byman K, Sroczynski E, Guberski DL (1986) Prevention of diabetes in BioBreeding/Worcester rats with monoclonal antibodies that recognize T lymphocytes or natural killer cells. J Exp Med 164: 1145-1159

Mordes IP, Desemone J, Rossini AA (1987) The BB rat. Diabetes/- Metab Rev 3: 725-750

Rothe H, Fehsel K, Kolb H (1989) Assoziation von erhöhter Tumornekrosefaktor-Produktion und Diabetesrisiko bei BB Ratten. Akt Endokrin Stoffwechsel, in press (Abstract)

Shinzato M, Burkart V, Kolb H (1989) Erhöhte Permeabilität in den Langerhansschen Inseln von diabetischen BB Ratten. Akt Endokrin Stoffwechsel, in press (Abstract)

DISCUSSION

TROWSDALE: Can you prevent lysis with anti TNF antibodies?

KOLB: Its very difficult at present to draw any final conclusions. There appears to be a synergy between various cytokines including TNF. At present we cannot say which is the dominant molecule

EISENBARTH: I think your data address very nicely the potential role for macrophages. Where do you see T cells fitting in would be my question namely do antibodies to T cells prevent disease? Can you transfer disease with macrophages as you can with T cells, what is your view of what the T cells are doing?

KOLB: There are two roles for macrophage and one may be T cell dependent and one may be T cell independent. In one macrophages do what T cells want. There are several situations where you can transfer disease with T cell lines and still can prevent organ destruction by inhibiting macrophage activity so an organ specific T cells might activate the macrophage and the macrophage might do the organ destruction this is the classical view of the role of the macrophage as a cell doing what the T cell wants and probably the majority of the audience would agree that this is the role of macrophages in type I diabetes. On the other hand at least in the BB rat and possibly in the NOD mouse as well macrophages present in the target organ precede the T lymphocyte infiltration. When you deplete macrophages by silica treatment you don't have any T lymphocyte infiltration in the islets in the NOD mouse as well as in the BB rat so we wonder whether macrophages in this peculiar situation have a second role that would be the secondary signals Dr Janeway speculated on yesterday. So our hypothesis at present is that something is peculiar about the islet which attracts macrophages and gives rise to a macrophage mediated inflammation and the macrophage mediated inflammation would never by itself go on to develop insulitis because the cytotoxic activity may not be strong and long enough but would create a condition which attracts T lymphocytes and provides the ability to stimulate the organ specific autoimmune T cells so the hypothesis is that a macrophage goes first and provides the conditions for T cell activation.

WILCOX: I thought I saw on your quantitative slides that where you have early macrophage infiltration you also have about 5 or 10% T cells so do you really have the macrophages first or could a very few T cells have a role?

KOLB: The real figure for macrophages is the class II positive cell number or the CD4 positive cell number and this gives a ratio of 30 macrophages per one lymphocyte and you of course could argue and its not excluded that there is one single autoantigen specific lymphycyte which is wondering around and giving the signals for all these macrophages coming in but what puzzles us is that once the macrophage is attracted you would expect that immediately more T lymphocytes come in and that is not the case.

LOHSE: Like the two persons asking questions before me I have difficulty in understanding how the macrophage finds its way into the islet. Don't you think that the quantitative data may be misleading you know from all sorts of inflammatory processes that the actual antigen specific T cells have a very very low frequency so that the T cells actually telling the macrophage to go into the islet may not be found by immunofluorescent studies and it may in fact even have gone by the time you look at the islet but the macrophage which is slower and more non-specific stays there then later on attracts the non-specific inflammatory infiltrate which we then define as insulitis?

KOLB: There is a long delay between macrophage infiltration and more T lymphocyte infiltration but it could be that there is a single specific T cell initially starting off everything. I don't know. Then the macrophage would be the effector cell and not the inductor cell. As regards the question why would the macrophage bind to the islet there are two speculations presently, a very good one is that insulin is chemotactic through macrophages so that could attract the macrophage and the second at least in some animal models there is retrovirus-like protein expression on islet cells again and this is chemotactic for macrophages.

COOKE: I'm going to go back to the T cell macrophage question. Did you just say Hubert that you were using class II as a marker for your macrophage because you felt you weren't getting a true representation by using ED1?

KOLB: In the early stages almost all class II positive cells are macrophages its different in late stages.

COOKE: I was going to say that class II is an activation molecule of T cells. It comes up transiently following activation of T cells so I don't think class II is really the best marker for you to use in that situation.

SYNOPSIS OF PAPER ENTITLED "Ir GENE EXPRESSION, ANTIGEN PROCESSING AND AUTOANTIGEN CHARACTERIZATION IN AUTOIMMUNE DISEASES OF THE NERVOUS SYSTEM"

H. Wekerle
Max-Planck Institute for Psychiatry
MPG Klinische Forschungsgruppe fur Multiple Sklerose
Josef-Schneider-StraBe 11
Postfach 6120
D-8700 Wurzburg 1
Federal Republic of Germany

Dr Wekerle began by highlighting the problems associated with the investigation of patients with multiple sclerosis. Whilst he thought it very likely that the disease was an autoimmune one, he reminded the audience that we still do not know what the target autoantigen is, have almost no access to the target tissue and, are as yet, unable to transfer the disease with human material. He suggested therefore that most of our knowledge on multiple sclerosis, to date, had to rely on animal models of the disease. He went on to highlight the two animal models that he had worked with; the first is the EAE Lewis rat in which the disease is inducible with myelin or myelin basic protein (MBP) in complete Freund's adjuvant. He pointed out that the T cells and the pathogenesis of this disease were CD4+ T cells which were specific for MBP. In the mouse models that he has worked with, he reported that differences in haplotypes in mice lead to differences in the epitopes of the MBP autoantigen that they recognize so that, for example, the PL/J mice see the 1-11 amino acid sequence of the autoantigen, whereas the SJL/J mice see the 90-101 amino acid sequence. In contrast, the Lewis rat encephalytogenic T cell clones seemed to be seeing the amino acid sequence 68-88

NATO ASI Series, Vol. H 38
The Molecular Biology of Autoimmune Disease
Edited by A. G. Demaine et al.

of MBP. Using these T cell clones it was possible to show that they transferred disease.

A major interest in the group currently is in the role which cells within the central nervous system may play in the process of antigen presentation. In this context, he pointed out that astrocytes and microglial cells can both express class I and class II antigens and, in addition, have antigen presenting capacity. In contrast, oligodendroglial cells, whilst expressing low levels of class I, neither express class II nor have the ability to function as antigen presenting cells with or without the addition of gamma interferon. He showed evidence of MBP specific T cells killing MBP-presenting astrocytes.
Using their panel of encephalytogenic T cell lines and clones in their PLJ mouse model and in the Lewis rat, they demonstrated that all T cell clones which recognize MBP have in common the presence of the V beta 8.2 determinant. Interestingly, despite the sequence homology between the mouse and rat V beta 8.2, the two species seem to recognize different epitopes of MBP.

In a different set of experiments, Dr Wekerle reported on work in the Lewis rat model in which an autoantigen specific CD8 positive T cell population were detectable in mice which had recovered from experimental allergic encephalomyelitis following innoculation with pathogenic CD4 positive T cell lines. These CD8 positive T cells were then allowed to proliferate in vitro in response to irradiated CD4 positive and CD8 positive lines and clones were generated. CD8 positive T cell line were shown when injected simultaneously with the CD4 line to prevent the induction of the EAE seen when CD4 cells were injected alone. They had demonstrated therefore a clonotypic specific counter regulatory T-T pathway with down-regulation of the CD4 positive T cell clones. There remains uncertainty as to the cell target of the CD8 positive cells. The therapeutic significance of these observations is currently under investigation.

Finally, Dr Wekerle reported on studies with T cell lines and clones which had been derived from patients with multiple sclerosis. They had apparently achieved a very high success rate in generating these T cells against human MBP. In summarising the data he said that there was really no good rule as to epitope recognition when one compared normals with patients with multiple sclerosis, but he emphasized that in the initial experiments there had been no attempt to group individuals according to their HLA status. To try to answer questions relating to the contribution which HLA class II makes to the process of antigen recognition, they had cloned out relevant class II genes and transfected them into mouse L cells to use as antigen presenting cells. Using the T cell line EB-BP6 they could show that this line recognizes the whole MBP molecule on L cells transfected with the alpha beta 2 genes of the HLA DR2 DW2 haplotype. These studies are still preliminary and as they have extended them into the examination of various fragments of MBP, Dr Wekerle pointed out how disappointing the results had been with peptide fragments which seemed to overlook the dominant epitopes and they had therefore resorted to using enzymatically digested MBP fragments with much more success, particularly using the fragment 76-91.

DISCUSSION

NEWSOM DAVIS: Those are very nice studies Helmut. Do you think that those MBP lines that you have are parallels of the CD4+cytotoxic lines in your experimental animals or do you think they are later lines such as helper cells for antibody production?

WEKERLE: This is a question which it is very difficult to answer conclusively. These cells in no way are distinguishable from those lines which we pull out from rats and mice. They recognize well epitopes on MBP. Some of them but not all of them are very strongly cytotoxic and hence I would think they would qualify as potential encephalitogenic clones.

NEWSOM-DAVIS: Your human clones are obviously from DR2 positive patients but what about the DR2 negative patients, do you have any clones from those patients?

WEKERLE: We have clones from a relatively large spectrum of patients but as I tried to stress its a very big enterprise to get together whole ranges of appropriately transfected antigen presenting cells and to go through them. We are not yet that far but we trust we will be in that situation soon.

QUESTION: When one raises T cell clones from PBM, which I understand you don't, one tends to select for DR restricted clones because the expression of DQ is rather low in PBM at least in monocytes. Have you tried to raise clones that recognise MBP with DQ?

WEKERLE: We did not really try to raise DQ clones but I take your point. There may be a bias towards DR which may perhaps leave DQ restricted cells under represented I should however stress that exactly the same situation seems to be the case for T cells which are isolated from thymuses of myasthenic patients.

QUESTION: Recent studies have suggested that the T cell repertoire may play a role in the establishment of EAE. Have you examined whether the Brown Norwegian rat expresses the V beta 8.2 gene?

WEKERLE: No we have not examined that. I would be cautious about placing too much emphasis on the differing ability of strains to respond to MBP. Remember that the C57 black mouse was traditionally thought to be the non-responder to MBP and to encephalomyelitis induction. We have regularly established encephalitogenic T cell clones in that strain.

QUESTION: You said that you don't know about the mechanism of activation of your CD8 positive clonotypic T cell line. Do you know something about the T cell receptor of this line?

WEKERLE: No, we were not able to clone them and hence T cell analysis has not been pursued.

QUESTION: Have you been able or did you try to block activation of this CD8 positive line by incubating your CD4 pathogenic line with the V beta 8 antibody?

WEKERLE: Unfortunately, none of the mouse anti V betas reacts with the rat so we have not done it.

QUESTION: You have shown very nicely that the Lewis rat uses the same set or a similar set of V beta genes as the PLJ mice, that is the V beta 8.2, however, it has also been shown that the SLJ mice uses a completely different set of V beta genes and we also know that the clones from this strain of mice recognize a different epitope so what is your opinion of this?

WEKERLE: Well the question is what is normal and what is abnormal. We heard that SJL mice have a large deletion in the V beta gene and they cannot use V beta 8 because its not there. I have no explanation for your question.

QUESTION: Have you tried to prevent or cure the disease by injecting monoclonals to V beta 8.2?

WEKERLE: We don't have these antibodies yet in the rat.

MECHANISMS OF RESISTANCE TO AUTOIMMUNE DISEASE INDUCED BY T-CELL VACCINATION

Ansgar W. Lohse
I. Medizinische Klinik und Poliklinik
Johannes Gutenberg-Universität Mainz
Langenbeckstr. 1
6500 Mainz
West Germany

Irun R. Cohen
Dept. of Cell Biology
Weizmann Institute of Science
Rehovot 76100
Israel

NATO ASI Series, Vol. H 38
The Molecular Biology of Autoimmune Disease
Edited by A. G. Demaine et al.

Many human autoimmune diseases tend to progress slowly. Phases of rapid progression may come to a halt and may be followed by transient or even permanent remissions. Autoimmune diseases in animals either arise spontaneously or are induced. The former tend to be slowly progressive, the latter mostly acute to subacute, and usually followed by spontaneous remissions. The mechanisms at work that prevent rapid disease progression and can effect remissions are poorly understood, but they may provide us with a clue both to natural self-tolerance and to the therapeutic induction of self-tolerance.

T-Cell Vaccination

Ben-Nun et al. were the first to isolate an autoreactive T cell line capable of mediating autoimmune disease in vivo (Ben-Nun et al. 1981a). This Z1a line recognizes an epitope on the amino acids 68-88 of myelin basic protein (BP) (Beraud et al., 1986). Upon passive transfer into naive Lewis rats activated Z1a cells cause severe experimental autoimmune encephalomyelitis (EAE) that is distinguished from active (antigen-induced) disease only by the more rapid onset. Animals that survive either active EAE or passive EAE were resistant to subsequent attempts of disease inductions (Ben-Nun et al. 1981b). The BP-reactive T cells were thus shown to be the agents responsible for the induction of EAE and for the subsequent resistance against EAE. While disease induction required functionally intact activated T-cells, resistance could also be achieved with irradiated or otherwise attenuated T lymphocytes (Ben-Nun et al. 1981b; Cohen 1986). The attenuated pathogenetic agent had become the inducer of disease resistance. This analogy to infectious disease and vaccination against infectious agents led to the term "T-cell vaccination" (Cohen et al. 1983). The principle of T cell vaccination has hence been extended successfully by us and by others to a number of different animal models of autoimmune diseases: adjuvant arthritis (AA) (Holoshitz et al. 1983), experimental autoimmune thyroiditis (EAT) (Maron et al. 1983), collagen II arthritis (Kakimoto et al. 1988) and experimental autoimmune neuritis (Taylor and Hughes 1988).

Anti-idiotypic T-cells induced by T-cell vaccination

The protection following T-cell vaccination is specific: a Lewis rat vaccinated with the BP-specific Z1a lymphocytes is protected from EAE, but is still susceptible to adjuvant arthritis. Vaccination with the clone A2b, which recognizes an epitope in mycobacterium tuberculosis (van Eden et al. 1988), is cross-reactive with cartilage proteoglycan (van Eden et al. 1985) and capable of inducing adjuvant arthritis in Lewis rats, similarly leads to efficient resistance to AA, but leaves the animals susceptible to EAE. The T-cell clones Z1a and A2b are both $CD4^+CD8^-$ cells derived from female Lewis rats. As far as we know they only differ in their T-cell receptor.

Ofer Lider, Evelyne Beraud and others have examined the specific protective response induced by T-cell vaccination in more detail. They found that subencephalitogenic doses of Z1a cells were also capable of inducing resistance to EAE (Beraud et al. 1989). While 10^5 or more activated Z1a cells or cells from its subclone D9 led to clinical disease, 10^4 or 10^3 cells caused no clinical disease, but nonetheless rendered the animals resistant. Resting Z1a cells even at doses of 10^7 cells induced neither disease nor resistance. Vaccination with 10^4 Z1a cells was found to follow similar kinetics as the recovery from clinical disease. Lider et al. could show that 6 days after injection of 10^4 Z1a cells into the hind footpads of naive Lewis rats the protective cell population was established and localized in the popliteal lymph nodes (Lider et al. 1988; Lider et al. 1989). When these popliteal lymph nodes (PLN) were left untouched the animals became resistant. Removal of the PLNs on day 6 resulted in failure to acquire resistance. Transfer of these removed PLNs to naive recipients rendered them resistant to EAE. In other words the PLN on day 6 carried the protective cell population induced by T cell vaccination. PLN cells from vaccinated animals showed a proliferative response against irradiated activated Z1a cells. This response was markedly stronger than the response against A2b cells and peaked around day 6. By day 9 this response was also present in the cervical lymph nodes. Thus the specific proliferative response was detected at the same time in the same places as was the protective cell population. We assume that the protective cells, or at least some of them, account for this proliferative response.

The responding cell population was examined further on a clonal level. PLN cells removed on day 6 after vaccination with Z1a cells were cultured in limiting dilution together with irradiated Z1a cells. Seven clones that proliferated specifically in response to Z1a cells but not in response to A2b cells could be established. Four of the seven clones were $CD8^+$ and were found to specifically suppress the proliferation of Z1a cells to their antigen (BP) but not of A2b cells to their antigen (M. tuberculosis). They thus seemed to be specific, probably anti-idiotypic, suppressor cells. The other three clones were $CD4^+$ and had little effect on the antigen-specific proliferation of either Z1a or A2b. However, these cells were able to stimulate resting Z1a cells, but had no effect on resting A2b cells. This clone-specific helper function suggests activation via the T-cell receptor. It seems reasonable to assume that these cells were truly anti-idiotypic: their T-cell receptors were mirror-images of the mirror image of BP (the T-cell receptor of Z1a) and thus mimicked BP. T-cell vaccination therefore seems to induce anti-idiotypic suppressor and anti-idiotypic helper cells.

Anti-idiotypic suppressor cells seem to be able to suppress disease in vivo as demonstrated by experiments performed in Hartmut Wekerle's laboratory in Würzburg (Sun et al. 1988). The role of the anti-idiotypic helper cells is at present speculative, but may lie in stabilising the immune response (Cohen and Attlan, 1989).

Anti-ergotypic T-cells

Non-activated T-cells were not capable of mediating disease, nor of inducing resistance. It was clear that in addition to the T-cell receptor an activation signal is required to induce a response against the vaccinating T lymphocytes. In addition several observations suggested that this activation signal in itself can trigger a response that is directed against any activated T-cell: Animals vaccinated with one T-cell clone exhibited a marked DTH reaction against other activated T-cell clones. Similarly, lymphocytes from vaccinated animals showed a varying degree of proliferative responses against unrelated activated T-cells. Although T-cell vaccination was found to be highly specific, animals vaccinated with control clones were sometimes less susceptible to disease than naive control animals. We could recently define these effects as due to T-cells that react to the activation state of other T-lymphocytes. In analogy to anti-idiotypic cells we named these cells anti-ergotypic (from ergon = work, action) (Lohse et al. 1989).

When naive animals were injected with $2x10^6$ activated A2b cells and the PLNs removed six days later, the PLN cells showed a very marked proliferative response to activated A2b cells, activated D9 cells or activated splenocytes. However, no proliferative response against resting D9 or normal splenocytes was detectable. This anti-ergotypic response could be induced by dead activated cells killed by shock-freezing, but supernatant of activated cells was ineffective. Thus the anti-ergotypic response is directed against a structural component of activated cells not present or not recognizable on resting cells.

Anti-ergotypic cells can also be detected in an antigen-induced immune response. Injection of mycobacteria in oil (CFA) induced a marked anti-ergotypic response (Lohse et al. 1989). It seems likely that these cells are part of any T-cell response in which activated T-cells trigger anti-ergotypic T-cells. Anti-ergotypic T-cells seem to be both $CD4^+CD8^-$ and $CD4^-CD8^+$ cells (Lohse et al. 1989).

Their role in T-cell vaccination could be demonstrated by testing their effect in vivo: anti-ergotypic lymph node cells induced by injecting $2x10^6$ activated A2b cells, removing the PLNs on day 6 and stimulating the PLN cells in vitro with irradiated Con A activated splenocytes, were capable of suppressing both active and passive EAE in vivo (Lohse et al. 1989). It seems likely that anti-ergotypic cells are responsible for the certain degree of non-specific protection seen after T-cell vaccination. However, their main role will probably be found in the initiation of the specific immune response. They may be the explanation why only activated cells vaccinate. Presumably an anti-ergotypic response is required in order to be able to mount an anti-idiotypic response.

Ben-Nun A, Wekerle H, Cohen IR (1981[a]) The rapid isolation of clonable antigen-specific T lymphocyte lines capable of mediating autoimmune encephalitomyelitis. Eur J Immunol 11: 195-199

Ben-Nun A, Wekerle H, Cohen IR (1981[b]) Vaccination against autoimmune encephalomyelitis with T lymphocyte line cells reactive against myelin basic protein. Nature 292: 60-61

Beraud E, Reshef T, Vandenbark A, Offner H, Fritz R, Chou CHJ, Bernard D, Cohen IR (1986) Experimental autoimmune encephalomyelitis mediated by T lymphocyte lines: Genotype of antigen presenting cells influences immunodominant epitope of basic protein. J Immunol 136:511-515

Beraud E, Lider O, Baharav E, Reshef T, Cohen IR (1989) Vaccination against experimental autoimmune encephalomyelitis using a subencephalitogenic dose of autoimmune effector cells. I. Characteristics of vaccination. J Autoimmunity, in press

Cohen IR (1986) Regulation of autoimmune disease; physiological and therapeutic. Immunol Rev 94:5-21

Cohen IR, Ben-Nun A, Holoshitz J, Maron R, Zerubavel R (1983) Vaccination against autoimmune disease with lines of autoimmune T lymphocytes. Immunol Today 4:227-230

Cohen IR, Attlan H (submitted) Network regulation of autoimmunity: an automaton model.

Holoshitz J, Naparstek Y, Ben-Nun A, Cohen IR (1983) Lines of T lymphocytes mediate or vaccinate against autoimmune arthritis. Science 219:56-58

Kakimoto K, Katsuki M, Hirofuji T, Iwata H, Koga T (1988) Isolation of T cell line capable of protecting mice against collagen-induced arthritis. J. Immunol. 140: 78-83

Lider O, Reshef T, Beraud E, Ben-Nun A, Cohen IR (1988) Anti-idiotypic network induced by T cell vaccination against experimental autoimmune encephalomyelitis. Science 239: 181-183

Lider O, Beraud E, Reshef T, Friedman A, Cohen IR (1989) Vaccination against experimental autoimmune encephalomyelitis using a subencephalitogenic dose of autoimmune effector cells. II. Induction of a protective anti-idiotypic response. J Autoimmunity; in press.

Lohse AW, Mor F, Karin N, Cohen IR (1989) Control of experimental autoimmune encephalomyelitis by T cells responding to activated T cells. Science (in press)

Maron R, Zerubavel R, Friedman A, Cohen IR (1983) T lymphocyte line specific for thyroglobulin produces or vaccinates against autoimmune thyroiditis in mice. J Immunol 131:2316-2322

Sun D, Quin Y, Chluba J, Epplen JT, Wekerle H (1988) Suppression of experimentally induced autoimmune encephalitomyelitis by cytolytic T-T cell interactions. Nature 332: 842-4

Taylor WA, Hughes RAC (1988) Responsiveness of P_2 of blood- and cauda equina-derived lymphocytes in experimental allergic neuritis in the Lewis rat: preliminary characterization of a P_2 specific cauda equina derived T-cell line. J Neuroimmunol 19:279-289

Van Eden W, Holoshitz J, Nevo Z, Frenkel A, Klajman A, Cohen IR (1985) Arthritis induced by a T lymphocyte clone that responds to mycobacterium tuberculosis and to cartilage proteoglycans. Proc Natl Acad Sci USA 82:5117-5120

Van Eden E, Thole JER, van der Zee R, Noordzij A, van Embden JDA, Hensen EJ, Cohen IR (1988) Cloning of the mycobacterial epitope recognized by T lymphocytes in adjuvant arthritis Nature 331:171-173

DISCUSSION

WEKERLE: May I perhaps stress that you don't have to have primed cells to get this back stimulation effect against activated cells. A cell population which is completely naive will show the same amplitude of proliferation against the activated T cell line of whatever specificity, self or foreign, and the T cells which are activated are CD8+

LOHSE: No, it is difficult to test whether naive cells will actually proliferate in response to activated cells because what is going to be your control?

WEKERLE: Its very easy to test. You irradiate the line and co-incubate it with a freshly groundup lymph node. You select the proliferating cell in the traditional way.

LOHSE: Yes, but you don't have the control. You can't say that a non-activated cell will stimulate less than an activated cell because you may have interleukins or other factors. The responses that I described were all in primed lymph nodes so by injecting activated cells of whatever idiotype you get a very strong response but this of course was in order to make the response more marked and to get very high counts and to just get a clearer picture of this particular component of the response. In the CD8+ experiments I think we show very clearly that a naive animal also has these cells and the capacity to activate them.

KOLB: These were exciting data. I wonder whether you have any information on whether the effect in the NOD mouse is specific. The development of diabetes in the NOD mouse is rather readily prevented by disturbing the immune system by injecting all types of substances.

LOHSE: Again, its extremely difficult to get the right control for NOD mouse because we don't have an MHC compatible strain that does not get diabetes so we don't really have the right controls to inject. We did inject PBS of course as a sham injection because as you know stress has an influence on the development of diabetes, so we could control for that. We don't have controls for the rest of the specificity, partly because we didn't want to kill any of the animals to test their responses against the cells we injected. I should stress again that we did not use glutaaldehyde to fix cells but we fixed them with a much more gentle cross linker and probably what we inject is not quite as crudely immunogenic as glutaldehyde fixed cells, but I agree with you we don't have the immunological controls for the specificity.

WILCOX: I was going to ask about specificity too because when you treat the patients you don't really want to do total immunosuppression because you can do that with steroids, so in your system where you use the total lymph node cells to vaccinate, does that in fact induce a sort of generalised immunosupression or is it selective for the adjuvent arthritis or for the diabetic response?

LOHSE: I think I may have confused some people in a way by stressing the non-specific effect that we have been able to characterise more clearly lately. T cell vaccination has a very high degree of specificity and normally an animal that is vaccinated either with the encephalitic clone or with the arthritis clone will only be protected from the disease that it was vaccinated against and you don't get a suppression of any other responses that you measure, so if you vaccinate with the arthritis clone you only get suppression of the response against mycobacteria not against any of the other immune responses. That is true for the lymphnode cells as well.

WILCOX: So how did you test that? Did you assay the response to PPD or something and show that was unaffected?

LOHSE: Well most of these studies were done by taking the cells from the animals irradiating them and adding them to the various clones and they suppressed the response of the mycobacteria reactive clones but not the response of other clones.

T CELL REACTIVITY TO ACETYLCHOLINE RECEPTOR IN MYASTHENIA GRAVIS

John Newsom-Davis, Gillian Harcourt, David Beeson, Norbert Sommer, Angela Vincent, Nick Willcox.

Neurosciences Group

Institute of Molecular Medicine

John Radcliffe Hospital

Headington

Oxford

OX3 9DU

England

Myasthenia gravis (MG) is an antibody-mediated autoimmune disease of neuromuscular transmission, characterised by fatiguable weakness of striated muscle. Patients with MG show heterogeneity in clinical features, thymus pathology and HLA associations. For example, young onset cases are typically female, show hyperplasia of the thymus medulla and are very likely to have HLA-B8 and -DR3, the association being somewhat stronger with -B8 (Compston, Vincent, Newsom-Davis and Batchelor 1980). Weakness is caused by IgG antibodies to the nicotinic acetylcholine receptor (AChR) that lead to receptor loss through complement-mediated lysis (Engel, 1980) and down-regulation secondary to cross-linking (Drachman, Adams, Stanley and Pestronk, 1980). The AChR has five subunits ($\alpha_2\beta\gamma\delta$), the γ subunit present in fetal and denervated muscle being replaced by an ε in innervated muscle. About 60% of MG antibodies bind to a region on the α subunit designated the main immunogenic region, and localised to residues 61-76 (Tzartos and Lindstrom, 1980). By analogy with experimental autoimmune myasthenia gravis, in which myasthenia is induced by immunising with electric fish <u>(Torpedo)</u> or autologous AChR, it is highly likely that

NATO ASI Series, Vol. H 38
The Molecular Biology of Autoimmune Disease
Edited by A. G. Demaine et al.

the pathogenic antibodies in MG are T cell-dependent. We have therefore begun to investigate AChR T cell epitopes in MG patients and in controls.

Reactivity with Torpedo AChR

Amounts of AChR available from amputated human muscle are very limited, and in our initial studies we used AChR from the electric organ of Torpedo marmorata (T-AChR) purified by affinity chromatography. The T-AChR and human AChR α subunits show about 75% homology in their extracellular domain. T cell lines were raised from peripheral blood lymphocytes (PBL) by alternate stimulation with T-AChR and rIL2 in the presence of antigen presenting cells, as first described by Hohlfeld, Toyka, Heininger, Grosse-Wilde and Kalies (1984).

T cell lines were raised from five MG patients and when tested in a proliferation assay (^{3}H-thymidine incorporation) showed stimulation indices (SI) of 4.8-14.0 [(SI = CPM (cells + antigen) $\div$ CPM (cells alone)]. One of these lines, from an HLA-DR2,4 donor, was cloned by limiting dilution, the SI values of the three T-AChR responsive clones ranging from 32-106 (Newsom-Davis, Harcourt, Sommer, Beeson, Willcox and Rothbard, 1989). The responses were apparently HLA class II restricted, in this case by the DR4 haplotype. However, very similar class II restricted T cell lines and clones were also raised from two healthy individuals.

The main immunogenic region, against which most MG antibodies are directed, is on the α subunit, and the response of T cell lines raised to T-AChR was matched by that to the purified α subunit, suggesting that T cell reactivity is principally to sequences in this subunit. However, responses to other subunits have not yet been tested.

Reactivity to synthetic peptides of the human α subunit

Because of the strong response of the T-AChR-specific T cell lines to the α subunit, we have tested the responses of PBL from MG patients and from controls to a number of α subunit synthetic peptides. These have been selected for the presence of motifs, deduced by Rothbard and Taylor (1988) as being common to many T cell epitopes (glycine or charged followed by 2 or 3 hydrophobic residues and ending with a charged or polar residue). PBL from 34 MG patients and 17 controls were tested for responsiveness to 11 human α subunit synthetic peptides in the proliferation assay. (Harcourt, Sommer, Rothbard, Willcox and Newsom-Davis, 1988). Most of the peptides failed to elicit a response. With some (eg p1-15) there were weak responses both in MG patients and controls, as Hohlfeld, Toyka, Mine, Walgrave and Conti-Tronconi (1988) have also found. Relatively strong stimulation by p125-143 was found in MG patients, but also in controls. By contrast, responses to p257-269 were present in 18% of MG patients but in no controls. This sequence lies extracellularly between the second and third transmembrane segments, and shows complete homology with T-AChR in this region. However, none of the MG T cell lines raised against T-AChR responded to this peptide or indeed to any of the other peptides except in the case of p125-143 to which one control and one MG line responded. This sequence differs from T-AChR at two residues. We found no clear association between HLA type and the response to a particular peptide.

<u>Reactivity to recombinant human AChR α subunit</u>

The above results imply that T-AChR was not an ideal antigen for studying AChR reactivity in MG. Because of limiting quantities of native human AChR available, we have adopted a recombinant approach to obtain expression of milligram quantities of human AChR α subunit polypeptides. A cDNA clone containing the full coding region of the human α subunit has been isolated, and restriction fragments coding for an almost full length fragment (r37-437) and for smaller polypeptides have been ligated into a plasmid vector pkk233-2 (Beeson, Brydson, Wood, Vincent and Newsom-Davis 1989). Expression of the recombinant polypeptides, and of the fusion protein f10-124, was obtained in <u>E. coli</u>, and identified by Coomassie blue staining and by Western blotting with anti-peptide antibodies. The polypeptides were purified by preparative gel electrophoresis, SDS being removed by dialysis against 0.2% cholate/PBS or by cryoprecipitation.

PBL responses to r37-437 at concentrations of 1-4 ug/ml were first compared with those to native T-AChR. With T-AChR, they were positive in 21/129 (16%) of MG patients compared to 11/23 (47%) with r37-437, SI values ranging from 2.5-10 and 2.5-15 respectively. Among controls, responses to T-AChR (SI 2.5-3.6) were positive in 2/23 (9%) and to r37-437 in 3/18 (17%). These results support the view that human AChR is a more appropriate antigen for studying T cell reactivity in MG than T-AChR.

T cell lines have been raised from PBL of 4 MG patients to r37-437, and have shown SI values of 3.5-22.0. In two of the patients a second line was similarly established from

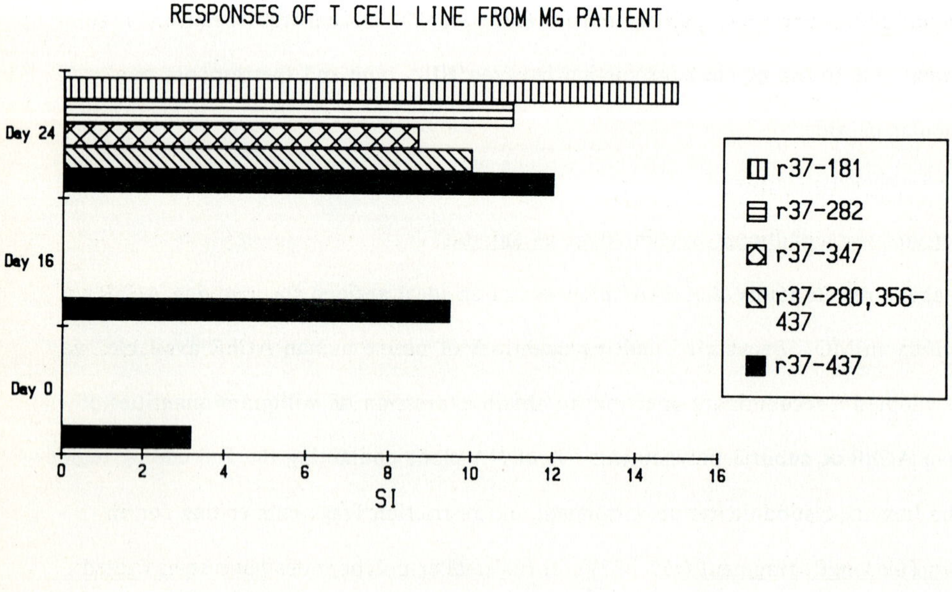

Figure. Proliferative responses of T cell line from MG patient, raised to human recombinant alpha-subunit r37-437. Note similar stimulation indices (SI) to the different recombinant polypeptides, indicating that the line response is dominated by epitopes lying within the smallest of these (r37-181)

another blood sample taken several months later. One patient, interestingly, showed almost identical response characteristics in her two lines, being very similar when tested with r37-437 and with various smaller recombinant fragments, as illustrated for one of the lines in Fig. 1. This suggests that most of the dominant T cell epitopes were similar in the two lines.

The T cell lines from 3 of the 4 patients have been cloned by limiting dilution, and a number of r37-437 reactive clones obtained from them.

Several clones from two of these patients have been studied in detail. All had the $CD3^+$, $CD4^+$, $CD8^-$ phenotype and their response to r37-437 was clearly HLA class II restricted. In one of the patients who had a relatively short history of MG, all the clones responded to the same extracellular region of the α -subunit as did the original cell line (Fig. 1), and showed the same HLA class II restriction. In another patient, whose history was much longer, the clones were more heterogeneous. Some resembled those of the first patient, whereas others responded to a cytoplasmic region in the C terminal half of the α -subunit, and showed a different class II restricting element.

Summary and conclusions

These studies indicate that recombinant human AChR is a more appropriate antigen for testing T cell responses in MG than the partially homologous Torpedo AChR, and have begun to define AChR T cell epitopes in MG patients. Interestingly, we have so far seen no overwhelming bias towards HLA-DR3 either as a marker of good responders or as a restricing element.

This approach should enable the full range of T cell epitopes to be defined in MG patients and in healthy individuals, not only for the α subunit but in due course for the other subunits too. Importantly, it should allow identification of the 'pathogenic' T cell epitopes that can provide help for anti-AChR antibody production, and thus elucidate the relationship between T cell and B cell epitopes in MG. Finally, if the search for pathogenic T cell epitopes is successful, the way would be open to investigate methods for selectively controlling the aberrant immune response.

Beeson D, Brydson M, Wood H, Vincent A, Newsom-Davis J. (1989) Human muscle acetylcholine receptor: cloning and expression in E. coli of cDNA for the alpha-subunit. Biochem Soc Trans 17:219-220

Compston DAS, Vincent A, Newsom-Davis J, Batchelor JR. (1980) Clinical, pathological, HLA antigen and immunological evidence for disease heterogeneity in myasthenia gravis. Brain 103:579-601

Drachman DB, Adams RN, Stanley EF, Pesronk A. (1980) Mechanisms of acetylcholine receptor loss in myasthenia gravis. J Neurol Neurosurg & Psychiatr 43:6

Engel AG. (1980) Morphologic and immunopathologic findings in myasthenia gravis and in congenital myasthenic syndromes. J Neurol Neurosug Psychiat 43:577-598

Harcourt GC, Sommer N, Rothbard J, Willcox HNA, Newsom-Davis J. (1988) A juxtamembrane epitope on the human acetylcholine receptor recognized by T cells in myasthenia gravis. J Clin Invest 82:1295-1300

Hohlfeld R, Toyka KV, Heininger H, Grosse-Wilde H, Kalies I. (1984) Autoimmune human T lymphocytes specific for acetylcholine receptor. Nature 310:244-246

Hohlfeld R, Toyka K, Miner L, Walgrave S, Contri-Tronconi B. (1988) Amphipathic segment of the nicotinic receptor alpha-subunit contains epitopes recognized by T lymphocytes in myasthenia gravis. J Clin Invest 81:657-660

Newsom-Davis, Harcourt G, Sommer N, Beeson D, Willcox N, Rothbard J. (1989) T cell reactivity in myasthenia gravis. J Autoimmunity 2 (Supplement):101-108

Rothbard JB, Taylor WB. (1988) A sequence pattern common to T cell epitopes. EMBO J 7:93-100

Tzartos SJ, Lindstrom JM. (1980) Monoclonal antibodies used to probe acetylcholine receptor structure: localization of the main immunogenic region and detection of similarities between subunits. Proc Natl Acad Sci 77:755-759

DISCUSSION

QUESTION: What are the implications of both the species differences and limited homology of alpha receptors in the fish and man? What about the differences between the main immunogenic regions of sih and human alpha sub-unit?

NEWSOM-DAVIS: There are a number of differences between the torpedo and the human in 37 to 87. I think 12 or 13 residues are different so it is not a surpise that the torpedo does not stimulate any of our T cell clones and althougth of course its tempting to think that the epitope in the region 37 to 87 may be important for generating antibodies because it is close to the main immunogenic region it would be quite premature at this point to say that is in fact the region that is going to be important.

QUESTION: The last thing you suggested was that clone A3 is stimulated by peptides within the sequence of 282 to 437. How do you explain the relevance of this in myasthenia gravis since this peptide region is inside not on the outside of the receptor.

NEWSOM-DAVIS: That's absolutely the case. Well one has to postulate there that damage to cells releases acetylcholine receptor and that as a consequence those particular sequences become exposed to the immune system. It is difficult and I wouldn't argue that those particular epitopes were necessarily primary in the pathogenesis of the disease unless some other process destroys the cell thereby releasing cytoplasmic receptor sequences.

SCHERBAUM: I would like to know if there is evidence that the locally infiltrating lymphocytes recognize more restricted epitopes of antigen, for example, have you cloned T lymphocytes derived from the thymus?

NEWSOM-DAVIS: No we haven't done that but others have. The clones responded to the region 85 to 144. Its early days, they don't have too many T cell lines and clones and neither do we at this moment and I think one doesn't want to base a very great deal on a limited number of epitopes but it will be intriguing to see whether they are the same.

MOUTSOPOULOS: Is the response in normal people DR restricted?

NEWSOM-DAVIS: No and the reason we didn't say that is that we haven't yet raised clones from control individuals. I think its likely that we shall be able to do so. By analogy with torpedo receptor it will be interesting to see whether its more difficult and of course its very important to know whether the epitopes are the same as in myasthenics and whether they have similar class II restriction.

TYPE I DIABETES AS A "MENDELIAN" AND "REGULATED" IMMUNE PROCESS

E. Russo, R.A. Jackson, F. Dotta, M.A. Lipes, L. Castano, J. Zielasek, D. Bleich, R.J. Keller, R. Ziegler, M. Hattori, R.C. Nayak, R.D. Herskowitz and G.S. Eisenbarth
Joslin Diabetes Center
One Joslin Place
Boston, Massachusetts 02215 U.S.A.

INTRODUCTION

From studies of non-organ specific autoimmune diseases such as Lupus Erythematosus the concept has developed that autoimmunity is characterized by marked variation over time reflected by clinical remission and exacerbation. Our family studies of the development of Type I diabetes is providing us with a very different picture of the autoimmunity associated with Type I diabetes. In addition studies of NOD mice indicate that the Mendelian inheritance of a series of necessary but not sufficient diabetes associated alleles (H-2 NOD, theta linked, and the autosomal recessive gene determining anti-polar antibodies) create diabetes susceptibility. We will review our studies indicating that Type I diabetes is an autoimmune process in which there is remarkable quantitative stability of autoantibody levels amongst prediabetics (at times extending to more than a decade). Individual prediabetics have characteristic differences in the levels of autoantibodies and the rate of progression to diabetes. This stability of the process has allowed us to develop a dual parameter linear regression model to aid in the prediction of the time of onset of Type I diabetes. As will be discussed this model utilizes the concentration of insulin autoantibodies as a marker of the rate of the autoimmune process and therefore speed of progression to overt diabetes.

AUTOANTIBODIES

A series of autoantibodies appear prior to the development of Type I diabetes (Jackson 1982; Tarn 1988; Bonifacio 1987; Baekkeskov 1987). Antibodies which we have evaluated in our family studies include anti-cytoplasmic islet cell antibodies (target antigen appears to be a monosialo ganglioside) (Colman

NATO ASI Series, Vol. H 38
The Molecular Biology of Autoimmune Disease
Edited by A. G. Demaine et al.

1988a; Colman 1988b; Nayak 1985), anti-insulin autoantibodies (Vardi 1987; Vardi 1988), antibodies to a 64K islet protein (measured by Baekkeskov and colleagues), antibodies (termed anti-polar) to a protein antigen at the secretory pole rat insulinoma cells (Dotta 1988), antibodies reacting with a 75Kd protein of RIN extracts and antibodies reacting with a lambda GT11 clone derived from a rat islet library. With the assays currently employed less than 30% of pre-Type I diabetics express the latter three antibodies, while the initial three are each present in more than 60% of pre-Type I diabetics. Insulin autoantibodies are unique in that the percentage of individuals expressing these antibodies as well as the concentration of the antibodies inversely correlate with the age at which Type I diabetes develops (Vardi 1988). None of the other antibodies show such an age relationship, and it is insulin autoantibodies which correlate with the rate of progression to overt Type I diabetes while none of the other antibodies show such a correlation. Individual patients can express any combination of the above autoantibodies in the prediabetic phase, but within the limits of the sensitivity of the assays always express the same combination of antibodies over long periods of time (We have observed one patient to develop antibodies to the lambda GT11 clone (termed DG-1) approximately two years after initial detection of cytoplasmic islet cell antibodies and a year prior to the development of overt diabetes. He is very unusual and in the few individuals with conversion to active autoimmunity which we have sequentially followed all antibodies which were present on followup appeared at the same time (e.g. anti-insulin, anti-64K, anti-cytoplasmic ICA) (Soeldner 1985).

To date we have screened approximately 6,000 first degree relatives of patients with Type I diabetes for cytoplasmic islet cell antibodies and 2,000 for insulin autoantibodies. Eighty cytoplasmic islet cell antibody and 60 insulin autoantibody positive relatives have been identified over the past 6 years. Twenty-seven antibody positive relatives have progressed to overt diabetes and for 21 of these relatives we have a minimal evaluation with measurement of anti-insulin autoantibodies, cytoplasmic ICA and intravenous glucose tolerance testing prior to diabetes.

We determine insulin autoantibodies with a fluid phase competitive radioassay. The levels of insulin autoantibodies in individual sera (measured in nU/ml of insulin precipitated) directly correlate with the product of affinity and capacity by Scatchard analysis. All prediabetic autoantibodies we have studied react equally well in competition studies with human, porcine, bovine, rat, sheep and chicken insulin, but fail to react with isolated A or B chains of the insulin molecule. The above species insensitivity, inability to react with isolated A chain, as well as direct workshop comparisons indicate that the insulin autoantibodies measured by current ELISA assays (Wilkin 1987; Diaz 1987) where insulin is bound to plastic wells are unrelated to those detected with the above radiobinding assay.

To date our studies of insulin autoantibodies indicate that they have a high (>50% with 5 years of followup) positive predictive value for the development of Type I diabetes (independent of the presence of cytoplasmic islet cell antibodies), they correlate inversely with the age at which Type I diabetes develops [log linear correlation (9)] but not simply chronologic age e.g. we have followed for the past 1.5 years three children under the age of 5, one with no insulin autoantibodies but cytoplasmic islet cell antibody positive, and two with extremely elevated levels of insulin autoantibodies, they fluctuate within ranges characteristic for each prediabetic (Fig. 1) and they correlate with the time to overt diabetes of individual islet cell antibody positive prediabetics. The ability to maintain characteristic levels of insulin autoantibodies over long periods of time suggest that either the concentration of the antibodies or the autoimmune process which results in the production of such antibodies are regulated. In our studies of NOD mouse, similar to man a subset of mice have such antibodies and those expressing insulin autoantibodies have a higher progression to diabetes (Ziegler 1989). The manner in which insulin autoantibodies are generated is not understood. We have found that non-islet cells (fibroblast or pituitary cell lines) transfected with the rat insulin II gene (sequence of rat insulin is identical to mouse insulin) when transplanted and rejected by mice give rise to insulin autoantibodies in several but not all murine strains (Ziegler to be published). This suggests that insulin autoantibodies may be secondary to the destruction of islet cells with resulting presentation of insulin as an antigen and abrogation of humoral tolerance. Nevertheless, the marked correlation with the rate of development of overt diabetes with insulin autoantibodies and earlier studies indicating that insulitis could be induced with homologous insulin lead us to hypothesize (with minimal evidence at present) that insulin may be the primary target of the autoimmunity leading to Type I diabetes.

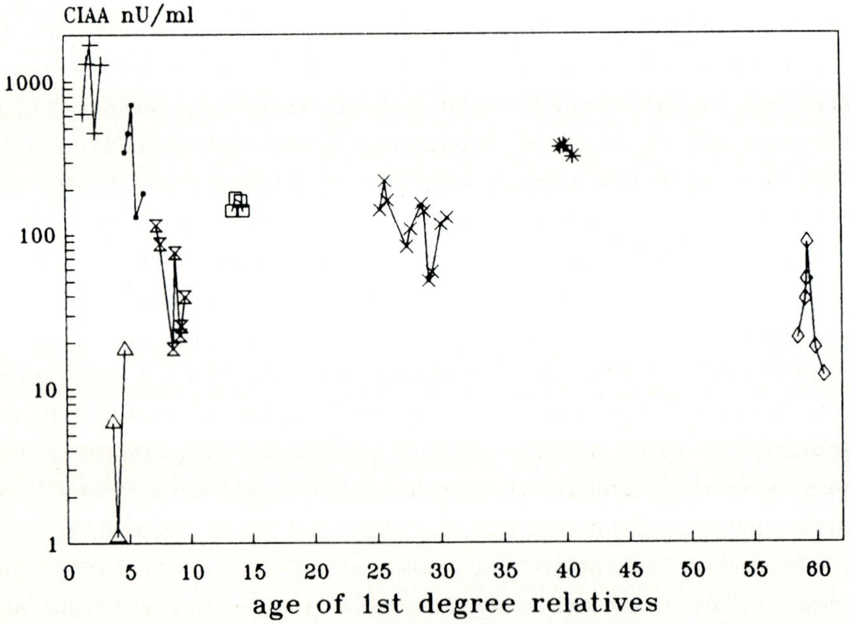

Figure 1: Level of insulin autoantibodies versus age at testing in seven autoantibody positive (ICA and/or CIAA) initially non-diabetic first degree relatives of patients with Type I diabetes.

INSULITIS

It is unlikely that antibodies mediate the immune destruction leading to Type I diabetes as no one has been able to transfer Type I diabetes with antibodies, neonates born to mothers with anti-islet and anti-insulin antibodies transiently express the maternal autoantibodies but do not develop diabetes, the disease is transferred in animal models by T cells (Koevary 1983; Appel 1988) and insulitis characterizes islet lesions (Foulis 1987). It is probably the plaque like nature of the insulitis process which underlies the long prodromal phase of Type I diabetes. Normal islets, inflamed islets, and islets in which all insulin secreting beta cells have been destroyed (and in which lymphocytes are not longer present) occur in the pancreas at the same time prior to the development of diabetes. We hypothesize that the progressive destruction of beta cells in different islets which leads to an impairment of insulin secretion which is reflected by loss of first phase insulin secretion to intravenous glucose and is then followed by overt diabetes. We have found that a combination of first phase insulin secretion and level of insulin autoantibodies are correlated with the time it takes islet cell antibody positive first degree relatives to develop overt diabetes (years to diabetes =2.5*(IVGTT insulin)/(level of insulin autoantibodies; r=.0##, p<.0#) (Jackson 1988).

The genes determining susceptibility to Type I diabetes have not been definitively identified in any species. It is noteworthy that studies in NOD mice indicate that bone marrow stem cells carry the genetic information to produce diabetes (Serreze 1988) in normal mice, suggesting as transplantation studies have indicated (Prowse 1986) that normal islets can be the target of autoimmunity. In the NOD mouse we have been unable to identify class II positive beta cells, their presence in BB rats has been questioned (Pipeleers 1987), and in normal human pancreas, pancreatic ductal cells express class II antigens (Dib 1988). The above observations coupled with the results of studies of transgenic mice (Sarvetnick 1988) make it less likely that class II positive beta cells contribute to anti-islet autoimmunity. Nevertheless the mechanism underlying Foulis and coworkers observation (Foulis 1987) of alpha interferon containing and class II positive beta cells in the pancreas of patients who have destroyed the bulk of their islet cells (studies at the time of autopsy after diabetes onset) remains to be elucidated. Whether environmental or non-Mendelian genetic factors such as somatic mutations trigger the development of autoimmunity (e.g. approximately 50% of identical twin pairs are concordant for Type I diabetes) is currently unknown.

GENETICS

In the NOD mouse and the BB rat a series of genes inherited in simple Mendelian fashion contribute to diabetes susceptibility. In the BB rat both a severe T cell immunodeficiency gene (Rabinowe 1984; Colle 1986) which leads to an absence of RT6 positive T lymphocytes (Grenier DL 1986) as well as class II RT1-U (Colle 1981; Buse 1984) underlie a major portion of diabetes susceptibility. It is noteworthy that in a diabetes resistant strain of BB rats which lack the autosomal recessive immunodeficiency gene but which have RT1-U, depletion of RT6 positive lymphocytes with the RT6 antibody induces diabetes (Grenier 1987).

In the NOD mouse we found that homozygosity for H-2 of the NOD was essential for the development of diabetes (Hattori 1986). In similar breeding studies of Leiter and coworkers homozygosity for H-2 of the NOD was also essential for diabetes (Porchazka 1987), while in the studies of Wicker and coworkers (backcrosses with an I-E negative strain) a rare H-2 heterozygous mouse developed diabetes (Wicker 1987). The class II I-A beta gene of the NOD mouse is unique and lacks an aspartic acid at position 57 (Todd 1987) of the molecule while I-A alpha of NOD is identical to Balb/c mice whose H-2 is not diabetogenic. In addition NOD mice do not express I-E (Hattori 1986) and Nishimoto and coworkers have reported that the breeding of an I-E transgene into NOD mice prevents insulitis (Nishimoto 1987). The above results have led to the hypothesis that the diabetogenic effect of the NOD mouse's H-2 results from its unique I-A beta and lack of I-E expression. We have sequenced the I-A beta of a strain related to the NOD mouse (CTS) and it has an identical I-A beta and does not express I-E, but differs from the NOD at class I alleles (Ikegami 1986). Until the diabetogenicity of the H-2 of recombinant chromosomes are assessed it will remain an unanswered question as to whether the class II genes of the NOD mouse or other H-2 linked genes are diabetogenic.

In backcrosses of NOD mice with a series of strains, the majority of mice homozygous for H-2 NOD do not develop diabetes, do not express anti-polar antibodies, and do not have insulitis. H-2 homozygosity appears to be necessary but not sufficient for the development of diabetes. Prochazka and coworkers have described linkage of diabetes to the theta T cell marker (Prochazka 1987), a finding confirmed by Hattori and coworkers (Hattori 1987). In addition Hattori's studies indicate that insulitis is closely associated with homozygosity for the theta linked gene. In studies in collaboration with Wicker and coworkers, Michael Appel, and Leiter and coworkers we have found that in a series of backcrosses that expression of an antibody reacting with the secretory pole of a rat insulinoma cell line is inherited in an autosomal recessive manner with approximately 98% penetrance, is inherited independent of H-2, and is highly associated with the development of diabetes (Dotta 1989). Antibodies to the polar antigen appear as early as 3 days in NOD mice. The above studies indicate that a series of genetic loci, functioning as AND gates determine susceptibility to the autoimmunity that results in diabetes. An understanding of the generation of autoimmunity in these animal models (and probably man) is unlikely until the "simply inherited" Mendelian genes determining susceptibility are characterized.

The dramatic manner in which these Mendelian genes can create autoimmunity despite major perturbations in the immune system is illustrated by studies indicating that the introduction of a rearranged V beta T cell receptor transgene which suppresses the endogenous V beta repertoire of NOD mice is unable to suppress the development of anti-polar antibodies, anti-insulin antibodies, and insulitis. Despite what is probably a thousand fold reduction in V beta repertoire marked insulitis occurs in transgene expressing NOD mice (Lipes 1989).

SUMMARY

Type I diabetes is rapidly becoming one of the most intensively studied autoimmune disorders. The disease remains one of marked morbidity and mortality despite the introduction of insulin therapy more than 6 decades ago. Studies of immunotherapy to date, with intervention after almost total beta cell destruction at the time of onset of diabetes have provided important scientific information but from a clinical standpoint long term maintenance of non-insulin requiring remissions has not been possible (Stiller 1983; Bougneres 1988; Shar 1989). It is likely with our current laboratory based ability to predict the development of diabetes that immunologic therapies to prevent the diabetes will be rapidly evaluated. The Mendelian nature of the disorder in man and animal models and the stability of the autoimmune process suggest that the study of this disease will lead to enhanced understanding of the generation and maintenance of tolerance to self.

REFERENCES

Appel MC, O'Neil JJ, Wicker LB, Kurnick JT (1988) Both the Lyt-2+ and L3T4+ T cell subsets are required for the transfer of diabetes in nonobese diabetic mice. J Immunol 140:52-58

Baekkeskov S, Landan M, Kristensen JK, Srikanta S, Bruining GJ, Mandrup-Poulsen T, Beaufort C, Soeldner JS, Eisenbarth GS, Lindgren F, Sundquist G, Lernmark A (1987) Antibodies to a 64,000 Mr human islet cell antigen precede the clinical onset of insulin dependent diabetes. J Clin Invest 79:926-934

Bonifacio E, Dawkins RL, Lernmark A (1987) Immunology and diabetes workshops: report of the second international workshop on the standardisation of cytoplasmic islet cell antibodies. Diabetologia 30:273

Bougneres PF, Carel JC, Castano L, Boitard C, Gardin JP, Landais P, Hors J, Mihatsch MJ, Paillard M, Chaussain JL, Bach JF (1988) Factors associated with early remission of Type I diabetes in children treated with cyclosporine. N Engl J Med 318:663-670

Buse JB, Ben-Nun A, Klein KA, Eisenbarth GS, Seidman JG, Jackson RA (1984) Class I, II and III major histocompatibility complex gene polymorphisms in BB rats. Diabetologia 22:77-79

Colle E, Guttmann RD, Seemayer T (1981) Spontaneous diabetes mellitus syndrome in the rat. I. Association with the major histocompatibility complex. J Exp Med 154:1237-1242

Colle E, Guttmann RD, Fuks A, Seemayer TA, Prud'homme GJ (1986) Genetics of the spontaneous diabetic syndrome. Interaction of the MHC and non-MHC associated factors. Mol Biol Med 3(1):13-23

Colman PG, DiMario U, Rabizadeh A, Dotta F, Anastasi E, Eisenbarth GS (1988) A prozone phenomenon interferes in islet cell antibody detection: direct comparison of two methods in subjects at risk to develop diabetes and in insulin dependent diabetes at onset. J Autoimmunity 1:109-117

Colman PG, Tautkus M, Rabizadeh A, Cahill C, Eisenbarth GS (1988) Assay for islet cell antibodies with rat pancreas and peroxidase protein A. Diabetes Care 11:367-368.

Diaz J-L, Wilkin T (1987) Differences in epitope restriction of autoantibodies to native human insulin (IAA) and antibodies to heterologous insulin (IA). Diabetes 36:66-72

Dib SA, Vardi P, Bonner-Weir S, Eisenbarth GS (1988) Selective localization of Factor VIII. Antigenicity to endothelial cells and expression of class II antigens by normal human pancreatic ductal epithelium. Diabetes 37:482-487.

Dotta F, Bonner-Weir S, Cahill C, Appel M, Nayak RC, Eisenbarth GS (1988) Immunoreactivity of islet tumor cells: a new diabetes associated antigen ("polar" antigen). Clin Res 36:480A

Dotta F, Wicker L, Peterson L, Pressey A, Appel M, Eisenbarth GS (to be published) Inheritance of anti-"polar" antibodies in NOD mice: evidence for a single recessive gene. Diabetes

Foulis AK, Farquharson MA, Meager A (1987) Immunoreactive alpha-interferon in insulin-secreting beta cells in Type I diabetes mellitus. Lancet 1423-1427

Grenier DL, Handler ES, Nakano K, Mordes JP, Rossini AA (1986) Absence of the RT6 T cell subset in diabetes-prone BB/W rats. J Immunol 136:148-151

Grenier DL, Mordes JP, Handler ES, Angelillo M, Makamura N, Rossini AA (1987) Depletion of RT6.1+ T lymphocytes induces diabetes in resistant BioBreeding/Worcester (BB/W) rats. J Exp Med 166(2):461-475

Hattori M, Buse JB, Jackson RA, Glimcher L, Makino S, Moriwaki K, Dorff M, Minami M, Kuzuya H, Imura H, Seidman JG, Eisenbarth GS (1986) The NOD mouse: recessive diabetogenic gene within the major histocompatibility complex. Science 231:733-735

Hattori M, Ikegami H, Eisenbrth GS, Makino S (1987) "Thy-1" linked diabetogenic gene but no "MHC" linked gene causes the primary destruction of beta cells of the NOD mouse. Diabetes suppl 1:82A

Ikegami H, Jackson RA, Makino S, Satt DE, Eisenbarth GS, Hattori M (1986) Homozygosity for two genes (H-2: chromosome 17 and Thy-1: chromosome 9) linked to development of Type I diabetes of the NOD mouse. Clin Res 34:683A

Jackson RA, Morris MA, Haynes BF, Eisenbarth GS (1982) Increased circulating Ia-antigen-bearing T cells in Type I diabetes mellitus. N Engl J Med 306:785-788

Jackson RA, Vardi P, Herskowitz R, Soeldner JS, Eisenbarth GS (1988) Dual parameter linear model for prediction of onset of Type I diabetes in islet cell antibody positive relatives. Clin Res 36:585A

Koevary S, Rossini A, Stoller W, Chick W (1983) Passive transfer of diabetes in the BB/W rat. Science 220:727-728

Lipes MA, Fenton RG, Zhou LZ, Seidman JG, Eisenbarth GS (to be published) Autoimmunity occurs in transgenic T cell receptor (TCR) beta gene non-obese diabetic (NOD) mice. Clin Res

Nayak RC, Omar MAK, Rabizadeh A, Srikanta S, Eisenbarth GS (1985) "Cytoplasmic" islet cell antibodies: evidence that the target antigen is a sialoglycoconjugate. Diabetes 34:617-619

Nishimoto H, Kikutani H, Yamamura K, Kishimoto T (1987) Prevention of autoimmune insulitis by expression of I-E molecules in NOD mice. Nature 328:432-434

Pipeleers DG, In't Veld PA, Pipeleers-Marichal MA, Gepts W, Van De Winkel M (1987) Presence of pancreatic hormones in islet cells with MHC-class II antigen expression. Diabetes 36:872-876

Prochazka M, Leiter ED, Serreze DV, Coleman DG (1987) Three recessive loci required for insulin dependent diabetes in nonobese diabetic mice. Science 237:286-289

Prowse SJ, Nomikoa IN, Pratt PF, Lafferty KJ (1986) Islet allografts are destroyed by disease recurrence in diabetic NOD mice and BB rats. Diabetes 55:243

Rabinowe SL, Eisenbarth GS (1984) Immunotherapy of Type I (insulin dependent) diabetes mellitus. In: Andreani D, DiMario U, Federlin KF, Heding LG (eds), Immunology in Diabetes. Kimpton Medical Publications, London p 171-175

Sarvetnick N, Liggitt D, Pitts SL, Hansen SE, Stewart TA (1988) Insulin-dependent diabetes mellitus induced in transgenic mice by ectopic expression of class II MHC and interferon-gamma. Cell 52:773-782

Serreze DV, Leiter EH, Worthen SM, Shultz LD (1988) NOD marrow stem cells adoptively transfer diabetes to resistant (NOD x NON) F1 mice. Diabetes 37:252-255

Shar SC, Malone JI, Simpson NE (1989) A randomized trial of intensive insulin therapy in newly diagnosed insulin-dependent diabetes mellitus. N Engl J Med 320:550-554

Soeldner JS, Tuttleman M, Srikanta S, Ganda OP, Eisenbarth GS (1985) Insulin dependent diabetes mellitus and initiation of autoimmunity: islet cell autoantibodies, insulin autoantibodies and beta cell failure. N Engl J Med 313(14):893-894

Stiller CR, Laupacis A, Dupre J, Jenner MR, Keown PA, Rodger W, Wolfe BMJ (1983) Cyclosporine for treatment of early Type I diabetes: preliminary results. N Engl J Med 308:1226-1227

Tarn AC, Thomas JM, Dean BM, Ingram D, Schwarz G, Franco-Bottazzo G, Gale EAM (1988) Predicting insulin-dependent. Diabetes April 16:845-850

Todd JA, Bell JI, McDevitt HO (1987) HLA-DQ beta gene contributes to susceptibility and resistance to insulin dependent diabetes mellitus. Nature 329:599-604

Vardi P, Dib SA, Tuttleman M, Connelly JE, Grinbergs M, Rabizadeh A, Riley WJ, Maclaren NK, Eisenbarth GS, Soeldner JS (1987) Competitive insulin autoantibody RIA: prospective evaluation of subjects at high risk for development of Type I diabetes mellitus. Diabetes 36:1286-1291

Vardi P, Ziegler AG, Matthews JH, Dib S, Keller RJ, Ricker AT, Wolfsdorf JI, Herskowitz RD, Rabizadeh A, Eisenbarth GS, Soeldner JS (1988) Concentration of insulin autoantibodies at onset of Type I diabetes: inverse log-linear correlation with age. Diabetes Care 11:736-739

Wicker LS, Miller BJ, Coker LZ, McNally SE, Scott S, Mullen Y, Appel MC (1987) Genetic control of diabetes and insulitis in the non-obese diabetic (NOD) mouse. J Exp Med 165(6):1639-1654

Wilkin T, Palmer J, Bonifacio E, Diaz JL, Kruse V (1987) First international workshop on the standardization of insulin autoantibodies. Diabetologia 30:676-677

Ziegler AG, Vardi P, Ricker AT, Hattori M, Soeldner JS, Eisenbarth GS (1989) Radioassay determination of insulin autoantibodies in NOD mice: correlation with increased risk of progression to overt diabetes. Diabetes 38:358-363

Ziegler AG, Vardi P, Gross DJ, Bonner-Weir S, Villa-Kamaroff L, Halban P, Ikegami H, Soeldner JS, Eisenbarth GS (to be published) Production of insulin antibodies by mice rejecting insulin transfected cells. J Autoimmunity

DISCUSSION

KOLB: In the experiments where you used transfected cell lines and injected them into the mouse you said that you have autoimmunity against the rat insulin because the sequence of the rat insulin is identical to mouse insulin. If I recall correctly normally those transfected cell lines have pro-insulin in them. So how could there be autoimmunity in the mice?

EISENBARTH: The sequences of the insulin molecules are identical and the antibodies are directed at the insulin molecule so I think that's an autoimmune response.

SCHERBAUM: I do not quite agree with your notion that the ICA levels are not predictive for type I diabetes because with your protein A assay your limit of detectability is poor?

EISENBARTH: High titres of ICA are highly predictive of subsequent development of diabetes what I meant to stress was that the quantitative level of ICA does not correlate with the rate of progression.

SCHERBAUM: Seeing this close correlation of the insulin autoantibody titres and the age of onset are you sure that you are not just lliking at age of onset when you express your formula?

EISENBARTH: Sure, we've done the linear aggression with age as a co-correlate and basically it has no influence so if you have an old person with high anti insulin autantibodies levels then he progresses faster than a younger one with low levels.

PAPEDOPOULOS: What is the role of cyclosporin?

EISENBARTH: Basically cyclosporin A has only been studied after the onset of type I diabetes and what has been found is quite interesting. The levels of C peptide are preserved for as long as the cyclosporin A is given but individuals actually progress from a non-insulin requiring remission to insulin even though they are maintaining beta cell function at least as measured by C peptide secretion.

PAPEDOPOULOS: Last September in the European Association for the Study of Diabetes Meeting all the cyclosporin studies were put together. After two years, one year on cyclosporin, one year off, remission is only 5-15%.

EISENBARTH: Even on cyclosporin A after onset almost all patients lose their non-insulin requiring remission and we've just actually had a meeting of the immunotherapy diabetes study group a week ago in Italy and the general consensus I think is that immunotherapy after onset will not leave patients in a non-insulin requiring remission.

THE CLONING ROAD TO THE TSH RECEPTOR AND AUTOIMMUNE GRAVES' DISEASE

Leonard D. Kohn, Takashi Akamizu, Motoyasu Saji, Shoichero Ikuyama, Shashikumar Bellur, and Kazuo Tahara
Section on Cell Regulation
Laboratory of Biochemistry and Metabolism
NIDDK
National Institutes of Health
Bethesda, MD 20892 USA

THE TSH RECEPTOR IS NOT THE SOLE AUTOANTIGEN IN GRAVES' PATIENTS NOR IS IT A WELL DEFINED AUTOANTIGEN

Graves' disease, the major form of autoimmune thyroid disease, is believed to be caused by autoantibodies to the thyrotropin (TSH) receptor. How these antibodies develop is still unknown; it is also not clear whether this is a thyroid disease or one of abnormal lymphocyte control. It can be presumed that the TSH receptor is structurally related to the receptors for other glycoprotein hormones; yet its relatively unique role as an autoantigen is unexplained. Further, it is increasingly evident that the sera of patients with Graves' disease have a multiplicity of antibodies to thyroid antigens in addition to the TSH receptor and that these may be relevant to understanding the expression of the disease or its pathogenesis.

The structure of the TSH receptor remains an enigma despite the efforts of a host of laboratories. Binding and purification studies in our own laboratory (Kohn, 1978; Kohn et al., 1983; Kohn et al., 1986a; Chan et al., 1987) have suggested that the high affinity binding site of the thyrotropin (TSH) receptor is a membrane glycoprotein; however, a glycolipid has also been implicated in receptor structure and function (Kohn, 1978). Studies with monoclonal antibodies to the TSH receptor (Kohn et al., 1983; Kohn et al., 1985; Kohn et al., 1986a; Chan et al., 1987) support the concept that multiple autoantigen domains exist. Thus the studies indicated there were antibodies which increased cAMP levels but only minimally inhibited TSH binding (stimulators, TSAbs),

NATO ASI Series, Vol. H 38
The Molecular Biology of Autoimmune Disease
Edited by A. G. Demaine et al.

others which inhibited TSH binding but did not increase cAMP levels (inhibitors, TBIAbs), and still others with both activities (mixed). The monoclonal antibody studies also indicated that (a) antibodies within each group can have different activities in assays related to thyroid cell growth, exophthalmos, and pretibial myxedema and (b) the TSH receptor is coupled to multiple transducers, for example the phosphoinositide-Ca-arachidonic acid as well as the adenylate cyclase signal system (Kohn et al., 1986a). The monoclonal antibody studies have been interpreted to delineate a TSH receptor structure with multiple domains; they do not exclude the existence of multiple TSH receptors or binding proteins.

A CLONING APPROACH TO GRAVES' AUTOANTIGENS

A human thyroid carcinoma lambda gt11 expression library has been immunoscreened with an IgG preparation from a patient with active Graves' disease (Chan et al., 1989). The IgG preparation was highly positive in assays measuring thyroid stimulating antibodies (TSAbs), thyrotropin binding inhibiting antibodies (TBIAbs) and thyroid growth promoting antibodies (TGPAbs). Although the IgG preparation contained no detectable microsomal or thyroglobulin antibodies, it was presumed that the IgG preparation would react to a multiplicity of autoantigens other than the TSH receptor. It is not surprising, therefore, that this approach identified 25 different human cDNA clones. The problem, then, was to define these cDNAs and relate their gene products to Graves' disease.

IDENTIFICATION OF A cDNA CODING FOR A PROTEIN REACTIVE WITH AUTOANTIBODIES TO THE TSH RECEPTOR

In a separate approach (Kohn et al., 1989abc),a FRTL-5 rat thyroid cell lambda gt11 expression library was immunoscreened with a polyclonal rabbit antibody developed against FRTL-5 thyroid cell TSH receptor preparations purified by affinity chromatography on TSH-Sepharose and reactive with monoclonal TSH receptor antibody-Sepharose (Kohn et al., 1986a; Chan et al., 1987: Chan et al.,

1988). This rabbit antibody immunoprecipitated the same multiplicity of TSH-binding proteins as did the monoclonal antibodies to the TSH receptor and could inhibit TSH-induced increases in cAMP levels and thymidine incorporation into DNA (growth) in FRTL-5 cells. Imunoscreening with the rabbit antibody to the TSH receptor preparation resulted in a single rat cDNA clone which cross-hybridized and was identical in size, 1.25 Kb, and restriction mapping to one of the 25 cDNA clones identified with the Graves' IgG preparation. These results suggested the cDNA coded for an autoantigen which might be related to the TSH receptor.

The 1.25 kb cDNA insert from both clones identified a 2 Kb mRNA in human, rat, ovine, and rat thyroid tissues or cells, in guinea pig adipocytes and human IM9 lymphocytes but not in human or rat tissues such brain, liver, kidney or muscle. Although the presence or absence of demonstrable mRNA in poly A+ RNA preparations thus appeared to correlate with the presence or absence of TSH receptor expression in tissues, it was evident that the level of expression in different tissues did not relate to functional expression of TSH receptor. Thus, the IM9 lymphocyte transcript was detectable in total RNA preparations whereas poly A+ RNA was required for Northern analysis in thyroid cells.

The full length sequence of this human thyroid cDNA clone, together with its predicted amino acid sequence, is presented in Figure 1. Several important features can be discerned. First, there are two potential N-linked glycosylation sites (Asn-X-Ser/Thr, underlined). Second although a hydrophobicity plot of the sequence reveals multiple hydrophobic areas (Fig. 2), only one is compatible with a membrane spanning domain, residues 374-390 (Fig. 1). Third, the clone has an open reading frame of 1827 nucleotides which encodes a protein of 69,812 daltons.

The radiolabeled protein product of the full length clone, obtained after in vitro transcription/translation experiments was an autoantigen in that it reacted with the sera of a multiplicity of Graves' patients, not simply the screening antisera, but not with normal sera similarly diluted (Chan et al., 1989; Kohn et al., 1989abc). The radiolabeled protein was also able to bind to Sepharose-TSH; this binding was inhibited by free TSH but not by free insulin, ACTH, prolactin, cholera toxin, or even hCG (Kohn et

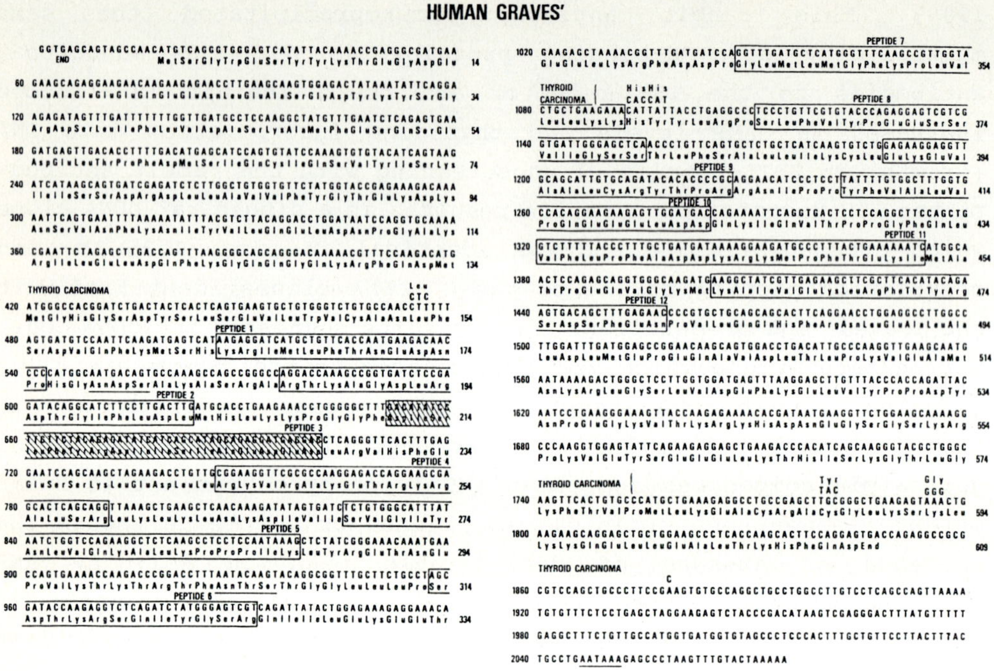

Figure 1. The complete nucleotide and deduced amino acid sequence of a cDNA isolated from a human thyroid library and identifying a novel 70 Kd thyroid autoantigen (Chan et al., 1989). The polyadenylation signal AATAAA is underlined. Two potential glycosylation sites are also underlined. A substitution of T for G (arrow) in the sequence of the comparable cDNA from a human Graves' thyroid library defines an in-frame stop codon and the full length sequence. The blocks denote sequences which were used to synthesize peptides for use in the studies measuring the interaction of the protein with TSH or antibodies to the TSH receptor (Kohn et al., 1989abc). The block denoting the sequence of the bioactive peptide 3, as determined in those experiments (Kohn et al., 1989abc) is cross-hatched.

al., 1989abc). The radiolabeled protein could also be immunoprecipitated by a monoclonal antibody to the human TSH receptor, 52A8; immunoprecipitation by 52A8 was specifically inhibited by free TSH (Kohn et al., 1989abc).

Monoclonal antibody 52A8, made against the human TSH receptor (Kohn et al., 1985; Kohn et al., 1986; Chan et al., 1987), is a "mixed" antibody since it can be both a competitive antagonist (inhibiting TSH binding) and a competitive agonist (stimulating adenylate cyclase and growth activities) of TSH in FRTL-5 rat thyroid cells. These are a strain of continuously cultured cells which maintain many of the functional properties of the thyroid in vitro, including TSH regulation of growth and function (Ambesi-Impiombato, 1986; Kohn et al., 1986b). The 52A8 antibody binds to rat FRTL-5 thyroid cells; this binding can be inhibited by TSH but not by the same concentrations of insulin or hCG (Kohn et al., 1989abc). Twelve peptides representative of different portions of the amino acid sequence predicted were synthesized (Fig. 1) and tested for reactivity with monoclonal 52A8 (Kohn et al., 1989abc). Peptide 3, residues 212 through 228, was able to inhibit the ability of TSH to increase cAMP levels in FRTL-5 thyroid cells as well as the ability of TSH to increase tritiated thymidine incorporation into FRTL-5 cell DNA (Kohn et al., 1989abc). In both cases, the peptide activity was concentration dependent.

Using 3T3 cells and L cells, measurements of transient expression of TSH binding were detected with radiolabeled TSH 48 hours later using "sense" but not "antisense" constructs of the full length clone with an SV 40 promotor (Kohn et al., 1989abc). Increases to 350 to 940 TSH binding sites per cell could be measured, with an affinity as high as 10^{-9} M. In no case, however, was there an associated ability for TSH to increase cAMP levels when tested 15 min to 3 hours after exposure to TSH (1×10^{-10} or 1×10^{-9} M). The TSH binding did, however, appear to be specific (Kohn et al., 1989) in that TSH binding was not inhibited by prolactin, albumin, thyroglobulin, insulin, or glucagon.

This clone thus defines a TSH-binding glycoprotein which has a single transmembrane domain and a binding site for TSH and a monoclonal antibody to the TSH receptor which lies between the two glycosylation sites (Fig. 2). The binding site is negatively

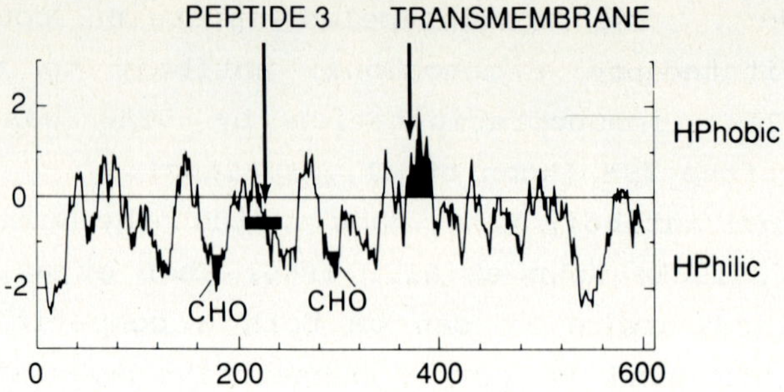

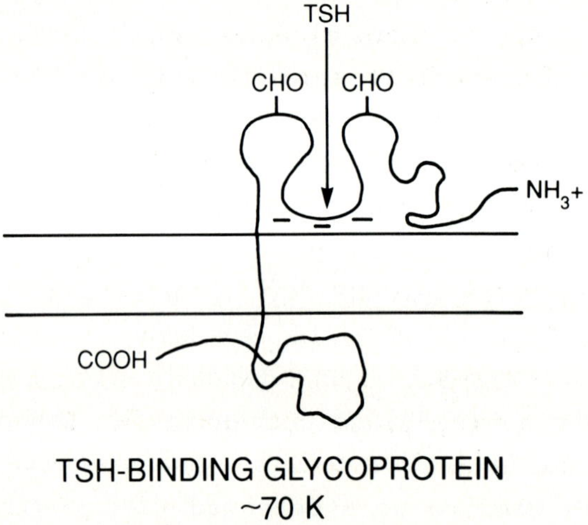

Figure 2. Model of TSH-binding transmembrane glycoprotein predicted from the data in Figure 1 and reported in Kohn et al., 1989abc. The hydrophobicity plot at the top is derived from the data of Figure 1. The two glycosylation sites (CHO) are noted as is the transmembrane domain. The region of peptide 3 which interacts with TSH and monoclonal antibodies to the TSH receptor is noted. The model at the bottom places this in the context of the lipid bilayer. A TSH-binding protein with a single transmembrane domain is predicted; the TSH binding site, which is negatively charged, is between the glycosylation sites.

charged, in line with studies which suggest that the TSH-binding domain in the receptor is negatively charged and salt sensitive (Kohn, 1978) in its reactivity with the positive charge on TSH. Its size, 70K, is compatible with a major TSH-binding protein seen in FRTL-5 thyroid cells (Kohn et al., 1986a; Chan et al., 1987; Chan et al., 1988) and in cross-linking studies (Kohn et al., 1983). The absence of G-protein binding domain evident in studies of adrenergic receptors (Lefkowitz and Caron, 1988) is of concern in defining this as a TSH receptor as is the absence of coupling to the adenylate cyclase signal. This is particularly true given work defining the cloning of the hCG receptor where such a domain is evident (D. L. Segaloff et al., 1989). Nevertheless, coupling to G proteins in this case could reflect a requirement for a coupling component such as the thyroid specific ganglioside or a missing subunit. The possibility that there is more than one TSH-binding component in cells, that not all are coupled to the adenylate cyclase signal system, and that these other proteins are important bioactivators and/or autoantigens will be explored briefly in studies to be described below.

Recombinant Autograhpha californica nuclear polyhedrosis virus containing the thyroid cDNA was produced by standard methods (Allaway et al., 1989). Insect cells transfected with the recombinant virus produced a 70K protein in large amounts; surprisingly, however, immunofluorescence and fractionation data indicate that the 70K protein is predominantly present in the nuclei of the infected insect cells and has undergone little or no glycosylation. At this point it is not clear whether these data represent evidence of complex processing in the insect virus system which is not a reflection of the protein in mammalian cells or whether these data indicate the TSH binding protein defined by this cDNA is a DNA binding protein and can act as a transgenic agent.

Using somatic cell human-hamster hybrids (Chan et al., 1988; Kohn et al., 1989abc), 6 loci were identified on 5 different human chromosomes, namely 22q11-13, Xq, 1q, 8, and 10. The presumptive functional chromosome, 22q11-13, is associated with the Sis proto-oncogene. In mice (Chan et al., 1988), the gene is mapped to a single locus on chromosome 15, also appears to be associated with the Sis proto-oncogene, and is on the same chromosome as the thyroglobulin and c-myc genes.

These results are intriguing with respect to the possibility that the clone is an important TSH-binding autoantigen in Graves' disease. Thus, recent work (Kendall-Taylor et al., 1988) in patients with Graves' disease and exophthalmos suggests there is a significant risk of exophthalmos in patients with P blood group by comparison to patients with Graves' disease who do not have exophthalmos. P blood group antigen is associated with the P_1 antigen and in particular to the alpha-4-Gal transferase converting paragloboside to the P_1 antigen. Current studies (W. O. McBride, personal communication) indicate that it maps to the same locus 22q11-13 and is probably near and closely linked, but not identical to, the gene coding for the cDNA described in these studies. Paragloboside and the P_1 antigen are glycolipids which can be viewed as structural analogs of higher order gangliosides implicated (Kohn, 1978) in TSH receptor structure and function. This association and these data are very exciting in that they offer the first clue, at a molecular level, as to the potential relationship of Graves', its ophthalmopathy, the glycolipid, and the TSH-binding membrane glycoprotein identified by the cDNA in these studies and by TBIAb assays clinically. The TSH binding component of the TSH receptor, rather than the receptor domain important in adenylate cyclase stimulation has been linked to exophthalmos in vitro (Rotella et al., 1986).

Second, the identification of genomic material on the X chromosome is obviously provocative with respect to the dramatically increased frequency of Graves' in females. Whether this is more than fortuitous will, however, require much more understanding of the genomic significance of these multiple gene copies.

The cDNA coding for the autoantigen defined above was cloned from a Graves' thyroid lambda gt11 expression library and sequenced. The sequence is nearly identical to the human thyroid carcinoma clone. These results would support the preliminary conclusion that a grossly abnormal protein structure is not the causative factor in forming Graves' autoantibodies.

Graves' disease has been argued to reflect an immune system irregularity at the lymphocyte level. In this respect, the identification of the 2 Kb mRNA in IM9 lymphocytes (Chan et al., 1988; Kohn et al., 1989abc) was not only compatible with the identification of TSH receptor activity in lymphocytes but also raised the possibility that this might be an autoantigen common to thyroid and lymphocytes. This appears to be true. Thus, although low levels of transcript are evident in normal tonsilar T cells, phytohaemagglutinin (PHA) increases the expression nearly 10 fold. Maximal increases were evident 16 hours after PHA and were blocked by cyclosporin. Transformed T cell lines had a high level of transcript without PHA stimulation and expression of the transcript in transformed lines was not changed by PHA.

Normal tonsillar B cells express even higher levels of the 2 Kb transcript than normal T cells; and mitogen stimulation by Staphlococcus aureus Cowan Strain 1 and phorbol myristate acetate (PMA) further elevates transcript levels, approximately 3 fold. Once again transformed B cell lines have higher levels of the transcript and mitogen stimulation does not increase transcript levels in the transformed lines.

Sequencing of the cDNA coding for the autoantigen after its isolation from an IM9 lymphocyte lambda gt11 expression library indicates that the lymphocyte and thyroid autoantigens are again effectively identical. This result, plus the existence of a single gene in the mouse, makes it likely that the same gene codes for the transcript in thyroid and immune cells.

Lymphocytes have TSH receptors as defined in binding studies but the receptor is not coupled to the cyclase signal system. This would be compatible with the thesis that TSH receptor binding involves a glycoprotein membrane component but coupling requires a second factor (Kohn, 1978; Kohn et al., 1986a; Chan et al., 1987), that this TSH-binding glycoprotein is coupled to a different signal transduction system, and/or there is more than one TSH-binding site or receptor important in autoimmune disease. One must question why this protein exists in lymphocytes; is its presence key to the development of autoimmune Graves'? The transfection studies in the insect virus system which define a nuclear form of the transcript may be relevant. The observation that transcript expression in thyroid and lymphocytes increases with mitogen stimulation or in transformed cells could suggest the autoantigen has an important role in growth as evidenced in other receptor-oncogene relationships.

ANOTHER IMPORTANT THYROID AUTOANTIGEN DEFINED BY CLONING

As noted above, the screening approach using the active Graves' sera identified 25 separate cDA clones. We have characterized another of these clones (Zarrilli et al., 1989) and found it has very interesting properties. This clone defined a 3.6 Kb transcript in human thyroid tissues and rat thyroid cells. Its tissue specificity was different from the TSH-binding autoantigen characterized above in that it could be detected at lower levels in liver and differentiated myoblasts but not in lymphocytes such as IM9 cells. Expression of the transcript was TSH regulated in rat thyroid FRTL-5 cells and cell cycle or, possibly, growth related. The cDNA hybridized with a single copy genomic sequence on human chromosome 10. Based on sequence derived from cDNA clones obtained from rat FRTL-5 thyroid cell, human thyroid carcinoma, and Graves' thyroid expression libraries, a highly conserved 1.05 Kb open reading frame was defined (Fig. 3). Most exiting, however, was the observation that the predicted amino acid sequence of this autoantigen exhibited a strong homology with the mitochondrial ADP/ATP translocator and two other mitochondrial carrier proteins, the phosphate carrier and the hydrogen ion carrier.

These results are exciting since they, for the first time, define a mitochondrial protein as an autoantigen in Graves' disease. This autoantigen has been recognized to be important in autoimmune myocarditis and liver disease (Schultheiss et al., 1986) and is an important modulator of thyroid hormone action in mitochondria (Sterling, 1986). We currently speculate that autoantibodies to this autoantigen may contribute to the myopathy of Graves' disease and account for the failure to correlate thyroid hormone levels with myopathy.

```
     TyrAlaLysGluGlyGlyPhePheGlyPheTyrArgGlyLeuMetProThrIleLeuGly
Hum  TATGCAAAGGAAGGTGGTTTCTTTGGATTTTACAGAGGTCTGATGCCTACTATTTTAGGA  778
Rat       C               C       C                       A
                          Leu

     MetAlaProTyrAlaGlyValSerPhePheThrPheGlyThrLeuLysSerValGlyLeu
Hum  ATGGCTCCATATGCAGGTGTTTCATTTTTTACTTTTGGTACCTTGAAGAGTGTTGGGCTT  838
Rat       C         A       C        C
                    Ser

     SerHisAlaProThrLeuLeuGlySerProSerSerAspAsnProAsnValLeuValLeu
Hum  TCCCATGCTCCTACCCTTCTTGGCAGTCCTTCATCAGACAATCCTAATGTCTTAGTTTTG  898
Rat     T       C     G      C A  A  G  C     C  C  C        C
        Tyr                  Arg

     LysThrHisValAsnLeuLeuCysGlyGlyValAlaGlyAlaIleAlaGlnThrIleSer
Hum  AAAACTCATGTAAACTTACTTTGTGGTGGTGTTGCTGGAGCAATAGCGCAGACAATATCC  958
Rat          CA                                     A     G
              Ile

     TyrProPheAspValThrArgArgArgMetGlnLeuGlyThrValLeuProGluPheGlu
Hum  TACCCATTTGATGTGACTCGTCGGCGAATGCAATTAGGAACTGTTCTGCCGGAATTTGAA  1018
Rat                 A  C      A       G  G  GG A  C  A     G     G
                                            Ala

     LysCysLeuThrMetArgAspThrMetLysTyrAspTyrGlyHisHisGlyIleArgLys
Hum  AAGTGCCTTACCATGCGGGATACTATGAAGTATGACTATGGACACCATGGAATTCGAAAA  1078
Rat                 A    G  C          T               G     G G
                                      Val                     Arg

     GlyLeuTyrArgGlyLeuSerLeuAsnTyrIleArgCysIleProSerGlnAlaValAla
Hum  GGACTCTATCGTGGTTTATCTCTTAATTACATTCGCTGTATTCCCTCTCAAGCAGTGGCT  1138
Rat     T G  C     C        G  C     C                    T

     PheTyrAsnIleArgThrTyrGluAlaValPheSerProGlnLeuLysLysAsnTyrGly
Hum  TTCTACAACATACGAACTTATGAAGCAGTTTTTTCACCTCAACTAAAAAAAAATTATGGT  1198
Rat     ............3'end of rat clone

     TrpPhePheLeuIleHisSerGlnArgGluLysEnd
Hum  TGGTTTTTCTTAATACATTCTCAGAGGGAGAAATGAAACATTACTATAATTGTGGGGGA  1258

Hum  ACATTACTTGAATGGGGATATTTACCCTGTCACAGAGCCATGGTATTTTAGTACTTGATT  1318

Hum  ATTTTTCTTTAGTCAGATCAGAACTGCTTACCATACTTTTTAGATGCGCCAAACATTATA  1378

Hum  CCTTAGAACATTGAAGAAAATATCGCAGCTAAGCTGATGCCTGGCTAAACCGCTTTAATG  1438

Hum  TTTTATTTGGAAGTAGAAACTAGCTTTACGGGGTTCAAGAGGTTGGCCATTAGCTTTCGT  1498

Hum  CATGCTGTTCAAAGTTTTTAATTGTTATCGGTTTTTAAAAGACTGACAGTGTTTATTATA  1558

Hum  TTAAAATAAGGTTATATTGCAATAGAATAATAGAGAATTGAATTTTTAAGTTGCTATGAA  1618

Hum  ACAGTCCAGCCATTGACATTTTATTTTTGTTATCTCTCTTCTCACAATTATGCTCCACTG  1678

Hum  GATAATAGGAAAAACACTTCTTTCCTTCATTTTTTAAATAAAAATTAATGTTTGATTTAA  1738
```

```
Hum    ........CCTATGGTCCCGTCCGGTGTTCTGTAAGTTGGCAACCTAGGCTCCTGACG  58
Rat    CGGCAACAG C    G TTC TA      T            G GG       GG

                   MetAlaAlaAlaThrAlaAlaAlaAlaLeuAlaAlaAlaAspPro
Hum  CGACCCTGGTCCTGATGGCGGCGGCGACGGCCGCGGCAGCCCTGGCGGCGGCCGATCCC  117
Rat  T G G A      G        CCT GT    T  A  G                 G  T
                            LeuVal

     ProProAlaMetProGlyAlaAlaGlyAlaGlyGlyProThrThrArgArgAspPheTyr
Hum  CCTCCCGCAATGCCAGGGGCGGCAGGGGCCGGAGGGCCCACAACCCGCAGAGACTTCTAC  177
Rat    A     GG    C CA     G   AG    G  C  G CT  T   C
              Val   Ala         Ser            Ser

     TrpLeuArgSerPheLeuAlaGlyS
Hum  TGGCTGCGCTCCTTTCTGGCCGGGAGAAGAAGAGGAGGTTACTTCAAACAGAACCTGGCAG  238
Rat          T     CT A       ...................................

Hum  TTGGATTAATACCTTGAAGTGTCTGTCTCCATAACCACATTTTAGCAAGATTCCCAGCCT  298
Rat  ............................................................

            erIleAlaGlyCysCysAlaLysThrThrValAlaProLeuAspArgValLys
Hum  TCCTCAGGTATTGCTGGATGCTGTGCCAAAACAACAGTTGCTCCATTGGATCGAGTAAAG  358
Rat  .......                         C            C

     ValLeuLeuGlnAlaHisAsnHisHisTyrLysHisLeuGlyValPheSerAlaLeuArg
Hum  GTTTTATTACAAGCTCACAATCACCATTACAAGCATTTAGGAGTATTTTCTGCATTGCGT  418
Rat                      C            A        G   C    C  C    C
                                                  Leu   Pro

     AlaValProGlnLysGluGlyPheLeuGlyLeuTyrLysGlyAsnGlyAlaMetMetIle
Hum  GCTGTTCCTCAAAAAGAAGGATTCCTTGGATTGTATAAAGGAAATGGTGCAATGATGATT  478
Rat          C     G     C A          A           C
                          Tyr

     ArgIlePheProTyrGlyAlaIleGlnPheMetAlaPheGluHisTyrLysThrLeuIle
Hum  CGAATCTTTCCCTATGGTGCAATCCAGTTTATGGCATTTGAGCATTATAAAACGTTAATT  538
Rat                C               C     C                    C
                                                           Phe

     ThrThrLysLeuGlyIleSerGlyHisValHisArgLeuMetAlaGlySerMetAlaGly
Hum  ACTACGAAGCTGGGAATTTCAGGTCATGTGCACAGATTAATGGCTGGATCCATGGCAGGT  598
Rat       A         G    T           T
                    Val

     .........MetThrAlaValIleCysThrAspProValAspMetValArgValArgLeu
Hum  .........ATGACAGCAGTTATCTGTACTGACCCTGTTGACATGGTTAGGGTCCGCCTA  658
Rat  AAGATGAGC                 C   T     C G  TG    C     G     G
     LysMetSer                     Tyr   Leu   Val

     AlaPheGlnValLysGlyGluHisArgTyrThrGlyIleIleHisAlaPheLysThrIle
Hum  GCATTCCAGGTGAAAGGGGAACACCGCTATACAGGAATTATTCATGCTTTCAAAACAATT  718
Rat    C     A        T      AC    T    G  C  C     G     G     C
                             Thr   Ser
```

Figure 3. Nucleotide and predicted amino acid sequence of a thyroid cDNA which codes for an autoantigen related to the family of mitochondrial carrier proteins including the ADP/ATP carrier. The nucleotide sequences of the cDNA from a Graves' thyroid expression library and from a rat thyroid expression library are presented in Rows 2 and 3 respectively; their derived amino acid sequences are presented in Rows 1 and 4 respectively. Similarity of the amino acid sequence of this thyroid autoantigen (HUM 7) with itself and with the human ADP/ATP carrier (AAC), the rat uncoupling protein (UCPr) and the inorganic phosphate carrier (PHOS), sequence conservation of critical residues, as well as conservation of the tripartate structure seen in this family of proteins are noted in Zarrilli et al., 1989.

OTHER TSH BINDING PROTEINS MAY BE IMPORTANT AUTOANTIGENS IN GRAVES' DISEASE

To complement and extend cloning studies, we used a microsequencing approach. Membrane components from FRTL-5 rat thyroid cells were solubilized and purified by affinity chromatography on TSH-Sepharose. Proteins binding to the TSH column and eluted by high salt concentrations or low pH were further identified by reactivity with different monoclonal antibodies to the TSH receptor. Two peptide fragments from one such protein, approximately 43 kd, were microsequenced and found to match the sequence of gamma-actin (Fig. 4 top). One of these sequences, a sequence not found in beta-actin, is similar to a sequence on the clone defined in Figure 1 (Fig. 4 bottom). The significance of this is not clear. The identification as gamma-actin was confirmed by antibodies to gamma-actin.

Separate studies using monoclonal antibodies to immunoscreen a thyroid carcinoma expression library identified elongation factor 2 (Usala et al., 1988).

SUMMARY

All the proteins above appear to be important molecules in the bioactivity of the thyroid cell and implicated as autoantigens Graves' diseas. Their existence and the apparent multiplicity of TSH-binding proteins raise important questions as to the basic nature of Graves' disease. Perhaps we should reexamine previous presumptions concerning the structure of the TSH receptor, its mechanism of action in effecting cell processes, and its role as an autoantigen causing Graves' disease.

The authors are grateful to their collaborators in the National Institutes of Health, particularly Drs. Bellur Prabhakar, Edward Oates, Graham Allaway, Michael Lerman, Abner Notkins, Wesley O. McBride and John Kehrl, for their involvement in and key contributions to studies which made some of this work possible.

A

γ ACTIN → MET Glu Glu Glu Ile Ala Ala Leu Val Ile Asp Asn

γ ACTIN → MET	Glu	Glu	Glu	Ile	Ala	Ala	Leu	Val	Ile	Asp	Asn						
									10								
Gly	Ser	Gly	Met	Cys	Lys	Ala	Gly	Phe	Ala	Gly	Asp	Asp	Ala	Pro	Arg	Ala	Val
							20										30
Phe	Pro	Ser	Ile	Val	Gly	Arg	Pro	Arg	His	Gln	Gly	Val	Met	Val	Gly	Met	Gly
									40								
→ Asp	Ile	Lys	Glu	Lys	Leu	Cys	Tyr	Val	Ala	Leu	Asp	Phe	Glu	Gln	Glu	Met	Ala
									220								
Thr	Ala	Ala	Ser	Ser	Ser	Ser	Leu	Glu	Lys	Ser	Tyr	Glu	Leu	Pro	Asp	Gly	Gln
	230					234a						240					

PEPTIDE A

PEPTIDE B

B

Comparison of the Amino Acid Sequence of Peptide A and Different Actins

Residue No.	2	3	4	5	6	7	8	9	10	11	12	13	14	15	16	17	18	19
peptide A			Glu	Ile	Ala	Ala	Leu	X	Ile	Asp	Asn	Gly	X	Gly	Met	X	Lys	Ala
human γ actin	Glu	Glu	Glu	Ile	Ala	Ala	Leu	Val	Ile	Asp	Asn	Gly	Ser	Gly	Met	Cys	Lys	Ala
human β actin			Asp	Ile	Ala	Ala	Leu	Val	Val	Asp	Asn	Gly	Ser	Gly	Met	Cys	Lys	Ala
γ at β actin			Asp	Ile	Ala	Ala	Leu	Val	Val	Asp	Asn	Gly	Ser	Ala	Met	Cys	Lys	Ala
TSH-BINDING GLYOPROTEIN	Glu	Lys	Glu	Val	Ala	Ala	Leu											
	391	392	393	394	395	396	397											

Figure 4. (TOP) Micro sequences of peptides from protein which binds to TSH-Sepharose and is measurable by a monoclonal antibody to the TSH receptor compared to gamma-actin sequences. (BOTTOM) One of the peptide sequences determined above, which is different from beta-actin and helps define gamma-actin as a unique protein, has a sequence similarity to a portion of the protein defined by the clone in Figure 1.

REFERENCES

Allaway GP, Prabhakar BS, Vivino AA, Chan JYC, Kohn LD, Notkins AL (1989) Characterization of a novel 70 kilodalton thyroid autoantigen produced in the baculovirus expression system. In: Proceedings 23rd Annual Meeting European Society for Clinical Investigation. Springer, Berlin Heidelberg New York

Ambesi-Impiombato FS (1986) Living, fast-growing thyroid cell strain, FRTL-5. US Patent 4,608,341

Chan J, DeLuca M, Santisteban P, Isozaki O, Shifrin S, Aloj S, Grollman EF, Kohn LD (1987) Nature of thyroid autoantigens: the TSH receptor. In: Pinchera A, Ingbar SH, McKenzie JM (eds) Thyroid Autoimmunity. Plenum Press, New York, 11-26

Chan J, Lerman MI, Prabhakar B, Isozaki O, Santisteban P, Kuppers R, Oates EL, Notkins L, Kohn LD (1989) Cloning and characterization of a cDNA that encodes a 70-kDa novel human thyroid autoantigen. J Biol Chem 264:3651-3654

Chan J, Santisteban P, DeLuca M, Isozaki O, Grollman EF, Kohn LD (1987) TSH receptor structure. Acta Endocrinologia (Copenh), Suppl 281, 115:166-172

Chan JYC, Santisteban P, Kozak CA, Kuppers R, Kohn LD (1988) Genomic organization and chromosomal mapping of a mouse lymphocyte gene: its cDNA sequence is homologous to a thyroid autoantigen. In: 63rd Annual Meeting American Thyroid Association. Endocrinology 121 (Supplement):T52

Kendall-Taylor P, Stephenson A, Stratton A, Papiha SS, Perros P, Roberts DF (1988) Differentiation of autoimmune ophthalmopathy from Graves' hyperthyroidism by analysis of genetic markers. Clinical Endocrinology 28:601-610

Kohn LD (1978) Relationships in the structure and function of receptors for glycoprotein hormones, bacterial toxins and interferon. In: Cuatrecassas P, Greaves MF (eds) Receptors and Recognition, Series A, Vol 5. Chapman and Hall, London 133-212

Kohn LD, Aloj SM, Tombaccini D, Rotella CM, Toccafondi R, Marcocci C, Corda D, Grollman EF (1985) The thyrotropin receptor. In: Litwak G (ed) Biochemical Actions of Hormones. Marcel Dekker, New York 457-512

Kohn LD, Alvarez F, Marcocci C, Kohn AD, Chen A, Hoffman WE, Tombaccini D, Valente WA, DeLuca M, Santisteban P, Grollman EF (1986a) Monoclonal antibody studies defining the origin and properties of autoantibodies in Graves' disease. Ann NY Acad Sci 475:157-173

Kohn LD, Isozaki O, Chan J, Akamizu T, Bellur S, DeLuca M, Santisteban P, Varutti AM, Grimaz A, Ikuyama S, Saji K, Owens G (1989a) The thyrotropin receptor in FRTL-5 thyroid cells: a cloning approach. In: Perrild H, Ambesi-Impiombato FS (eds) FRTL-5 Today. Elsevier, Amsterdam, in press

Kohn LD, Isozaki O, Chan JY, Akamizu T, Bellur S, Santisteban P, Ikuyama S, Saji M, Doi S, Tahara K, Kosugi S, Sabe H, Mori T (1989b) Characterization of the thyrotropin receptor and other Graves' disease autoantigens. In: Chin W, Boime I (eds) Proceedings of International Symposium on Glycoprotein Hormones. Plenum Publishing Corp, New York in press

Kohn LD, Saji M, Akamizu T, Ikuyama S, Isozaki O, Kohn AD, Santisteban P, Chan JYC, Bellur S, Rotella CM, Alvarez FV, Aloj SM (1989c) Receptors of the thyroid: the thyrotropin receptor is only the first violinist of a symphony orchestra. In: Ekholm R, Kohn LD, Wollman S (eds) Control of the Thyroid: Regulation of its Normal Growth and Function. Plenum Publishing Corp, New York in press

Kohn LD, Valente WA, Grollman EF, Aloj SM, Vitti P (1986b) Clinical determination and/or quantification of thyrotropin and a variety of thyroid stimulatory and inhibitory factors performed in vitro with an improved thyroid cell line FRTL-5. US Patent 4,609,622

Kohn LD, Valente WA, Laccetti P, Cohen J, Aloj SM, Grollman EF (1983) Multicomponent structure of the thyrotropin receptor: relationships to Graves' disease. Life Sciences 32:15-30

Lefkowitz R, Caron MG (1988) Adrenergic receptors: models for the study of receptors coupled to guanine nucleotide regulatory proteins. J Biol Chem 263:4993-4996

Rotella CM, Zonefrate R, Toccafondi R, Valente WA, Kohn LD (1986) Ability of monoclonal antibodies to the TSH receptor to increase collagen synthesis in human fibroblasts, an assay which appears to measure exophthalmogenic immunoglobulins in Graves' sera. J Clin Endocrinol Metab 62:357-367

Schultheiss HP, Schulze K, Kuhl U, Ulrich G, Klingenberg M (1986) The ADP/ATP carrier as a mitochondrial autoantigen - facts and perspective. Ann NY Acad Sci 488:44-64

Segaloff DL, Sprengel R, McFarland KC, Rosemblit N, Kohler M, Nikolics K, Seeburg PH (1989) The structure of the LH/hCG receptor as determined by cDNA cloning. In: Chin W, Boime I (eds) International Symposium on Glycoprotein Hormones. Plenum Publishing Corp, New York, in press

Sterling K (1986) Direct thyroid hormone activation of mitochondria: the role of adenine nucleotide translocase. Endocrinology 119: 292-295

Usala SJ, Wondisford FE, Yoshida T, Ichikawa Y, Weintraub BD (1988) Isolation and characterization of a human TSH receptor gene: evidence for at least one intervening sequence. In: 63rd Annual Meeting American Thyroid Association. Endocrinology 121 (Supplement):T57

Zarrilli R, Oates EL, McBride OW, Lerman MI, Chan JY, Santisteban P, Ursini MV, Notkins AL, Kohn LD (1989) Sequence and chromosomal assignment of a novel cDNA identified by immunoscreening of a thyroid expression library: similarity to a family of mitochondrial solute carrier proteins. M o l Endocrinology submitted

DISCUSSION

EISENBARTH: There have been other claimants for having cloned the TSH receptor. Could you summarise the field?

KOHN: I think there was one other claim which was made by a consortium of a Japanese group and Bruce Weintraub at the NIH. The receptor was identified by screening with monoclonal antibodies developed by the Japanese group but the clone turned out to be elongation factor 2.

QUESTION: Has the ganglioside component of the receptor been characterised, what ganglioside is it? Is it specific for the thyroid, or it can be found in other tissue?

KOHN: We showed some years ago that there is a very specific thyroid ganglioside. Its that ganglioside which is identified by the monoclonal antibodies which are stimulating antibodies. Its not clear what relevance that has, in other words whether that is a true anti-ganglioside antibody.

WILCOX: Can I ask two things; firstly, does this recombinant antigen give you a better diagnostic assay for Graves' Disease?

KOHN: Yes.

WILCOX: Secondly, what is the significance of having multiple chromosomal sites?

KOHN: We don't know, obviously they could be all pseudo genes, obviously the presence on the X chromosome gives one pause for thought. Could it be that the X chromosome is under some regulatory control and is real and that is why females have a much higher preponderance of the disease.

THYROID PEROXIDASE: STUDIES ON AUTO-ANTIBODY RECOGNITION, GENE EXPRESSION AND SECONDARY STRUCTURE PREDICTION

Kate S Collison, D Mahadevan, P S Barnett, Nan D Doble, R W S Tomlinson, J-P Banga, A M McGregor

Department of Medicine
King's College Hospital Medical School
Denmark Hill
LONDON SE5 8RX, UK

NATO ASI Series, Vol. H 38
The Molecular Biology of Autoimmune Disease
Edited by A. G. Demaine et al.

INTRODUCTION

The spectrum of autoimmune thyroid diseases (AITD) are common, being seen in 2-4% of the population in areas of adequate dietary iodine intake and are increasing well characterised clinically and immunologically (Weetman et al 1984). The recognition of the likely immunological basis of AITD dates back to 1956 with the observations of Rose and Witebsky in animal models and Roitt and Doniach in man on antibody activity against thyroglobulin (TG). The subsequent demonstration of autoantibody activity against thyroid cell cytoplasmic constituents (Roitt et al 1964), despite the frequency with which this autoantibody activity is associated with AITD, left unresolved the question of how an intracellular determinant might be accessible to the immune system and therefore questioned the clinical relevance of these autoantibodies. Attempts to characterise and localise the relevant auto-antigen were limited to its recognition as the thyroid "microsomal" auto-antigen (TMA) and as a constituent of thyroid exocytotic vesicles involved in the transfer of TG from the cell to its site of storage in the central colloid space of thyroid follicles. Understanding of the TMA remained unchanged until the early 1980's when developments in technology including improved assay systems for the detection of autoantibodies to the TMA (Weetman et al 1983) coupled with the use of poly- and monoclonal antibodies led to the demonstration that; (i) the TMA is expressed on the thyroid cell surface (Khoury et al 1981), (ii) has a molecular weight of about 105,000 (Banga et al, 1985) and that (iii) monoclonal antibodies to the TMA, by binding to the surface of cultured human thyroid cells were able to kill these cells in the presence of complement (Weetman et al 1985; Banga et al 1986). The recent cloning and sequencing of the human gene for thyroid peroxidase (TPO) (Kimura et al, 1987), the key enzyme in the generation of thyroid hormone from their pro-hormone TG, has opened up a new era in our understanding of AITD with confirmation that the auto-antigen recognized for so long as the TMA is largely, if not entirely, TPO (Czarnocka et al 1985). With molecular characterisation of the auto-antigen, studies in the field of AITD will undoubtedly move rapidly. Dissection of the process of T cell recognition (Banga et al 1989a) of TPO and particularly of the relevant pathogenic epitopes of the molecule have begun in a number of laboratories. Whilst these may well have more relevance than autoantibodies in the pathogenesis of AITD a considerable literature has accumulated on autoantibodies to the TMA/TPO complex. It has proved difficult to prove beyond doubt their pathogenic role though in situations such as the transient syndromes of post-partum thyroid dysfunction (Fung et al 1988), a role seems likely.

Based on these observations, recent studies in our laboratories have focused on three main areas; (i) the antigenic determinants recognized by autoantibodies to the TMA/TPO, (ii) with the generation of oligonucleotide probes derived from the nucleotide sequence of the human TPO gene

(Banga et al 1990), the regulation of TPO gene expression. (iii) In trying to understand the process of recognition of autoantigenic determinants by T and B cells an understanding of the three dimensional structure of TPO will be essential. Crystals of TPO will be needed for these studies and are not yet available. Considerable developments have occurred in means for predicting the secondary structure of proteins and these are now being applied to TPO. The progress to date in these studies are presented in this chapter.

WHAT DO AUTOANTIBODIES TO THE TMA/TPO COMPLEX SEE?

Despite thyroid peroxidase being a large molecule the assumption has always been that the number of determinants on the molecule recognised by the immune system (epitopes) would be limited. In seeking to characterise the B cell epitopes we have been particularly interested to examine the possibility that autoantibodies might be directed towards the catalytic or active site of the enzyme. Using immunoblotting following SDS-PAGE under non-reducing and reducing conditions and assessment of TPO enzymatic activity by peroxidation of guaiacol and iodide (Doble et al, 1988) it is quite clear that autoantibodies to the TMA/TPO in the sera of patients with AITD are polyclonal and amongst the commonest epitopes recognized are those at or near the active site of the enzyme which, because of their presence, inhibit TPO enzymatic activity. Extending these studies, it has been interesting to examine the ability of autoantibodies to the TMA/TPO complex to cross-react with other peroxidase enzymes (Banga et al 1989b). Using purified preparations of myeloperoxidase (MPO), lactoperoxidase (LPO) and horseradish peroxidase (HRP) we have been able to demonstrate by ELISA and SDS-PAGE under reducing and non-reducing conditions followed by immunoblotting that autoantibodies to the TMA/TPO complex cross-react with these peroxidases. This cross-reactivity is real in the sense that TMA immobilised on Sepharose-4B absorbs out all the autoantibody activity against the TMA/TPO complex and sera treated in this way no longer cross-react with MPO, LPO or HRP.

REGULATION OF TPO GENE EXPRESSION IN HUMAN THYROID CELLS

With the recent successful cloning of the human TPO gene (Kimura et al 1987) we have prepared synthetic oligonucleotide probes derived from the nucleotide sequence of the gene. Using a 40mer oligonucleotide probe, shown by Northern blotting to hybridise specifically to a thyroid mRNA of 3kb, we have used the technique of slot-blot hybridization to examine the activiation of the TPO gene in cultured human thyrocytes (Collison et al 1989). Dose-response and time course studies have demonstrated clearly the role of thyrotropin (TSH) in switching on the TPO gene and inducing its mRNA expression. The TSH-induced response was mimicked by the adenylate cyclase activator forskolin but inhibited by the protein kinase C activating phorbol ester TPA. These preliminary studies provide a clear demonstration of the central role of TSH in thyroid cell regulation. In addition they offer an assay system which, in allowing quantification of the level of gene expression, will permit studies not only on the physiology of thyroid cell activition but also on thyroid cell modulation under pathogenic conditions such as occur in Graves' disease where autoantibodies interact with the TSH receptor to either activate or inhibit thyroid cell function.

SECONDARY STRUCTURE PREDICTION OF TPO

We are not yet able to purify human TPO in sufficient quantities and at a level of sufficient purity, though these studies are progressing well (Tomlinson et al 1989). In contrast MPO can be purified satisfactorily and in our initial studies on secondary structure prediction we have made use of this material since, as discussed earlier, (i) considerable sequence homology exists between TPO and MPO (Libert et al 1987) and (ii) autoantibodies to the TMA/TPO complex cross-react with MPO (Banga et al 1989b). Two approaches have been adopted. Firstly, circular dichroic (CD) spectroscopy has been carried out on MPO of greater than 90% purity as assessed by SDS-PAGE. This technique allows ascertainment of the alpha helical content of the protein. Secondly, multiple sequence alignments of human and porcine TPO, human MPO and the related eosinophil peroxidase (EP) have been performed using the algorithm of Barton and Sternberg and 4 different prediction methods have been applied to the multiple aligned sequences.

The 4 methods (i. Lim, ii. Chou and Fasman, iii. Robson and iv. Rose) applied to each sequence independently in conjunction with the data obtained from the CD spectra for MPO and the organisation of the exon/ intron genes of TPO and MPO have allowed a first prediction of the secondary structure of TPO. These structural prediction studies show the TPO molecule to be a predominantly alpha-helical protein, consisting of 12 domains, including the transmembrane and a cytoplasmic domain. The haem binding sites appear to reside in 3 extracellular domains D, E and F (Banga et al, 1989c). In addition, prediction of B and T cell epitopes have been attempted using the hydrophilicity scale of Hopp and Woods for antibodies and the T cell epitope motifs described by Rothbard and Taylor.

CONCLUSIONS

The 1980's have seen dramatic developments in our understanding of the "thyroid cytoplasmic antigen". Characterisation of this autoantigen as the key thyroid enzyme TPO has led rapidly to studies on the elucidation of the determinants of TPO seen by the immune system. The key to our understanding of the development of AITD lies in our understanding of T cell recognition of TPO as does our future ability to manipulate and abrogate the aberrant autoimmune response with immunological therapies. Studies which will characterise the interaction of T cells with TPO will undoubtedly follow very rapidly on the past decade's work.

REFERENCES

Banga, J-P., Pryce, G., Hammond, L. and Roitt, I.M. (1985). Structural features of the autoantigens involved in thyroid autoimmunity; the thyroid microsomal-microvillar autoantigen. Molec. Immunol. 22: 629-638

Banga, J-P., Mirakian, R., Hammond, L., Pryce, G., Bidey, S., Bottazzo, G.F., Weetman, A.P., McGregor, A.M. and Roitt, I.M. (1986). Characterisation of monoclonal antibodies directed towards the microsomal-microvillar thyroid autoantigen recognized by Hashimoto autoantibodies. Clin. Exptl. Immunol. 64: 544-554

Banga, J-P., Barnett, P.S., Mahadevan, D. and McGregor, A.M. (1989a). Immune recognition of antigen and its relevance to autoimmune disease: recent advances at the molecular level. European J. Clin. Invest. 19: 107-116

Banga, J-P., Tomlinson, R.W.S., Doble, N.D., Odell, E. and McGregor, A.M. (1989b). Thyroid microsomal/thyroid peroxidase autoantibodies show discrete patterns of cross-reactivity to myeloperoxidase, lactoperoxidase and horseradish peroxidase. Immunology. 67: 197-204

Banga, J-P., Mahadevan, D., Barton, G., Saldanha, J., Odell, E. and McGregor, A.M. (1989c). Secondary structure prediction on thyroid peroxidase, a potent human autoantigen involved in destructive autoimmune thyroid disease. J. Endocrinol. 121 Supplement. Abstract 114

Banga, J-P., Barnett, P.S., Ewins, D.L., Page, M.J., and McGregor, A.M. (1990). Analysis of auto-antigenic determinants of thyroid peroxidase antigen, generated using the polymerase chain reaction. In: Demaine A.G., Banga J-P. McGregor A.M. (eds) Molecular Biology of Autoimmune Disease. Springer, Berlin, Heidelberg, New York In press

Collison, K.S., Banga, J-P., Barnett, P.S., Kung, A.W.C. and McGregor, A.M. (1989). Activation of the thyroid peroxidase gene in human thyroid cells: effect of thyrotropin, forskolin and phorbol ester. J. Molec. Endocrinol. 3: 1-5

Czarnocka, B., Ruf, J. Ferrand, M., Carayon, P. and Lissitzky, S. (1985). Purification of the human thyroid peroxidase and its identification as the microsomal antigen involved in autoimmune thyroid disease. FEBS Lett. 190: 147-152

Doble, N.D., Banga, J-P., Pope, R., Lalor, E., Kilduff, P. and McGregor, A.M. (1988). Autoantibodies to the thyroid microsomal/thyroid peroxidase antigen are polyclonal and directed to several distinct antigenic sites. Immunology. 64: 23-29

Fung, H.Y.M., Kologlu, M., Collison, K., John, R., Richards, C.J., Hall, R. and McGregor, A.M. (1988). Post-partum thyroid dysfunction in Mid-Glamorgan. Brit. Med. J. 296: 241-244

Khoury, E.L., Hammond, L., Bottazzo, G.F. and Doniach, D. (1981). Presence of organ-specific microsomal auto-antigen on the surface of human thyroid cells in culture: its involvement in complement-mediated cytotoxicity. Clin. Exptl. Immunol. 45: 316-324

Kimura, S., Kotani, T., McBride, O.M., Umeki, K., Hirai, K., Nakayama, T. and Ohtaki, S. (1987). Human thyroid peroxidase. Complete cDNA and protein sequence, chromosome mapping and identification of two alternatively spliced mRNA's. Proc. Natl. Acad. Sci. (USA) 84: 5555-5559

Libert, F., Ruel, J., Ludgate, M., Swillens, S., Alexander, N., Vassart, G. and Dinsart, C. (1987). Thyroperoxidase, an autoantigen with a mosaic structure made of nuclear and mitochondrial gene modules. EMBO J. 6: 4193-4196

Roitt, I.M., Doniach, D., Campbell, P.M. and Hudson, R.V. (1956). Autoantibodies in Hashimoto's disease (lymphadenoid goitre). Lancet 2: 820-821

Roitt, I.M., Ling, N.R., Doniach, D. and Crouchman, K.G. (1964). The cytoplasmic autoantigen of the human thyroid; immunological and biochemical characteristics. Immunology. 7: 375-381

Rose, N.R. and Witebsky, E. (1956). Changes in the thyroid glands of rabbits following active immunisation with rabbit thyroid extracts. J. Immunol. 76: 417-427

Tomlinson, R.W.S., Banga, J-P. and McGregor, A.M. (1989). Purification of human thyroid microsome/thyroid peroxidase antigen by fast protein liquid chromatography (FPLC). J. Endocrinol. 121 Supplement. Abstract 117

Weetman, A.P., Rennie, D.P., Hassman, R., Hall, R. and McGregor, A.M. (1983). Enzyme-linked immunoassay of monoclonal and serum microsomal autoantibodies. Clin. Clinica Acta 138, 237-243

Weetman, A.P. and McGregor, A.M. (1984). Autoimmune thyroid disease; developments in our understanding. Endocrine Reviews 5: 309-355

Weetman, A.P., Gunn, C.A., Rennie, D.P., Hall, R. and McGregor, A.M. (1985). The production and characterisation of monoclonal antibodies to the human thyroid microsome. J. Endocrinol. 105; 47-56

DISCUSSION

WEETMAN: I would just like to make the comment that I think there may be an important consequence of the cross-reactivity that you have described between myeloperoxidase and thyroid peroxidase. Patients treated with anti-thyroid drugs rarely get agranulocytosis and its known that the drugs act as a substrate for the myeloperoxidase and thyroid peroxidase enzymes. We have recently seen a patient with Graves' Disease who developed agranulocytosis. She has myeloperoxidase and thyroid peroxidase antibodies. It seems possible that the drug is actually acting as a hapten and that the thyroid peroxidase and myeloperoxidase are acting as carriers and that is why these patients develop agranulocytosis.

WILKIN: I would like to extend a little bit with this cross-reactivity story and ask you if you have tested Wegener's sera with your method?

McGREGOR: We have not. Tony have you ever looked at Wegener's sera to see whether there is any cross-reactivity?

WEETMAN: Yes, there certainly is and what's more the entire reactivity in certain Wegener's sera can be absorbed out by thyroid peroxidase.

PUJOL-BORELL: Just a couple of brief questions Alan. First of all is there any evidence that the antibody can neutralise the effect of thyroid peroxidase and produce thyroid dysfunction independently of damage that might be produced by complement fixation?

McGREGOR: Those studies haven't yet been done by us.

PUJOL-BORELL: Is there any evidence that thyroid peroxidase can circulate and be a circulating antigen as opposed to simply an antigen in situ in the thyroid?

McGREGOR: I think that the data that is available is very controversial. We haven't really looked seriously. Others have claimed in the past that you can detect it in the circulation. I've never been really convinced by the data so my own feeling is no.

PAPADOPOULOS: Can you really base any reliability on the secondary structure prediction of thyroid peroxidase using the analysis of myeloperoxidase by circular dichroic (CD) spectroscopy?

McGREGOR: As I explained, we do not have access to sufficient highly purified thyroid peroxidase (TPO) of any species to perform CD spectroscopy on. Because of the access to highly purified myeloperoxidase and, in particular, its homology with TPO and the antibody cross-reactivities we have demonstrated between TPO and myeloperoxidase (MPO), we have felt comfortable in using the data on MPO CD spectroscopy. As I said too, we interpret the data with caution and will perform the analysis on TPO as soon as we have it available. However, we are reassured by the sequence alignment and computer prediction studies which confirm the high alpha helical content of both MPO and TPO.

SJOGREN´S SYNDROME, A MODEL TO STUDY AUTOIMMUNITY AND MALIGNANCY

H.M.Moutsopoulos
Department of Internal Medicine
School of Medicine
University of Ioannina
451 10 Ioannina-GREECE

P. Youinou
Centre Hospitalier Regional
et Universitaire de Brest
Laboratoire d´ Immunologie
9 Avenue Foch, Brest-FRANCE

Sjogren´s syndrome (Ss) is a chronic autoimmune disorder with strong female preponderance. The syndrome can occur alone (primary Ss,pSs), or in association with almost all autoimmune diseases. Histologically, up to 30% of unselected patients with connective tissue disease present features reminiscent of Ss in their labial minor salivary glands (SG),of whom only a small percentage expresses sicca manifestations. In this review, we will discuss the clinical and immunologic aberrations of the syndrome which support the view that pSs is a priviliged model for studying autoimmunity and lymphoid malignancy.

Diversity of clinical presentation

Primary Ss has a wide clinical spectrum, expanding from an exocrinopathy to a systemic process and to B-lymphocyte neoplasia.It should be emphasized though, that Ss is a very slowly progressing disease and from the initial symptoms to the full blown development of the syndrome 8-10 years elapse. The symptoms and findings from the exocrine glands relate to decreased or abolished gland function and include: keratoconjunctivitis sicca, xerostomia, parotid or major salivary gland enlargement,xerotrachea,dyspareunia, dry skin, atrophic gastritis and subclinical pancreatitis.Similar symptoms from the exocrine glands can be seen in patients with sarcoidosis, amyloidosis,lipoproteinemia IV and V,chronic graft versus host disease and recently, in patients with HIV infection.

Extraglandular manifestations (systemic) are seen in one third of pSs patients. Usually this group of patients complain of easy fatigue,low grade fever,myalgias,arthralgias and non-erosive systemic polyarthritis.Raynaud´s phenomenon is common and usually precedes sicca manifestations.Kidney involvement can present either as interstitial nephritis (manifesting with hyposthenuria, renal tubular dysfunction with or without acidosis and Fanconi´s syndrome) or membranous or membranoproliferative glomerulonephritis

NATO ASI Series, Vol. H 38
The Molecular Biology of Autoimmune Disease
Edited by A. G. Demaine et al.

(connoting systemic vasculitis and cryoglobulinemia or an overlap with systemic lupus erythematosus). Lung involvement presents with diffuse interstitial pattern or lung infiltrates. Pleurisy is very uncommon in pSs patients. Vasculitis usually presents with palpable purpura and sometimes with ulcerative leg lesions and digital gangrene. Myositis and peripheral neuropathy of mixed type (sensory-motor) or mononeuritis multiplex,are other clinical manifestations. Central nervous system manifestations,if any,should be extremely rare. Involvement of mesenteric arteries is responsible for nausea,vomiting, acute abdomen and hematochesia. Gallbladder perforation is also seen. Histologically the vessel patterns include leukoclastic and lymphocytic vasculitis,acute necrotizing angiitis and endarteritis obliterans involving small and medium size muscular arteries.

Frank lymphadenopathy and/or splenomegaly are not uncommon.Bunim and Talal, 20 years ago, first reported an increased incidence of non-Hodgkin's lymphoma in patients with Ss. They described three cases of lymphoma and one case of Waldenstrom's macroglobulinemia among 58 cases of Ss patients. Since then many other investigators substantiate this observation.Most of the lymphoma cases usually develop in patients with systemic Ss and affect lymph nodes as well as parenchymal organs. Lymphomatous involvement of the major salivary or lacrimal glands occur infrequently in Ss. Kassan et al studied the relative risk of lymphoid malignancy in a population consisting of 136 female patients with Ss (followed-up at the NIH for 8.1 years per patient) as well as an age,sex,race and time specific matched control population.It was found that Ss patients have 43 times higher relative risk compared to control group. The relative risk of lymphoma increased even more in patients with parotid gland enlargement,splenomegaly,lymphadenopathy or if they had previously received chemotherapy or radiation for their disease.

Zulman et al applying immunohistological techniques,to study lymphomatous tissues,found that most of them were of B-cell origin,and showed that the vast majority of the cells contained IgM kappa immunoglobulin in their cytoplasm. Schmid et al used the same technique to analyze the confluent lymphoid proliferating areas in minor SG from Ss patients and revealed that they contain monoclonal IgM kappa B-cell population. They suggested that these lesions represent "early lymphomas" analogous to carcinoma "in situ".

In the last 7 years, we have seen 8 lymphoma cases out of the 120 cases of pSs which followed in our Rheumatology Clinic.The lymphomatous lesions were affecting the exocrine glands in 5 patients (4 the labial minor salivary and 1 the lacrimal gland). All of these lymphomas were classified as immunocytomas.One patient developed a pharyngeal mass,while the remaining two presented with lymphadenopathy of the cervical and axillary nodes.The patient with the pharyngeal mass and one of the two patients with lymphadenopathy were classified as intermediate lymphomas (centrocytic-centroblastic) while the third as immunocytoma. All the patients with lymphoma exhibited systemic Ss and the majority had circulating autoantibodies directed to immunoglobulins and Ro(SSA) and/or La(SSB) antigens. None of the immunocytoma patients was treated. The patient with the cervical and axillary lymphadenopathy three months after the diagnosis had a spontaneous remission.

We are facing now a new spectrum of lymphoma in Ss patients which suggests that the initial site of clonal expansion is likely to be the exocrine glands; most of the cases are low grade lymphomas and spontaneous remission can occur. However,longer follow-up is necessary to substantiate these observations.

Benign to malignant lymphoproliferation

Significant progress has been accomplished in the understading of the pathogenesis of Ss. The two major autoimmune phenomena are: B-lymphocyte hyperreactivity and focal lymphocytic infiltration within the affected organs.

It has been known, for over 30 years,that the serologic hallmark of Ss patients is hypergammaglobulinemia. Further studies have revealed that the excess of immunoglobulins consists of autoantibodies directed to non-organ specific antigen such as immunoglobulins (rheumatoid factors,RFs) and cellular antigens such as Ro(SSA),La(SSB) and RAP(RANA,SSC),as well as organ-specific antigens such as SG,thyroid gland and gastric mucosa. All these antibodies are of IgG and IgM isotypes.The spectrum of autoantibodies differs in patients with pSs and those with secondary Ss (sSs) (Table 1).

Autoantibodies in pSs patients correlate with the intensity of the lymphocytic infiltration of the labial minor SG and with the presence of extraglandular manifestations. Thus the polyclonal B-cell hyperreactivity does not seem random and most probably is driven by antigen(s). That is suggested by the high amount of autoantibody to "nuclear" antigens,as opposed to the low number of autoreactive B-cells in the immune repertoire.Additional arguments are the presence of IgG autoantibodies,the high rate of mutations of germ-line genes,and the rather limited number of antigens recognized by Ss patient B-cells. There is no conclusive evidence,however,relating pathogenetically these autoantibodies to tissue destruction in Ss.

Table 1: Prevalence of various autoantibodies in patients with primary Sjogren´s syndrome (pSs) and patients with rheumatoid arthritis (RA) with and without secondary Sjogren´s syndrome (sSs)

Autoantibodies	pSs	RA-sSs	RA
	% positive		
Anti-Ro(SSA)	60	28	5-10
Anti-La(SSB)	46	5	0
RAP (RANA,SSC)	14	60	49
Anti-salivary duct	25	69	ND

ND= not done

From the early 1970´s,Anderson et al have pointed out that circulating monoclonal immunoglobulins are another manifestation of Ss.Using a high resolution agarose electrophoresis technique,combined with immunofixation,we have shown that systemic pSs patients possess in their serum and excrete in the urine monoclonal light chains and immunoglobulins.Moreover,the circulating cryoglobulins consist of a monoclonal IgM kappa immunoglobulin with RF activity.Other investigators,using immunoglobulin gene rearrangement,have come to the same conclusions. These indicate that such patients present a monoclonal B-cell expansion,long before they develop an overt lymphoid malignancy.This is reinforced by the presence of cross-reactive idiotypes in the kappa light chain of monoclonal RFs of patients with Ss and those with Waldenstrom´s macroglobulinemia and lymphoma.

The majority of lymphocytes infiltrating the SG of pSs patients express T-helper cells phenotype.T-suppressor cells are 3-5 times fewer,whereas B-cells make up approximately 20% of the infiltrating population.Monocytes-macrophages and NK cells are very scanty ($<$5%).The infiltrating T-helper cells carry of their surface HLA-DR antigens but not interleukin-2(IL-2) receptor. IL-2 and interferon-gamma (IFN-gamma) are found in abundance.Finally, epithelial cells express DR antigens inappropriately on the ducts and acini.Whether this expression is the consequence of IFN-gamma production by activated T-cells on the triggering event for T-cell activation is still a matter of debate.Nonetheless,taken together,these immunologic abnormalities support the view that the infiltrating T-helper cells are activated.

Other data have suggested that B-cells are activated as well,within the

SG. These cells secrete large amount of immunoglobulin with RF activity,"in vitro",and it has been demonstrated that monoclonal immunoglobulins are produced by B-cells eluted from the SG.By means of an immunoperoxidase staining technique,we showed that most of the B-cells infiltrating the minor SG of Ss patients with monoclonal cryoglobulin, belong to a single clone,whilst those infiltrating the glands of patients with polyclonal cryoglobulins or no cryoglobulins, are polyclonal (Table 2).

Table 2: The relationship between the characteristics of serum cryoglobulins and those of salivary gland-infiltrating B-cells in 16 patients with primary Sjogren´s syndrome

Minor salivary gland biopsies Patients	Number	Peroxidase-Antiperoxidase technique monoclonal kappa population Number
With monoclonal cryoglobulins	7	4
With polyclonal cryoglobulins	3	0
No cryoglobulins	6	0

These findings favour the concept that the initial site of clonal B-cell expansion of Ss in the exocrine tissue. The fact that the whole B-cell hyperactivity and proliferative ability cannot be accounted for by T-cell dysfunction,prompted us to further analyze these CD5 positive B-cells in the peripheral blood and SG of Ss patients.They were found increased in the circulation and present in exocrine tissue,and that indicates that CD5 positive B-cells may play a pivotal role in the physiopathology of Ss.These cells have been shown to produce most of the IgM RF and anti-DNA antibodies,while the proliferating cell in 80% of chronic lymphocytic leukemia(CLL) is the CD5 positive B-cells.Furthermore,B-cells obtained from patients with CLL and stimulated with phorbol-ester are able to produce multispecific autoantibodies.Thus, CD5 positive B-cells can bridge the gap between nonorgan-specific autoimmune disease and B-cell malignancy.

CD5 positive B-cells may be an important regulator of other cells, but the way the act is thus far unclear.The immune suppression observed in patients with multiple myeloma has been shown to be mediated by CD5 positive B-cells.In contrast,mouse CD5 positive B-cells seem to be involved in helper function,acting through the cross-reactive idiotype network.In humans, it has been reported that monoclonal antibodies directed to CD5 molecule, together with autologous CD4 positive T-cells,are able to markedly enhance B-cell differentiation.This "in vitro" model may mimic the lymphocyte cooperation in the SG of Ss patients.These cells can in turn activate other B-cell clones as well as T-cells,and induce HLA-DR expression on the glandular cells through IFN-gamma.This leads to further T-cell activation,tissue destruction and autoantibody formation.Finally,eventual exhaustion of the immune capability with defective IL-2 production and impaired NK cell function predispose to monoclonal B-cell proliferation and lymphoid malignancy.

As mentioned,susceptibility of Ss is under strong genetic control.It has been shown that pSs is closely associated with the HLA-DR3 and -DRw52 alloantigens and sSs in RA with the -DR antigen.Exceptions to the above have been reported in certain ethnic groups: HLA-DR5 is prominent in Greeks with pSs and -DRw53 in Japanese (Table 3).This may indicate that the Ss susceptibility gene(s) would be in linkage disequilibrium with various DR genes or belong to other locus than the DR.

Table 3:HLA-alloantigens in patients with primary Sjogren´s syndrome compared to healthy individuals.

HLA-alloantigens	Healthy	Primary Ss	Significance
	% positive		
B8	19	59	0.01
DR3	23	66	0.01
DR5 (Greeks)	31	68	0.05
DRw52	53	81	0.05
DRw53 (Japanese)	61	89	0.05

In spite of the above progress,Ss basically remains an incurable disease. This should not discourage patients and physicians.Patients with Ss may feel miserable,mainly because of symptoms originating from dry mucous membranes. The physicians must therefore keep in mind that there is nothing minor about these symptoms and that every attempt has to be made in order to alleviate them.For example,Cyclosporin-A and nandrolone decanoate have been tried in double blind studies,but unsuccessfully.It has been claimed that bromhexine given orally improves sicca complaints.Substitution or stimulation of the missing secretions,however,remains the basis of symptomatic management.Finally,steroids and/or cyclophosphamide and plasmapheresis should be reserved for the treatment of a life threatening major organ involvement.

In conclusion,Ss evolves throughout three phases (Table 4): initiation (glandular disease),promotion(systemic disorder) and progression(B-cell lymphoma. Remarkable progress has been accomplished in the understanding of these processes. The emphasis now should be placed on dissecting the initiating events and the connections between the phases.

Table 4: The evolution of Sjogren´s syndrome

S J O G R E N ´ S S Y N D R O M E				
? INITIATION	? ------>	Promotion	? ------>	Progression
GLANDULAR DISEASE	------>	SYSTEMIC DISEASE	------>	B-cell lymphoma
Polyclonal B-cell activity		poly-oligo-monoclonal B-cell activity		Monoclonal B-cell activity

REFERENCES

1. Dalavanga YA, Drosos AA, Moutsopoulos HM (1986) Labial salivary gland immunopathology in Sjogren´s syndrome.Scand J Rheumatol (Suppl),61:67-70
2. Dalavanga YA, Detrick B, Hooks JJ, Drosos AA,Moutsopoulos HM (1987) Effect of cyclosporine A on the immunopathological lesion of the labial minor salivary glands from patients with Sjogren´s syndrome. Ann Rheum Dis 46: 89-92
3. Dauphinee M, Tovar Z, Talal L (1988) B-cells expressing CD5 are increased in Sjogren´s syndrome. Arthritis Rheum 31: 642-647
4. Drosos AA,Skopouli FN, Galanopoulou CK, Kitridou RC,Moutsopoulos HM (1986) Cyclosporin A therapy in patients with primary Sjogren´s syndrome: results of one year.Scand J Rheumatol (Suppl.) 61:246-249
5. Lydyard PM, Youinou P,Cooke A (1987) CD5 positive B-cells in rheumatoid arthritis and chronic lymphocytic leukemia.Immunol Today 8: 37-39
6. Moutsopoulos HM, Andonopoulos AP (1988) Sjogren´s syndrome: a human model of autoimmunity and malignancy. Brit J Rheumatol 27: 253-257
7. Papasteriades CA, Skopouli FN, Drosos AA, Andonopoulos AP,Moutsopoulos HM (1988) HLA-alloantigen associations in Greek patients with Sjogren´s syndrome. J Autoimmunity 1: 85-90
8. Talal N, Moutsopoulos HM, Kassan SS (1988) Sjogren´s syndrome.Clinical

and Immunological aspects. Springer-Verlag, Heidelberg

9. Thomas Y, Geiclaman E, De Mentino J, Wang J, Goldstein G, Chess L (1984) Biological functions of the OKT1 cell surface antigen. I: The T1 molecule is involved in helper function. J Immunol 133: 724-728
10. Urisch RC, Jaffe ES (1987) Sjogren´s syndrome like illness associated with the AIDS-related complex. Human Pathology 18: 1063-1068
11. Youinou P, Mackenzie L, Le Masson G, Papadopoulos NM, Jouquan J,Pennec YL, Angelidis P, Katsikis P, Moutsopoulos HM, Lydyard PM (1988) CD5 expressing B-lymphocytes in the blood and salivary glands of patients with primary Sjogren´s syndrome. J Autoimmunity 1: 185-194.

INDEX

NATO ASI Series H

Vol. 1: Biology and Molecular Biology of Plant-Pathogen Interactions.
Edited by J.A. Bailey. 415 pages. 1986.

Vol. 2: Glial-Neuronal Communication in Development and Regeneration.
Edited by H.H. Althaus and W. Seifert. 865 pages. 1987.

Vol. 3: Nicotinic Acetylcholine Receptor: Structure and Function.
Edited by A. Maelicke. 489 pages. 1986.

Vol. 4: Recognition in Microbe-Plant Symbiotic and Pathogenic Interactions.
Edited by B. Lugtenberg. 449 pages. 1986.

Vol. 5: Mesenchymal-Epithelial Interactions in Neural Development.
Edited by J.R. Wolff, J. Sievers, and M. Berry. 428 pages. 1987.

Vol. 6: Molecular Mechanisms of Desensitization to Signal Molecules.
Edited by T.M. Konijn, P.J.M. Van Haastert, H. Van der Starre, H. Van der Wel, and M.D. Houslay. 336 pages. 1987.

Vol. 7: Gangliosides and Modulation of Neuronal Functions.
Edited by H. Rahmann. 647 pages. 1987.

Vol. 8: Molecular and Cellular Aspects of Erythropoietin and Erythropoiesis.
Edited by I.N. Rich. 460 pages. 1987.

Vol. 9: Modification of Cell to Cell Signals During Normal and Pathological Aging.
Edited by S. Govoni and F. Battaini. 297 pages. 1987.

Vol. 10: Plant Hormone Receptors. Edited by D. Klämbt. 319 pages. 1987.

Vol. 11: Host-Parasite Cellular and Molecular Interactions in Protozoal Infections.
Edited by K.-P. Chang and D. Snary. 425 pages. 1987.

Vol. 12: The Cell Surface in Signal Transduction.
Edited by E. Wagner, H. Greppin, and B. Millet. 243 pages. 1987.

Vol. 13: Toxicology of Pesticides: Experimental, Clinical and Regulatory Perspectives.
Edited by L.G. Costa, C.L. Galli, and S.D. Murphy. 320 pages. 1987.

Vol. 14: Genetics of Translation. New Approaches.
Edited by M.F. Tuite, M. Picard, and M. Bolotin-Fukuhara. 524 pages. 1988.

Vol. 15: Photosensitisation. Molecular, Cellular and Medical Aspects.
Edited by G. Moreno, R.H. Pottier, and T.G. Truscott. 521 pages. 1988.

Vol. 16: Membrane Biogenesis. Edited by J.A.F. Op den Kamp. 477 pages. 1988.

Vol. 17: Cell to Cell Signals in Plant, Animal and Microbial Symbiosis.
Edited by S. Scannerini, D. Smith, P. Bonfante-Fasolo, and V. Gianinazzi-Pearson. 414 pages. 1988.

Vol. 18: Plant Cell Biotechnology.
Edited by M.S.S. Pais, F. Mavituna, and J.M. Novais. 500 pages. 1988.

Vol. 19: Modulation of Synaptic Transmission and Plasticity in Nervous Systems.
Edited by G. Hertting and H.-C. Spatz. 457 pages. 1988.

Vol. 20: Amino Acid Availability and Brain Function in Health and Disease.
Edited by G. Huether. 487 pages. 1988.

NATO ASI Series H

Vol. 21: **Cellular and Molecular Basis of Synaptic Transmission.**
Edited by H. Zimmermann. 547 pages. 1988.

Vol. 22: **Neural Development and Regeneration. Cellular and Molecular Aspects.**
Edited by A. Gorio, J.R. Perez-Polo, J. de Vellis, and B. Haber. 711 pages. 1988.

Vol. 23: **The Semiotics of Cellular Communication in the Immune System.**
Edited by E.E. Sercarz, F. Celada, N.A. Mitchison, and T. Tada. 326 pages. 1988.

Vol. 24: **Bacteria, Complement and the Phagocytic Cell.**
Edited by F.C. Cabello und C. Pruzzo. 372 pages. 1988.

Vol. 25: **Nicotinic Acetylcholine Receptors in the Nervous System.**
Edited by F. Clementi, C. Gotti, and E. Sher. 424 pages. 1988.

Vol. 26: **Cell to Cell Signals in Mammalian Development.**
Edited by S.W. de Laat, J.G. Bluemink, and C.L. Mummery. 322 pages. 1989.

Vol. 27: **Phytotoxins and Plant Pathogenesis.**
Edited by A. Graniti, R.D. Durbin, and A. Ballio. 508 pages. 1989.

Vol. 28: **Vascular Wilt Diseases of Plants. Basic Studies and Control.**
Edited by E.C. Tjamos and C.H. Beckman. 590 pages. 1989.

Vol. 29: **Receptors, Membrane Transport and Signal Transduction.**
Edited by A.E. Evangelopoulos, J.P. Changeux, L. Packer, T.G. Sotiroudis, and K.W.A. Wirtz. 387 pages. 1989.

Vol. 30: **Effects of Mineral Dusts on Cells.**
Edited by B.T. Mossman and R.O. Bégin. 470 pages. 1989.

Vol. 31: **Neurobiology of the Inner Retina.**
Edited by R. Weiler and N.N. Osborne. 529 pages. 1989.

Vol. 32: **Molecular Biology of Neuroreceptors and Ion Channels.**
Edited by A. Maelicke. 675 pages. 1989.

Vol. 33: **Regulatory Mechanisms of Neuron to Vessel Communication in Brain.**
Edited by F. Battaini, S. Govoni, M.S. Magnoni, and M. Trabucchi. 416 pages. 1989.

Vol. 34: **Vectors as Tools for the Study of Normal and Abnormal Growth and Differentiation.**
Edited by H. Lother, R. Dernick, and W. Ostertag. 477 pages. 1989.

Vol. 35: **Cell Separation in Plants: Physiology, Biochemistry and Molecular Biology.**
Edited by D.J. Osborne and M.B. Jackson. 449 pages. 1989.

Vol. 36: **Signal Molecules in Plants and Plant-Microbe Interactions.**
Edited by B.J.J. Lugtenberg. 425 pages. 1989.

Vol. 37: **Tin-Based Antitumour Drugs.** Edited by M. Gielen. 226 pages. 1990.

Vol. 38: **The Molecular Biology of Autoimmune Disease.**
Edited by A.G. Demaine, J-P. Banga, and A.M. McGregor. 404 pages. 1990.

Vol. 39: **Chemosensory Information Processing.** Edited by D. Schild. 403 pages. 1990.